Biopsy Pathology of the Breast

Biopsy Pathology Series

General Editors

A. Munro Neville PhD, DSc, MD, FRCPath
Ludwig Institute for Cancer Research
London, UK

Professor F. Walker MD, PhD, FRCPath
Department of Pathology
University of Aberdeen, UK

Clive R. Taylor MD, PhD
Department of Pathology and Laboratory Medicine
USC School of Medicine
Los Angeles, CA, USA

Editor Emeritus

Leonard S. Gottlieb MD, MPH
Department of Pathology and Laboratory Medicine
Boston University Medical Center
Boston, MA, USA

Titles in the series

Biopsy Pathology of the Breast

Second Edition

J.P. Sloane

MB BS, FRCPath

Royal Liverpool University Hospital, Liverpool, UK

With a contribution by

P.A. Trott

FRCPath

Royal Marsden Hospital, London, UK

and edited by

S.R. Lakhani

BSc, MB BS, MD, FRCPath

Royal Free and University College Medical School, London, UK

A member of the Hodder Headline Group
LONDON
Co-published in the USA by Oxford University Press, Inc., New York

First published in Great Britain in 2001 by
Arnold, a member of the Hodder Headline Group,
338 Euston Road, London NW1 3BH

http://www.arnoldpublishers.com

Co-published in the United States of America by
Oxford University Press Inc.,
198 Madison Avenue, New York, NY10016
Oxford is a registered trademark of Oxford University Press

Whilst the advice and information in this book are believed to be true and
accurate at the date of going to press, neither the authors nor the publisher
can accept any legal responsibility or liability for any errors or omissions
that may be made. In particular (but without limiting the generality of the
preceding disclaimer) every effort has been made to check drug dosages;
however it is still possible that errors have been missed. Furthermore,
dosage schedules are constantly being revised and new side-effects
recognized. For these reasons the reader is strongly urged to consult the
drug companies' printed instructions before administering any of the drugs
recommended in this book.

British Library Cataloguing in Publication Data
A catalogue record for this book is available from the British Library

Library of Congress Cataloging-in-Publication Data
A catalog record for this book is available from the Library of Congress

ISBN 0 340 758767 (hb)

1 2 3 4 5 6 7 8 9 10

Commissioning Editor: Georgina Bentliff
Project Editor: Michael Lax
Production Editor: Anke Ueberberg
Production Controller: Iain McWilliams

Typeset in 9.5/12.5 Stones Serif by Scribe Design, Gillingham, Kent
Printed and bound in Italy by Giunti

Contents

JOHN P. SLOANE

It was with the most profound regret that the academic community and, in particular, those with an interest in protean aspects of breast cancer, learned of the death of John Sloane on 10 May 2000 while working at his microscope in his laboratory at the University of Liverpool.

His untimely passing at the age of 54 years is a great loss.

He was responsible for laying the foundations of our current approaches to improving the diagnosis and differential diagnosis of breast pathology. His individual published papers on the subject contain many novel data and concepts and will remain a cornerstone in our practice for years to come.

The thoughts of his colleagues are with Patricia and her family who should take great pride in John's many achievements.

This second edition of *Biopsy Pathology of the Breast* is dedicated to his memory, with grateful thanks from his colleagues that he was able to complete it before his death.

A. Munro Neville

Preface to the second edition

Although I have tried to be as concise as possible, the second edition of this book is much longer than the first. The most obvious reason is that much more has been learned about breast pathology in the intervening period. The role of pathologists has changed as a consequence of greater specialization and clinical involvement, and they are now key players in the multidisciplinary teams that diagnose and manage patients. Treatment options for patients with *in situ* and invasive carcinoma have increased, and this has led to a demand for more prognostic and predictive data in pathological reports. Mammographic screening has been extensively introduced since the first edition, including a national programme in the UK. This has also resulted in a demand for more pathological data and has significantly increased the complexity of examining breast specimens, both macroscopically and histologically. A greater emphasis on cancer prevention has led to a wider role for the pathologist in assessing the cancer risk of patients with borderline lesions. The present culture of quality assurance has driven up standards and made greater demands on all involved.

There is no separate section on mammographic screening despite its profound effect on the practice of diagnostic breast pathology. This book is concerned with examining breast specimens, and changes brought about by screening are consequently discussed in the appropriate places. There are thus expanded sections on specimen radiography, non-operative diagnosis, borderline lesions such as ductal carcinoma *in situ* and radial scar, and a new section on standardized datasets and quality assurance. The radiographic appearances of many lesions are described and illustrated.

There have been numerous studies of molecular pathological changes in the breast in recent years, mainly searching for tumour markers that predict prognosis or response to treatment. At the time of writing, only immunohistochemical staining for steroid receptors and c-erB-2 (neu, Her-2) have become incorporated into routine diagnostic practice, for predicting response to hormonal and antibody treatment, respectively. Others are discussed in the book if there have been claims about their usefulness or if they shed significant light on the pathology of breast disease. They have so far complemented rather than replaced traditional histological methods of assessment and have been beset with similar problems of reproducibility.

There are separate chapters dealing with histochemical and molecular methods of examining the breast, external quality assessment, including a brief account of kappa statistics, and premalignancy. They are separated from the remainder of the text in order to provide a general background to these topics. This avoids disrupting the accounts of specific lesions to which they are relevant with lengthy explanations.

Despite the greater length of the book, I hope it remains a useful practical guide for trainee and consultant pathologists as well as for the clinicians and radiologists who interpret their reports.

John P. Sloane

Acknowledgements

The cases used to illustrate this book are mainly those I have encountered in my routine diagnostic work or second-opinion practice, but some cases or illustrations have been specifically provided by colleagues. These colleagues include Professors John Azzopardi and Barry Gusterson and Drs Rosemary Millis, Nikiforos Apostolikas, Hugh Penman, Ian McGrath, Mary Petrelli and Caroline Smith. Some of the black and white photographs were prepared by Ray Stuckey and Philip Court of the Royal Marsden Hospital and the remainder by Alan Williams of the University of Liverpool. I am also indebted to Mr Williams for processing and digitizing all the new colour illustrations. I should like to thank Christine Jarvis, Lynn Hopwood and Andrew Dodson for their technical assistance, and Valerie Power and Patricia Whittaker for help in preparing the manuscript. I am especially indebted to Dr Sunil Lakhani for reading the manuscript and making valuable comments and criticisms. Finally, I thank my wife, Patricia, for her forbearance.

1 The normal female breast

ANATOMY

Breast tissue is contained entirely within the superficial fascia of the anterior chest wall and extends from the 2nd to the 6th or 7th intercostal space. It receives blood from branches of the axillary artery and from the anterior and lateral perforating branches of the intercostal artery. The nerve supply is derived from anterior and lateral cutaneous branches of the 4th, 5th and 6th thoracic nerves.

The lymphatic drainage of the breast has been the subject of many anatomical studies in view of its relevance to the spread of breast carcinoma. The breast skin contains a valveless subepithelial plexus from which tuft-like projections extend up into the papillary dermis. This plexus is confluent with that of the skin of the rest of the body and communicates via vertical channels with a coarser valvular labyrinth of subdermal lymphatics. Both these are confluent with the subareolar lymphatic plexus, which in turn communicates with the fine lymphatics around the breast ducts and lobules. The subareolar plexus also receives lymph from the areola and nipple. Lymph flow in the normal state tends to be from superficial to deep rather than centripetally to the subareolar plexus (Halsell *et al.*, 1965; Turner-Warwick, 1959).

Lymph drains mainly to the axillary and internal mammary nodes as well as to a posterior paravertebral group of intercostal glands (Spratt, 1979). This last mode of spread may be relevant to the development of ipsilateral pleural effusions in patients with

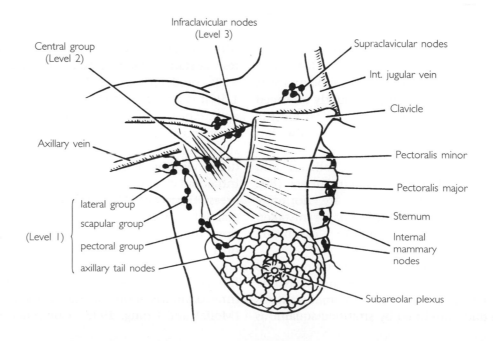

1.1 The major pathways of lymphatic drainage of the breast (modified after Spratt).

Infraclavicular nodes (Level 3)

Central group (Level 2)

Supraclavicular nodes

Int. jugular vein

Clavicle

Axillary vein

Pectoralis minor

Pectoralis major

Sternum

lateral group

scapular group

pectoral group

axillary tail nodes

(Level 1)

Internal mammary nodes

Subareolar plexus

breast carcinoma. These nodal groups do not drain specific zones of the breast. All parts of the breast drain into all groups, although the proportion of lymph derived from each quadrant will vary from group to group (Vendrell-Torne *et al.*, 1972).

In radical and extended simple mastectomy specimens, the axillary lymph nodes are often reported in three major groups (McDivitt *et al.*, 1968) (Fig. 1.1). Level 1 nodes are lateral and inferior to the pectoralis minor and include the lateral, scapular and pectoral groups as well as those in the axillary tail of the breast. Level 2 nodes lie posterior to the pectoralis minor and are essentially those of the central axillary group. Level 3 nodes are positioned medial and superior to pectoralis minor and form part of the infraclavicular group.

HISTOLOGY

Normality is difficult to define in the adult female breast as many of the so-called benign pathological changes are so common that they could be regarded as part of the normal spectrum. The description below may thus be seen as an idealized view of the normal state.

There is some variation in the terminology used to describe the parts of the duct system. The relative merits of different systems of nomenclature will not be discussed here, but one in common use will be adopted and used consistently throughout the book.

The nipple and areola have a distinctive histological appearance. The subcutaneous tissue contains numerous, irregularly arranged smooth muscle bundles that have an erectile function for the nipple. The areola also has numerous sebaceous glands, many of which are not associated with hair follicles and discharge directly on to the skin surface (Fig. 1.2). Apocrine sweat glands are normally present (Fig. 1.3) and should not be mistaken for superficial breast lobules exhibiting apocrine metaplasia.

About 15–20 collecting ducts empty onto the surface of the nipple through separate orifices (Fig. 1.4). The most proximal portions of these ducts are lined by stratified squamous

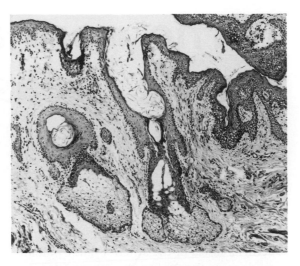

1.2 Sebaceous glands of areola discharging directly on to skin surface (H&E).

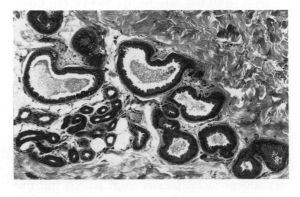

1.3 Apocrine sweat glands of areola (H&E).

epithelium continuous with that of the skin, but in the collecting ducts there is an abrupt transition to the two-layered epithelium characteristic of the remainder of the glandular tree. The collecting ducts are continuous with the lactiferous sinuses, which, in their resting state, exhibit marked infolding of their walls, producing a papillary appearance (Fig. 1.5); it is important to distinguish this normal appearance from papillary proliferations. The lactiferous sinuses receive the segmental and subsegmental ducts into which the lobules drain via the terminal ducts, which have intralobular and extralobular portions. The breast thus consists of a number of separate glandular trees or segments, each draining onto the nipple through its own collecting duct (*see* Fig. 1.4). Three-dimensional reconstruction using computer modelling of one human breast showed no interpenetration or intercommunication of the glandular trees (Moffat and Going, 1996). Computer graphic

1.4 Diagram showing the ductal and lobular system of the breast.

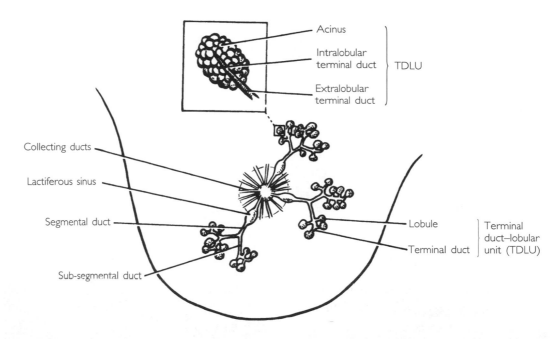

Acinus

Intralobular terminal duct

Extralobular terminal duct

TDLU

Collecting ducts

Lactiferous sinus

Segmental duct

Sub-segmental duct

Lobule

Terminal duct

Terminal duct–lobular unit (TDLU)

1.5 (Left) Normal lactiferous sinus in a resting breast. Note the papillary appearance produced by infolding of the wall (H&E).

1.6 (Right) Normal lobules. Small, uniform, two-layered acini are embedded in a loose cellular stroma. The intralobular terminal duct is seen in the middle of the lobule at the bottom left. The small duct seen at the extreme bottom left of the picture is probably the extralobular terminal duct of this lobule (H&E).

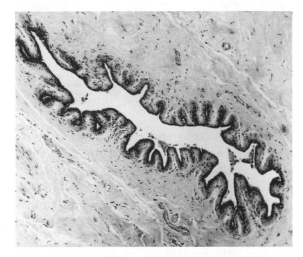

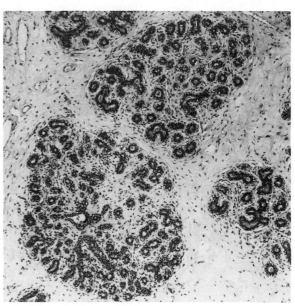

three-dimensional reconstruction of 20 quadrantectomy specimens undertaken by Ohtake *et al.* (1995), however, revealed ductal anastomoses connecting different mammary glandular trees, particularly near the nipple.

A lobule and its terminal duct are collectively known as a terminal duct–lobular unit. Lobules consist of a number of acini embedded in fine, vascular connective tissue (Fig. 1.6) and vary greatly in size from less than 10 to more than 100 acini. Normal limits are thus difficult to define. Some of the size variation results from the age of the subject and the plane of section (Bonser *et al.*, 1961).

An inner epithelial and an outer myoepithelial layer of cells line the entire duct system from the transitional zone in the collecting duct to the acini in the lobules. The myoepithelial layer is discontinuous so that some of the epithelial cells reach the basement membrane. Myoepithelial cells, on the other hand, do not reach the lumina. Adjacent epithelial cells are joined by watertight junctional complexes at the luminal ends of their lateral membranes and by desmosomes in

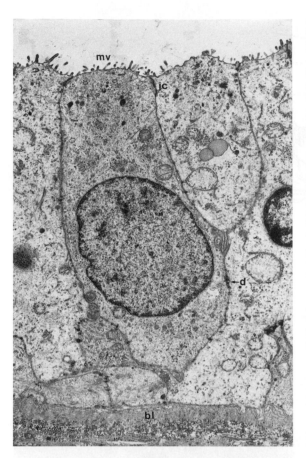

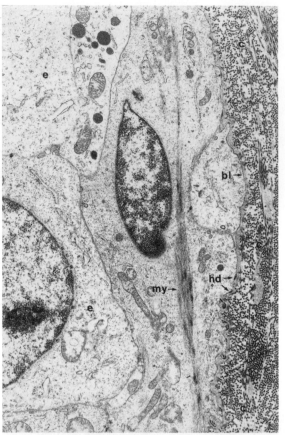

1.7 (Left) Electron micrograph of normal breast epithelium. The luminal membranes exhibit microvilli (mv). The lateral membranes are joined by junctional complexes (jc) at the luminal end and by desmosomes (d) in many other places. The basal lamina (bl) is seen at the bottom of the picture. The epithelial cell on the right of the photograph is in direct contact with the basal lamina, whereas the cytoplasm of a myoepithelial cell intervenes in the centre. Note the sparse cytoplasmic organelles. A few electron-dense granules are seen in the upper part of the cell (× 8357).

1.8 (Right) Electron micrograph of normal myoepithelial cell containing myofilaments (my) exhibiting focal densities. The cell is attached to the basal lamina (bl) by many hemidesmosomes (hd). Collagen (c) is seen to the right of the cell and epithelial cells (e) to the left. The epithelial cell cytoplasm contains a few electron-dense granules at the top of the picture. In some of these there is a suggestion of a double membrane, but the halo is insufficiently clear to regard them as true dense-core granules (× 13 648).

other areas. The epithelial cell cytoplasm exhibits sparse organelles with few mitochondria, scattered rough endoplasmic reticulum and an inconspicuous Golgi apparatus (Fig. 1.7). A few fine filaments may be present. A variety of intracytoplasmic membrane-bound vesicles have been described, which vary in their location, size, shape and electron density (Stirling and Chandler, 1976b) (Figs. 1.7 and 1.8), their function being unknown. True double membrane-bound neurosecretory (dense-core) granules have not been found in the normal breast despite extensive searching, although they may occur in some breast carcinomas (*see* p. 191).

Myoepithelial cells are joined by hemidesmosomes to the basal lamina and by desmosomes to the epithelial cells. They exhibit micropinocytotic vesicles and contain a large number of fine filaments and dense bodies resembling those of smooth muscle (Fig. 1.8). Cilia with a 9+0 structure have been identified on myoepithelial cells, and it has

been suggested that they may have a chemoreceptor or mechanoreceptor function (Stirling and Chandler, 1976a). Myoepithelial cells show, in general, greater development of myofilaments in the interlobular and terminal ducts than in the acini (Stirling and Chandler, 1976b, 1977).

Some cells are difficult to categorize, either because they lack distinguishing features or because they exhibit characteristics of both cell types. It has been suggested that these *indeterminate cells* are progenitors that can give rise to epithelial and myoepithelial cells, or represent a transition between the two (Ozzello, 1971).

The immunohistochemical characteristics of normal breast epithelial and myoepithelial cells are described in the relevant sections of chapter 3.

Lymphocytes and macrophages are present within the epithelium and are readily identified using immunohistochemical techniques with the appropriate antibodies. The intraepithelial

1.9 (Top) Formalin-fixed, paraffin-embedded section of an interlobular duct in which macrophages have been stained immunohistochemically using a CD68 antibody. Macrophages are present in the epithelium (upper half of picture) and surrounding stroma (lower half). The intraepithelial cells exhibit long dendritic processes (black arrow), which, because of their length, are often seen unaccompanied by cell bodies (red arrows).

1.10 (Middle) Formalin-fixed paraffin-embedded section of an interlobular duct stained immunohistochemically with a CD8 monoclonal antibody. The CD8+ T cells are more numerous in the epithelium than in the stroma.

1.11 (Bottom) Electron micrograph of normal breast demonstrating the epithelial–stromal junction (esj). The left-hand arrow points to the plasma membrane of a myoepithelial cell and the right-hand arrow to the plasma membrane of a delimiting fibroblast. The laminae lucida and densa are not clearly identified as there is multilayering of the basal lamina in this section (× 13 949).

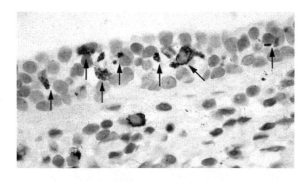

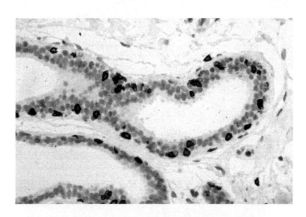

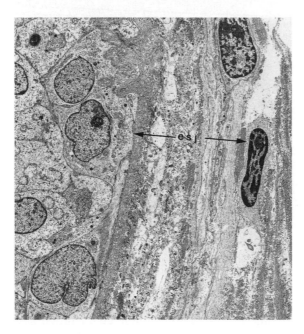

lobules, and their intraepithelial and stromal densities are approximately equal (Lwin *et al.*, 1985).

The stroma of the lobule has a much looser texture than that of the rest of the breast (*see* Fig. 1.6). It consists of irregular connective tissue fibres and a few fibroblasts, together with a number of histiocytes, lymphocytes, plasma cells and mast cells. Most of the plasma cells produce IgA, but some produce IgM.

The boundary zone between the epithelium and the stroma has been studied in some detail at the ultrastructural level. The plasma membranes of the epithelial and myoepithelial cells border on the basal lamina, which has an electron-lucent inner zone known as the lamina lucida and an outer electron-dense portion known as the lamina densa. There is then a zone of connective tissue fibres and a thin ring of delimiting fibroblasts with attenuated cytoplasm. The term epithelial–stromal junction (ESJ) has been coined to describe the zone extending from the epithelial and myoepithelial plasma membranes to the delimiting fibroblasts (Ozzello, 1970) (Fig. 1.11). The blood and lymphatic vessels lie outside the ESJ.

The periductal stroma differs from that in the lobules in that it contains elastin fibres. The collagen is also denser, and the basal lamina is often multilayered.

CHANGES IN PREGNANCY AND LACTATION

During the first trimester of pregnancy, the lobules exhibit little or no increase in size, but the epithelial cells show uniform cytoplasmic vacuolation, prominent nucleoli and occasional mitotic figures (Bailey *et al.*, 1982). Ultrastructurally, there is an increase in size and number of the mitochondria and hyperplasia of the rough endoplasmic reticulum (Salazar *et al.*, 1975). Lipid inclusions are present at the luminal pole. The myoepithelial cells show slight elongation.

By mid-pregnancy, the lobules become larger with an increase in the size and number of the acini, some of which are dilated with secretion (Fig. 1.12). Cytoplasmic vacuolation

lymphocytes are all T cells, almost exclusively CD8 positive (Figs 1.9 and 1.10). Lymphocytes are evenly distributed between the lobules and ducts, their density being greater in the epithelium than in the stroma. Macrophages tend to be found in greater number in ducts than in

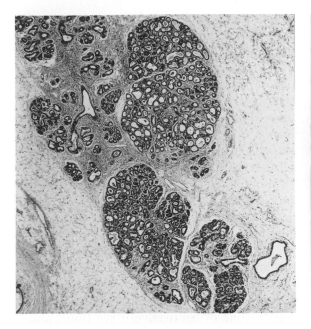

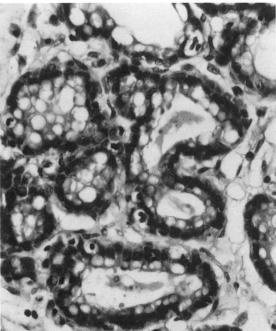

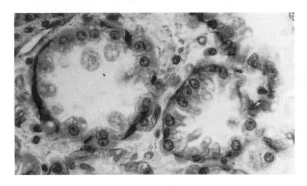

1.12 (Left) The breast in mid-pregnancy. The lobules are enlarged, but the intervening stroma is still plentiful. Many acini are dilated with secretion (H&E).

1.13 (Right) Higher-power view of Fig. 1.12 showing marked cytoplasmic vacuolation of the acinar epithelial cells (H&E).

1.14 (Left) Acini of pregnant breast stained immunohistochemically for myosin. The attenuated myoepithelial cells are seen best on the left of the picture.

1.15 (Right) Lactating breast exhibiting very marked lobular enlargement and distension of the acini. The interlobular stroma is almost completely obliterated, but thin septa still separate the individual lobules (H&E).

of the epithelial cells is more prominent, and there may be protrusions into the lumen (Fig. 1.13). Ultrastructurally, lipid inclusions are larger and more numerous, the rough endoplasmic reticulum more extensive and the Golgi apparatus dilated. The luminal membranes exhibit numerous microvilli.

Lobular secretory activity and size continue to increase so that there is in the last trimester extensive obliteration of both the intralobular and the interlobular connective tissue. Myoepithelial cells participate less in the proliferative process and become progressively elongated. They are difficult to identify in conventional sections but may be visualized with immunohistochemical techniques using antibodies to various cell constituents, including the contractile proteins smooth muscle actin and myosin (Fig. 1.14) (*see* Chapter 3). The stretching of the myoepithelial cells presumably enhances their contractile properties. Ultrastructurally, their myofilament bundles are markedly increased.

With the onset of lactation, there is an even greater distension of acini and obliteration of connective tissue (Fig. 1.15). The changes are not usually uniform, and secretion appears to be asynchronous. There are thus groups of

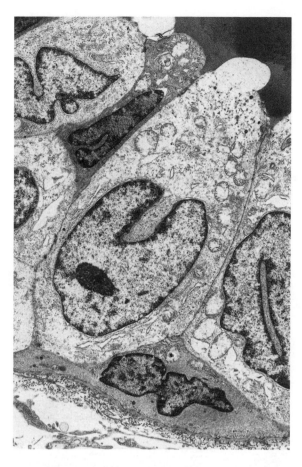

1.16 Electron micrograph of a lactating epithelial cell. A milk fat globule can be seen passing from the cell into the lumen at the top right. These globules acquire an envelope of luminal plasma membrane as they leave the epithelial cell ($\times$ 8690).

acini that are markedly distended with secretion and lined by flattened epithelial cells, whereas others are lined by taller cells and exhibit less distension. Interlobular ducts and lactiferous sinuses are markedly dilated.

Ultrastructurally, the rough endoplasmic reticulum is very prominent, presumably related to increased protein synthesis. The Golgi is also hypertrophied. Numerous fat globules are seen in the cytoplasm which, on passing into the lumen of the acinus, acquire an envelope of plasma membrane known as the milk fat globule membrane (Bargmann *et al.*, 1961) (Fig. 1.16).

CHANGES WITH THE MENSTRUAL CYCLE

There has been some dispute over whether there are discernible changes in the breast during different phases of the menstrual cycle. Potten *et al.* (1988) studied the proliferative

activity of the normal breast from six reduction mammoplasty specimens and 116 fibroadenoma excisions by thymidine labelling and counting mitoses. Maximum proliferative activity was observed on about the 21st day of the cycle and the minimum on the 7th, using either method. There was, however, a major variation in proliferative activity that could not be explained by menstrual status or age (see below). No significant effect of oral contraceptives was seen. The proportion of apoptotic cells did not change significantly in the menstrual cycle but was higher in parous women.

Anderson *et al.* (1989) have also shown that proliferative activity is higher in the second half of the cycle, with great variation from lobule to lobule and from case to case. They also reported increased activity with oral contraceptive use in nulliparous women. Russo *et al.* (1987) found that thymidine labelling was greatest in the intralobular terminal ducts.

INVOLUTION

Involution follows the cessation of lactation, but the return to the normal resting state is not always complete as well-developed lobules may persist for several years (Bonser *et al.* 1961). Isolated lobules exhibiting secretory changes similar to those seen in pregnancy and lactation may also be seen in otherwise normal breasts. Although these lobules could represent a failure of involution, there is evidence that they may arise in patients who have not been pregnant. Battersby and Anderson (1989) described an involutional change seen for up to 5 years after pregnancy and characterized by lobules with disorganized, irregular outlines and flattened epithelium. A crenated basement membrane was consistently found, and immunostaining for the basement component laminin showed strong diffuse reactivity around and between acini.

Involutionary changes also occur with advancing age. The acini become contracted as a result of the loss of lining cells. The basement membrane becomes thickened and the loose, intralobular connective tissue replaced by dense fibrous tissue. Involuting lobules may also assume a microcystic appearance (Hayward and Parks, 1958). Acini coalesce to form small cysts that later shrink and become replaced by dense fibrous tissue. These two forms of lobular involution may progress side by side (Fig. 1.17). Proliferative activity, as judged by mitotic count and thymidine labelling, decreases with age (Russo *et al.*, 1987, Potten *et al.*, 1988). The interlobular ducts are also affected, and many of the smaller ones may disappear completely. The ducts remaining show shrinkage, irregular loss of elastin and often a rather prominent myoepithelial layer (Fig. 1.18). Involution is not infrequently associated with the formation of psammomatous deposits of hydroxyapatite in the glandular lumina or stroma. This microcalcification may be detected by mammographic screening and lead to a needle or open localization biopsy (*see* Fig 4.32).

These changes are often not uniform and may vary from segment to segment or even within the same segment. Uneven involution may give rise to varying proportions of epithelium, fat and fibrous tissue in different parts of the breast, producing clinically palpable lumps.

The relationship of involutionary changes to the menopause is not clear cut. Bonser *et al.* (1961) found that, in breasts from premenopausal women, lobular development was regarded as good in 27%, average in 65% and poor or absent in 8%. Using the same criteria on breasts from postmenopausal subjects, they found that lobular development was good in none, average in 19% and poor or absent in 81%. A morphometric study (Hutson *et al.*, 1985) has shown that the amount of epithelial tissue in the breast declines steadily from the third to the sixth decade, indicating that involution is a largely premenopausal phenomenon. Mean lobular

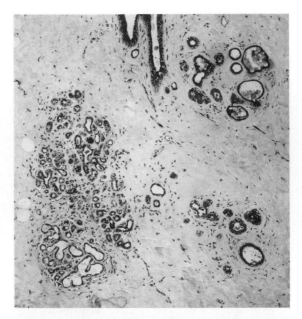

1.17 Lobular involution. The two lobules on the right exhibit a microcystic appearance, whereas most of the acini on the left are contracted (H&E).

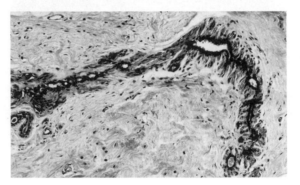

1.18 Ductal involution. The duct is shrunken and the epithelial cells atrophic. The myoepithelial cells are prominent, presumably because of the smaller dimensions of the duct (H&E).

volume also declines steadily over this period. There appears to be no correlation between the amount of epithelium in the breast and the number of previous pregnancies.

Lobular development is not simply determined by ovarian function. Bonser *et al.* (1961) also studied lobular development in castrated patients and found good lobular development in 20%, average in 60% and poor in 20%. Furthermore, good lobular development was seen more than 15 years after oophorectomy.

REFERENCES

Anderson T.J., Battersby S., King R.J.B., McPherson K., Going J.J. (1989) Oral contraceptive use influences resting breast proliferation. *Hum. Pathol.*, **20**, 1139–44.

Bailey A.J., Sloane J.P., Trickey B.S. and Ormerod M.G. (1982) An immunocytochemical study of alpha-lactalbumin in human breast tissue. *Pathology*, **137**, 13–23.

Bargmann W., Fleischauer K., and Knoop A. (1961) Uber die Morphologie der Milchsekretion. II Zugleich eine Kritik am Schema der Sekretionsmorphologie. *Z. Zellforsch.*, **53**, 545–56.

Battersby S., Anderson T.J. (1989) Histological changes in breast tissue that characterize recent pregnancy. *Histopathology*, **15**, 415–19.

Bonser G.M., Dossett J.A., and Jull J.W. (1961) *Human and Experimental Breast Cancer*. London, Pitman Medical.

Halsell J.T., Smith J.R., Bentlage C.R., Park O.K., Humphreys J.W. (1965) Lymphatic drainage of the breast demonstrated by vital dye staining and radiography. *Ann. Surg.*, **162**, 221–6.

Hayward J.L., Parks A.G. (1958) Alterations in the microanatomy of the breast as a result of changes in the hormonal environment. In Currie A.R. (ed.) *Endocrine Aspects of Breast Cancer*. Edinburgh, E. and S. Livingstone.

Hutson S.W., Cowen P.N., Bird C.C. (1985) Morphometric studies of age related changes in normal human breast and their significance for evolution of mammary cancer. *J. Clin. Pathol.*, **38**, 281–7.

Lwin K.Y., Zuccarini O., Sloane J.P., Beverley P.C.L. (1985) An immunohistochemical study of leucocyte localization in benign and malignant breast tissue. *Int. J. Cancer* **36**, 433–8.

McDivitt R.W., Stewart F.W., Berg J.W. (1968) Tumors of the breast. In *Atlas of Tumor Pathology, II*. Washington DC, Armed Forces Institute of Pathology.

Moffat D.F., Going J.J. (1996) Three dimensional anatomy of complete duct systems in human breast: pathological and developmental implications. *J. Clin. Pathol.* **49**, 48–52.

Ohtake T., Abe R., Kimijima I., *et al.* (1995) Intraductal extension of primary invasive breast carcinoma treated by breast-conservative surgery: computer graphic three-dimensional reconstruction of the mammary duct-lobular systems. *Cancer*, **76**, 32–45.

Ozzello L. (1970) Epithelial-stromal junction of normal and dysplastic mammary glands. *Cancer*, **25**, 586–600.

Ozzello L. (1971), Ultrastructure of the human mammary gland. *Pathol. Ann.*, **6**, 1–59.

Potten C.S., Watson R.J., Williams G.T. *et al.* (1988) The effect of age and menstrual cycle on proliferative activity of the normal breast. *Br. J. Cancer*, **58**, 163–70.

Russo J., Calaf G., Roi L., Russo I.H. (1987) Influence of age and gland topography on cell kinetics of normal breast tissue. *J. Natl Cancer Inst.*, **78**, 413–18.

Salazar H., Tobon H., Josimovich J.B. (1975) Developmental, gestational and postgestational modifications of the human breast. *Clin. Obstet. Gynecol.*, **18**, 113–37.

Spratt J.S. (1979) Anatomy of the breast. *Major Prob. Clin. Surg*, **5**, 1–13.

Stirling J.W., Chandler J.A. (1976a) Ultrastructural studies of the female breast. *Anat. Rec.*, **186**, 413–16.

Stirling J.W., Chandler J.A. (1976b), The fine structure of the normal, resting terminal ductal-lobular unit of the female breast. *Virchows Arch. (Pathol. Anat.)*, **372**, 205–26.

Stirling J.W., Chandler J.A. (1977) The fine structure of ducts and subareolar ducts in the resting gland of the female breast. *Virchows Arch.*, **373**, 119–32.

Turner-Warwick R.T. (1959) The lymphatics of the breast. *Br. J. Surg.*, **46**, 574–82.

Vendrell-Torne E., Setoain-Quinquer J., Domenech-Torne F.M. (1972) Study of normal mammary lymphatic drainage using radioactive isotopes. *Nucl. Med.*, **13**, 801–5.

2 Pathological examination and reporting of breast specimens

MACROSCOPIC EXAMINATION

Biopsies and mastectomy specimens are best cut into thin (about 5 mm) slices and then examined by careful visual inspection and palpation (Fig. 2.1). For mastectomy specimens, somewhat thicker slices (10 mm) may be necessary and may be arranged separately or left hinged to the skin. The latter makes reconstruction easier if the specimen needs to be re-examined at a later date but has the disadvantage of making it more difficult to detect small superficial lesions. Where the slices are separate, they should be arranged in order so that the exact location of any abnormality can be determined and the specimen reconstructed if necessary. In a good light, a remarkable amount of detail can be observed,

2.1 Diagram of slicing and orientation of a local excision specimen of the right breast. The long suture marks the lateral aspect, the short one the superior aspect. The 5 mm slices are allowed to fall to the right and are arranged in order from medial to lateral. The superior, inferior, superficial (S) and deep (D) margins of each slice can thus be identified and the tumour (T) located in relation to each of them. The slice numbers define the tumour's position in relation to the medial and lateral margins. This method also allows the anatomical relationship between the tumour and any other lesion, detected macroscopically or histologically, to be determined if the positions of the blocks (B1–9) are noted at cut up. The tumour size and the distance from the nearest margin (NM–supero-superficial in this case) should be measured.

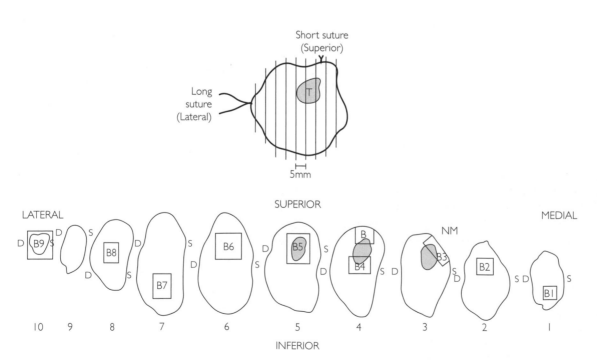

2.2 Slice of breast tissue immersed in a 0.0l% solution of methylene blue in formol saline overnight and examined under a dissecting microscope. The lobules are easily identified as dark blue structures against a pale blue background.

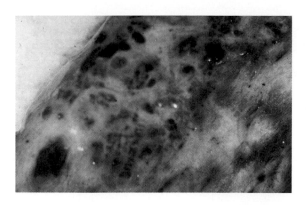

and even normal ducts and lobules can be identified as glistening grey structures against a white background. Straightforward visual inspection is all that is usually required, but if very small lesions are being sought, the tissue slices can be stained with methylene blue or other dye and then examined with a hand lens or even a dissecting microscope (Fig. 2.2).

Specimens may be examined in the fixed or fresh state. In the former case, some preliminary slicing should be undertaken within 2 hours of surgery to allow adequate penetration of the fixative. This should ideally be undertaken by the pathologist in order to minimize ensuing problems of orientation, but it may be necessary for the surgeon to incise the specimen in the operating theatre if there is likely to be significant delay in the specimen reaching the laboratory. The excision margins should be marked (see below) and the specimen reconstructed to maintain orientation, having placed absorbent paper between the slices. Some workers have injected formol saline into breast specimens in an attempt to fix them without producing distortion and disorientation, but this procedure has not been widely adopted, presumably because a very large number of injections is needed to achieve adequate penetration while minimizing tissue disruption.

The examination of specimens in the fresh state should be undertaken within 2 hours if a ligand-binding assay for oestrogen receptors is to be performed. Fresh specimens should ideally be sent to the laboratory immediately but can, if necessary, be left in sealed polythene bags in a refrigerator overnight without significant loss of histological detail

or immunostaining properties. Furthermore, specimens stored in this way become firm and easy to slice. In the author's experience, this method is preferable to leaving large unsliced specimens at room temperature in formol saline overnight. Good communication between operating theatres and pathology laboratories is critical, however, to ensure that fresh specimens are transported promptly and any possibility of autolysis avoided. Freezing should be avoided as this produces ice-crystal artefacts. Slicing is usually performed manually, but it can be carried out using a meat slicer (Davies *et al.*, 1973).

Manton *et al.* (1981) have described an automated technique for processing breast biopsies for subgross examination. Samples are fixed in formol saline, sliced, stained with haematoxylin, dehydrated in alcohols and cleared with methyl salicylate before being examined with a dissecting microscope. Marcum and Wellings (1969) examined entire human breasts by cutting them into 1–2 mm slices that were then defatted in acetone, hydrated, stained in haematoxylin, dehydrated, cleared in toluene and stored in plastic bags containing methyl salicylate. Detailed methods like these cannot be used routinely and are more suitable for research projects. They may be employed for diagnostic purposes, however, in identifying small lesions, such as lobular carcinoma *in situ* (LCIS), which would not otherwise be detectable macroscopically.

The size of any tumour should be measured and later checked on the histological sections to ensure that that it does not extend significantly beyond its macroscopically defined limits and that the whole of the area identified grossly comprises tumour down the microscope. The contour, consistency and location of the mass should be recorded, including the distance from the nearest excision margin. Several blocks should be taken from the tumour, especially around its periphery where *in situ* changes and vascular invasion are most easily appreciated and where the distance from the excision margins can be checked microscopically. The periphery of a carcinoma is also the most appropriate place to count mitoses when grading (*see* p. 216). Blocks should then be taken from any other macroscopic abnormalities and from the ostensibly normal areas. It is important to note the slice numbers from which these blocks are taken as well as their positions within the slices as this enables the anatomical relationship between the main mass and any microscopic tumour to be established. This clearly has implications for measuring tumour size, assessing multifocality and determining adequacy of excision. In mastectomy specimens, representative blocks should be taken from all four quadrants.

In re-excision specimens, where the tumour has already been removed, blocks should be taken from any abnormality in the cavity wall suspicious for residual disease. If no residual tumour is seen macroscopically, several blocks, preferably extending around the full circumference in one plane, should be taken to detect any remaining microscopic malignancy.

Blocks are best taken from the nipple in two planes: one in the sagittal and the other in the coronal plane at the junction with the areola. The former is useful for identifying Paget cells in the epidermis and investigating cutaneous pathology. The latter allows all the mammary ducts to be visualized as they converge on the nipple and is useful for assessing the extent of spread of ductal carcinoma *in situ* (DCIS), particularly to determine whether more than one glandular tree is involved (Fig. 2.3).

Excision margins

The greater use of breast-conserving surgery has increased the need for pathologists to determine the adequacy of excision of carcinomas. This is usually performed by coating the whole surface of the specimen with some material that will remain adherent to it during fixation, processing and section-cutting. India ink, coloured gelatins and dyes such as alcian blue are commonly used materials. Correction fluid, such as Tipp-Ex, has been used in a few centres, but like some other markers, it is radio-opaque and may interfere with specimen radiography. The specimen can then be sliced and blocks taken to include the excision margins nearest to the tumour borders. The

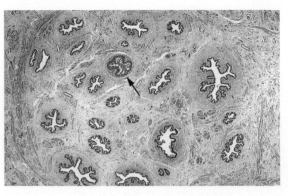

2.3 Coronal section of a nipple showing the lactiferous sinuses and terminal ducts cut in transverse section. One (arrowed) shows a ductal carcinoma *in situ* involving one of the glandular trees.

anatomical position of the nearest margin can be determined if the surgeon has marked the specimen in some way. A simple method is to insert a long suture in the lateral and a short suture in the superior aspect. If the side from which the specimen was taken is known, all the margins can then be identified (see above). In some centres, pathologists peel the specimen like an orange so that the whole of the excision margin can be embedded. Alternatively, the surgeon may 'shave' the inside of the cavity that is left after removing the tumour.

There is, however, an imperfect correlation between the adequacy of excision as determined by the pathologist and the presence of residual carcinoma in the breast, the reasons for which are discussed on p. 133. Nevertheless, if the excision margins are carefully sampled, the pathologist can give a reasonable assessment of the probability of tumour remaining in the breast, particularly if other important factors (e.g. vascular invasion and multifocality) are taken into account. Assessing the adequacy of excision is important in all types of primary malignant lesion. Complete local excision is potentially curative for DCIS, well-delineated invasive carcinomas without metastatic disease and malignant mesenchymal tumours. In more aggressive and extensive carcinomas for which the prognosis is poor, adequate surgery is necessary to prevent the distressing complication of local recurrence.

Extent of sampling

Pathological changes in the breast are often focal and may show considerable variation even within the same segment. Histological examination is thus subject to serious sampling problems, which are especially important in biopsies containing small carcinomas (either infiltrating or *in situ*) and lesions of possible precancerous significance. Thorough macroscopic examination is, therefore, essential to reduce sampling errors.

It is very difficult to determine what is an acceptable level of sampling of breast showing no obvious macroscopic abnormality. The more extensive it is, the greater the chance of detecting small carcinomas and risk lesions, but the probability of finding such changes has to be balanced against the cost of doing so. It is reasonable to expect the whole of small biopsies to be blocked but not large specimens, which would involve an enormous amount of work. It is an important question whether the pathologist's role is simply to diagnose a symptomatic or screen-detected abnormality or to screen for additional microscopic malignancies or precancerous lesions.

Schnitt and Wang (1989) investigated the problem of cost-effectiveness by reviewing 384 consecutive biopsies from symptomatic women in which gross examination revealed no abnormality. All tissue was submitted for histological examination, producing 3342 blocks. Carcinoma or atypical hyperplasia was detected in 26 cases (6.8%). There were 12 cases of LCIS, 4 of atypical lobular hyperplasia (ALH), 4 of DCIS, 3 of atypical ductal hyperplasia (ADH) and 3 of invasive carcinoma. They calculated that if the first 5 blocks only had been taken from each case, 1386 (41%) blocks would have been saved but 6 of the 26 malignant or borderline lesions would have been undetected. If sampling had been limited to 10 blocks per case, 610 fewer blocks would have been taken but all the lesions would have been detected with the exception of a single case of LCIS. A very useful observation was that in all but one case, the lesions were located in the fibrous part of the breast rather than the grossly fatty tissue. It was suggested that a cost-effective method of sampling grossly benign biopsies is to submit a maximum of 10 blocks of fibrous breast tissue per case and only examine the remainder if carcinoma or atypical hyperplasia is found. This view is supported by the author.

In a similar study of 157 biopsies from screened women (Schnitt *et al.*, 1989), 2183 blocks were required to sample the whole of each specimen (13 blocks per case). This resulted in the detection of carcinoma in 50 patients and atypical hyperplasia in 19. When sampling was initially restricted to areas containing radiological abnormalities and further tissue was taken only if carcinoma or atypical hyperplasia was found, 38% fewer blocks were required (leaving 9 blocks per case), but 1 of the 50 cancers and 4 of the 19 atypical hyperplasias would have been missed.

In the author's experience, it is best to sample all the mammographic abnormalities where there is any doubt about their representing a malignant process. In cases where malignancy has been diagnosed preoperatively on needle aspirates or cores, sufficient blocks should be taken to determine accurately the size of the tumour and the status of the excision margins. In sliced specimens, it is usually best to take tissue from the first and last slices for these purposes (see p. 10). Blocks of radiologically normal tissue from either side of the mammographic abnormality should always be taken as the extent of *in situ* or invasive malignancy is often underestimated by radiology alone.

Large blocks

Large blocks and sections can give impressive results, allowing the whole cross-section of a biopsy to be cut in many cases (Fig. 2.4). Sampling problems can be reduced, and the size, extent and adequacy of excision of carcinomas can be determined more easily. They facilitate orientation by obviating the need for a mental reconstruction of the overall picture from several separate sections. The number of blocks required to gain the relevant diagnostic and prognostic information is thus reduced.

The technique has not, however, gained general acceptance, partly because of the obvious problem of storage and partly because many technical staff experience difficulty in cutting large sections and find it hard to achieve adequate processing and good cytological detail. Although these problems can generally be overcome with perseverance, most laboratories do not feel that the effort is justified given that the same information can be obtained from several conventional sections, particularly if the location in the specimen from which the blocks were taken is accurately recorded (see above). Furthermore, large sections, like their smaller counterparts, are essentially two-dimensional and thus give no information about the pathological features of a lesion in the third dimension.

Regional lymph nodes

As many lymph nodes as possible should be dissected from all specimens that include an axillary dissection. In the author's experience, this is best achieved by cutting the specimen into very thin slices, which are then palpated and visually scrutinized. The lymph nodes can be divided into three levels (see Fig. 1.1), but only if the surgeon has marked the boundaries with stitches or clips. An attempt should be made to identify lymph nodes within simple mastectomy specimens as there are usually one or two in the axillary tail. Clearing agents have been used to facilitate the detection of lymph nodes in mastectomy and axillary dissection specimens, but the procedure is time consuming and can significantly delay reporting. Although some workers have found that these agents significantly increase lymph node yield, the author has found no or only minimal difference if conventional examination is performed carefully.

Sentinel lymph node biopsy involves identifying the most proximal axillary lymph node *in vivo* using a dye or radio-active tracer introduced preoperatively into the vicinity of the tumour. The former has the advantage of lower cost and the latter the ability to localize the node externally and reduce the size of the surgical incision. The node (or nodes if more than one is included in the specimen) is then removed and submitted for histological examination. The presence or absence of tumour determines whether or not an axillary dissection is performed. The node can be

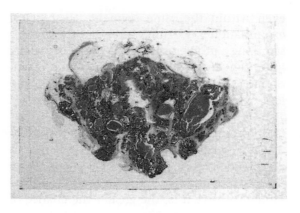

2.4 H&E-stained section prepared from a large block showing extensive ductal carcinoma *in situ* reaching the excision margin at the bottom of the illustration.

subjected to intraoperative frozen section examination so that the decision to perform an axillary dissection can be made while the patient is on the operating table, thus avoiding a second operation. This is an inefficient use of laboratory time but has to be balanced against the benefit for the patient and the considerable time saved examining unnecessary axillary dissection specimens.

There is currently much controversy surrounding the level of detail with which sentinel nodes should be examined. Cserni (1999) studied 70 cases in which blue dye was used to detect the sentinel node. In the 58 cases in which sentinel nodes were found (1–3 per case), they were serially sectioned at 3–5 μm intervals taking an H&E-stained section every 10th–20th level. Sections for immunohistochemistry with antibodies to cytokeratin and EMA were taken after every sixth H&E if they were negative. Of 39 node-positive patients, judged on the basis of all the nodes, 36 had positive sentinel nodes, and in 21 the sentinel node was the only one involved. Cserni estimated that simply taking one or two levels from close to the central area of the nodes would have resulted in failure to detect metastases in 31% of cases. Turner *et al.* (1999) evaluated the use of 8 step sections at 40 μm with cytokeratin immunohistochemistry in 60 sentinel nodes from 42 patients that were negative on frozen section, and permanent sections examined at two levels. The latter had shown micrometastases in nine nodes from eight of the patients. In the remaining 51 nodes, only 2 from one patient had metastatic carcinoma. As a consequence of these findings, they recommended that the sentinel node be examined using cytokeratin immunohistochemistry at two levels of the paraffin block.

Van Diest (1999) felt that there was a consensus that sentinel nodes should be examined more carefully than others should. He recommended that frozen section examination could be performed if desired. Nodes less than 5 mm in diameter could be embedded intact, those between 5 and 10 mm halved and those greater than 10 mm cut into slices not exceeding 5 mm. Where the initial H&E result is negative, four further sections should be cut at 250 μm and examined with H&E and immunohistochemistry for cytokeratins. In the light of present evidence, this seems reasonable advice.

In the opinion of the author, however, the crucial issue that needs to be addressed is the level of detail required to examine the sentinel node in order to detect axillary node metastases of known prognostic significance, as opposed to micrometastases, which have recently been shown to have prognostic significance. Some centres (including the author's own) have found sentinel node status to be a strong predictor of axillary node involvement (as determined by conventional examination), even if assessed by routine histological examination alone. At the time of writing, sentinel node biopsy is under extensive investigation, and a large multicentre trial is being conducted in the UK which will hopefully lead to a firm policy on sentinel node examination.

SPECIMEN RADIOGRAPHY

The use of this technique has increased enormously since the introduction of population-based mammographic screening and adds significantly to the length of time taken to examine a pathological specimen. Although its greatest value is in localizing and characterizing impalpable lesions detected by mammography, it has occasionally been used to detect small unsuspected carcinomas in biopsies from symptomatic women (Rosen *et al.*, 1970; Bauermeister and Hall, 1973). The low detection rate, however, makes it unnecessary to perform the procedure on a routine basis, and in most laboratories the use of specimen radiography is restricted to specimens containing impalpable lesions detected by mammography.

Techniques

A radiograph should first be taken of the whole sample to determine whether the mammographic abnormality has been excised and whether excision appears to be complete. This is usually the responsibility of the radiologist or surgeon. Pathologists should consult the radiologist who reported the clinical mammogram if they cannot identify the lesion confidently. The specimen should then be cut into thin slices. If a lesion obviously corresponding to the mammographic abnormality is seen, it can be sampled in the usual way (see above). If not, it is advisable to take a further radiograph of the sliced specimen, arranged on radiolucent material, in order to locate the lesion and direct the tissue sampling (Fig. 2.5). It is best to mark the sites from which the blocks are taken on the mammogram in order to enable precise correlation of the histological and radiological appearances. For the same reason, it is also advisable for the pathologist to provide a description of the radiographic as well as the macroscopic appearances in the report. Specimen radiography can be undertaken in the radiology department or the histopathology laboratory using a portable machine. The latter has the benefit of convenience, but the former usually results in higher-quality images.

Although this method is regarded as an ideal way of localizing mammographic abnormalities, it is a two-stage procedure regarded by some pathologists as too time consuming. A number of one-stage methods have therefore been developed, usually employing some form of grid. In one of these methods, biopsy specimens are securely mounted (usually using elastic bands) on pieces of Perspex inlaid with a wire grid (Champ *et al.*, 1989). Using the grid co-ordinates, the mammographic

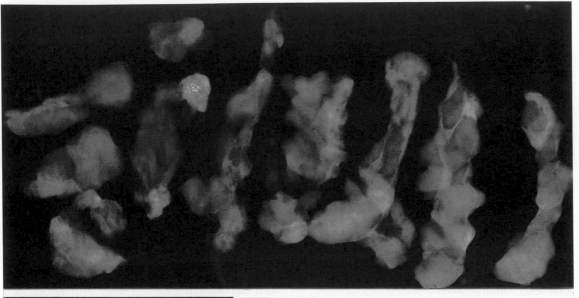

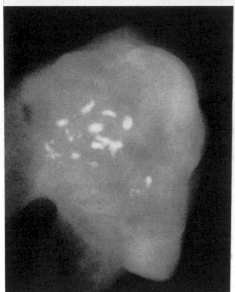

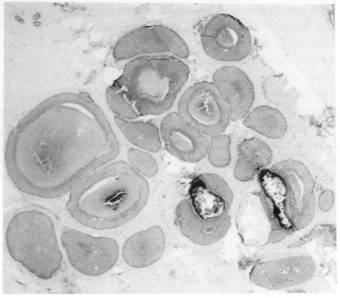

2.5 Radiograph of a sliced breast biopsy removed following the detection of a focus of coarse branching calcification by mammographic screening. The lesion was impalpable. The upper photograph shows the whole specimen, the calcification being restricted to the edge of one slice only. This area is magnified in the lower left illustration. At the lower right is the H&E-stained section prepared from the calcified zone, which shows high nuclear grade ductal carcinoma *in situ* with a comedo growth pattern. Coarse calcification is seen within the comedo necrosis in the lower half of the picture.

abnormality is mapped to a particular area which is then incised. Any macroscopically detectable abnormality on the cut surface is sampled. If no abnormality is seen, the tissue overlying the appropriate grid squares is blocked in its entirety.

In another method (Gauvin *et al.*, 1990), the specimen is placed in a plastic Petri dish containing paraffin wax and covered by a translucent and radiolucent plate containing numerous asymmetrically spaced holes 3–4 mm in diameter. The specimen is X-rayed and a pin is inserted through the hole nearest

the mammographic abnormality into the tissue and secured by the underlying paraffin. The plate is removed, and the specimen is sectioned. An area measuring 15–20 mm around the pin is processed separately.

In an even simpler method (Walker *et al.*, 1992), the radiologist, using the specimen radiograph as a guide, inserts a hypodermic needle into the tissue as close as possible to the centre of the suspicious lesion. The specimen is then transported to the histopathology department where the pathologist slices it along the plane of the needle. After fixation, several blocks are taken adjacent to the needle shaft.

The advantage of these methods and their variants is that time and money are saved in avoiding a second specimen radiograph. There are, however, several disadvantages. The specimen may move on the grid, or the localizing pin or needle may become dislodged. The pathologist is dependent on the surgeon or radiologist to undertake a procedure in a specified fashion in the operating theatre or radiology department. Sampling multiple abnormalities may be very difficult as the tissue loses its integrity when the first slice is cut. Finally, identifying lesions in thick specimens may be difficult given the two-dimensional nature of the radiograph.

A three-dimensional method of specimen radiography has been described in which the specimen is radiographed from four viewpoints by means of rotation in a radiolucent tetrahedral container. Although expensive and time consuming, this method enables a better radiological assessment to be made of surgical clearance and consequently a more appropriate selection of blocks for histological evaluation of the excision margins (Davies et al., 1997).

The method adopted in a particular laboratory will clearly depend on local resources and preferences, but pathologists must satisfy themselves that the pathological changes responsible for the mammographic abnormalities have been identified in the histological sections. If not, the residual tissue and/or blocks should be X-rayed again to determine whether the radiological lesion has not been blocked or whether it is present in the blocks deep to the plane of section. Any unblocked tissue should be stored until the mammographic changes have been characterized histologically. Tissue should not simply be taken from the vicinity of a guidewire introduced preoperatively as it may not be very close to the mammographic lesion.

Correlation between radiology and pathology

Two types of microcalcification have been identified by Frappart et al. (1984). The first is crystalline, amber, transparent material, birefringent under polarized light, with a pyramidal shape on scanning electron microscopy and containing wedellite – a particular form of calcium oxalate. The second is non-crystalline, opaque, grey-white, non-birefringent, and ovoid or fusiform on scanning electron microscopy, and contains hydroxyapatite – a form of calcium phosphate. The latter is by far the most frequently encountered in breast pathology and is generally detected easily in H&E stained sections as dense haematoxyphilic deposits (see Fig. 2.5 above). In this case, the correlation of histological and radiological features usually, therefore, presents little difficulty.

In contrast, wedellite is usually visible only under crossed polarizers, where it appears as large, angulated, birefringent crystals (Fig. 2.6). Consequently, it is often overlooked, and this may lead to difficulties in correlating the mammographic and pathological appearances. Wedellite is largely restricted to benign lesions. Gonzalez et al. (1991) found wedellite crystals in 13% of breast biopsies, typically within apocrine cysts that were sometimes associated with separate foci of lobular carcinoma in situ. The rupture of some of the cysts with extrusion of the crystals was accompanied by stromal inflammation that included multinucleate foreign-body type giant cells. Wedellite was rarely seen in association with invasive carcinomas. They concluded that calcium oxalate is a secretory form of calcification, in contrast to the dystrophic nature of hydroxyapatite.

It should be remembered that the size and extent of microcalcifications seen on

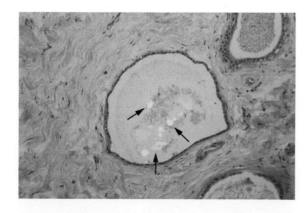

2.6 A section stained with H&E viewed under partially crossed polarizers to demonstrate the presence of a cyst in which there are a few crystals of birefringent wedellite (arrows).

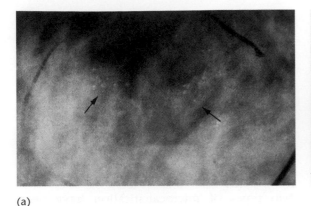

(a)

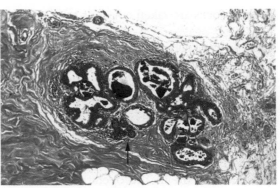

(b)

2.7 (a) Clinical radiograph showing fine granular calcification. (b) Histological sections of the calcified zone showing numerous terminal duct–lobular units with grossly dilated acini containing psammomatous deposits of hydroxyapatite. The normal acini are arrowed for comparison. The acini are lined by uniform small cells with hyperchromatic nuclei and a high nuclear-to-cytoplasmic ratio. Elsewhere the lobules exhibited intraluminal proliferation amounting to atypical ductal hyperplasia.

radiographs are often not the same as those seen down the microscope. The smallest particles may not be resolved in the radiograph, and many that are visualized represent the superimposition of several that are histologically visible. The Von Kossa stain may be useful in detecting occult deposits of hydroxyapatite but not oxalate, which appears to be unreactive (Symonds, 1990).

Specimen radiography is useful in assessing the adequacy of surgical excision when the abnormality reaches the margin of the specimen on the radiograph; that is, it has high positive predictive value and is consequently useful in selecting margins for histological assessment. The converse, however, is not true, margins apparently clear on radiological examination frequently being involved on histological examination. Graham *et al.* (1994) studied 56 specimens with margins tumour free by 1–16 mm on radiography and found margin involvement in 38 on histological examination. Specimen radiography thus has a low negative predictive value in this respect. Rarely, microcalcification may not be contained within the tumour but located next to it (Homer *et al.*, 1989)

Although the mammographic abnormality that led to the decision to biopsy is usually obvious in a specimen radiograph, this is not always the case, and discussion with the radiologist is sometimes necessary. It is nevertheless essential for pathologists to have a working knowledge of the radiological appearances of common breast lesions in order to ensure that diagnoses made down the microscope are

responsible for the mammographic abnormalities. For example, calcifications associated with high nuclear-grade DCIS are usually coarse and branched (*see* Fig. 2.5 above), whereas fine granular calcifications are more likely to be associated with low nuclear-grade DCIS or benign processes such as sclerosing adenosis, blunt duct adenosis and involutional change (Fig. 2.7). The size and shape of tumours detected as soft tissue densities should be compared in the radiographs and histological sections. Stellate lesions are usually invasive carcinomas (Fig. 2.8) but may be radial scars (*see* Fig. 6.34., p. 96), particularly if smaller and less dense.

INTRAOPERATIVE FROZEN SECTION DIAGNOSIS

The frequency with which intraoperative frozen sections are used has dramatically declined in recent years as a result of the marked improvement in non-operative diagnosis using the triple approach of clinical examination, imaging (usually radiology but

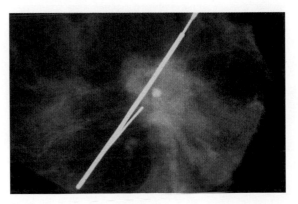

2.8 Localization biopsy in which the localization wire overlies an irregular soft tissue density that proved to be a grade 2 invasive ductal (no special type) carcinoma.

often including ultrasound) and fine needle aspiration cytology or needle core biopsy (see Chapter 4). This combined approach can lead to a definitive non-operative diagnosis of malignancy in a high proportion of cases, thus enabling the nature and extent of surgery to be determined in advance of the operation. Furthermore, oestrogen receptor status can now be determined immunohistologically on formalin-fixed paraffin-embedded sections and no longer requires the collection of frozen material.

There are many problems associated with intraoperative frozen section examination. The smooth and efficient working routine of the histopathology laboratory is disrupted, and operating theatre time and bed occupancy cannot be planned precisely if the nature of a patient's operation is not known until the surgical procedure is under way. Cytological assessment is difficult because frozen sections are usually thicker than those cut from paraffin blocks and are more likely to lift, fold and tear. Furthermore, some of the staining and processing methods employed may produce an appearance that is not comparable with that seen in paraffin-embedded material, with which pathologists are more familiar. The larger cell size can lead to an erroneous diagnosis of malignancy. Cytological detail may remain difficult to interpret even after thawing and fixation in formalin. The limitations of interpreting cytological detail make architectural features all the more important, and it is essential for frozen sections to be examined using a microscope with a high-quality, low-power objective lens.

A number of lesions present special difficulties in frozen section interpretation. Carcinoma *in situ*, of both the lobular and the ductal type, may be impossible to distinguish from hyperplasia, especially if atypical. Ashikari, Huvos and Snyder (1977) reported that only 18% of cases of *in situ* lobular carcinoma and 55% of those of DCIS were diagnosed correctly on frozen section examination. Sclerosing adenosis, microglandular adenosis and radial scar are notoriously difficult to distinguish from tubular carcinoma

because of their infiltrative appearances (*see* pp. 88–94). Infiltrating lobular carcinomas are likely to escape diagnosis because the malignant cells may be so widely dispersed in the stroma that they may be misinterpreted as benign or overlooked altogether.

Caution should always be exercised in interpreting papillary lesions, and some pathologists do not usually venture anything more precise than a diagnosis of papillary tumour. Although some of the papillary carcinomas can be identified with confidence, it is as well to be wary of lesions that appear benign as cytologically malignant zones may occasionally be found in other parts of the lesion in paraffin-embedded sections. This is especially true of multiple intraduct papilloma (*see* p. 113).

Frozen sections should not generally be used in the diagnosis of microdochectomy specimens removed from patients with nipple discharge unless there is an obvious tumour. Discharge from the nipple is often caused by small papillary tumours in the major ducts that are detectable only in histological sections. High-quality paraffin-embedded sections are necessary to make an accurate histological diagnosis.

If there is any doubt about the diagnosis of a frozen section, it is always better to defer diagnosis until paraffin-embedded sections are available. The underdiagnosis of malignancy is obviously preferable to its overdiagnosis, which can result in unnecessary and sometimes mutilating surgery. The pathologist should always insist that request forms be correctly completed, giving the relevant clinical findings as well as the mammographic and cytological data where available.

In a survey by Rosen (1978) of 556 frozen sections reported by eight pathologists of varying experience at the Memorial Hospital, New York, 145 were said to be malignant and 381 benign. Of the benign cases, eight were later found to be malignant, giving a false-negative rate of 3%. Six of these were lobular carcinoma *in situ*, one a DCIS and one a small infiltrating carcinoma. There were no false positives, but the diagnosis was deferred until paraffin-embedded sections were available in

5.4% of cases. These figures represent what is probably the maximal attainment of accuracy in an intraoperative frozen section service.

Despite these difficulties, there remain a handful of cases in which intraoperative frozen section examination is justifiable even where there are well-developed non-operative diagnostic services. In the guidelines issued by the UK and EC working groups on breast screening pathology (National Coordinating Group for Breast Screening Pathology, 1995; European Community, 1996), it was recommended that three essential criteria should be fulfilled before intra-operative frozen section diagnosis is undertaken:

1. The abnormality must be clearly and unequivocally identified on macroscopic examination.
2. It must be large enough (generally at least 10 mm) to allow an adequate proportion of the lesion to be fixed and processed without prior freezing.
3. It must have proved impossible to make a definitive diagnosis preoperatively.

THE MINIMUM DATASET

The reporting form illustrated in Fig. 2.9 is the standard proforma used by the Breast Unit at the Royal Liverpool University Hospital, UK. It is derived from and almost identical to that produced for European breast screening programmes, differing only in the order in which the pathological features are listed and in the inclusion of all three nuclear grades of DCIS. The diagnostic criteria are those adopted for the European breast screening programmes. Reporting by proforma using nationally or internationally agreed terminology and diagnostic criteria ensures that a standard set of data is given for each patient and that results are comparable from centre to centre, even in different countries. Published audits have shown that there is significant interlaboratory variation in reporting breast cancer (Dey *et al.*, 1997) and that proformas are very effective in ensuring that all necessary data are provided (Cross *et al.*, 1997a, 1997b).

The amount of information required in breast pathology reports has significantly increased in recent years. It is no longer sufficient for pathologists to make accurate and reproducible diagnoses of *in situ* and invasive breast cancer, and there is a requirement to report those features with prognostic significance. There are four main reasons for this. First, the number of treatment options has increased. Breast-conserving surgery is more widely employed but is suitable only for selected patients. Furthermore, local and radical surgery are often accompanied by adjuvant treatment with radiotherapy or cytotoxic or hormonally active drugs. The choice of therapy for an individual patient is to a large extent determined by the pathological characteristics of the cancer. Second, cancer registries monitor not only the incidence of specific cancers, but also changing patterns of disease, which are important for epidemiological reasons as well as for strategic purposes in planning health services. Third, prognostic features are useful in monitoring screening programmes as success in reducing mortality is reflected by more favourable characteristics of the cancers detected. Last but not least, prognostic data are important in counselling patients with breast cancer.

These changes in pathological reporting have, however, occurred in a culture of evidence-based medicine in which it is necessary to justify reporting data using two criteria:

1. They must be shown to have clinical value.
2. It must be possible, given the subjective nature of histological interpretation, to report them consistently.

The justification for including the data on the form using both criteria is given in the appropriate parts of this book (see particularly Chapter 12).

QUALITY ASSURANCE IN BREAST PATHOLOGY

The increasing demand for high-quality pathological data and the introduction of mammographic screening have been the main

Surname... ☐RIGHT   ☐LEFT
PATHOLOGIST.................................Date of reporting...........................Report No. ....
Specimen Type (More than one to be ticked)
☐ Localisation biopsy ☐ Open biopsy ☐ Segmental excision ☐ Mastectomy ☐ Wide bore needle core
☐ Lymph node dissection only ☐ Repeat excision to clear margins
Specimen weight ....g
Specimen radiograph seen? ☐ Yes ☐ No Mammographic abnormality present in specimen? ☐ Yes ☐ No ☐Unsure
Histological calcification   ☐Absent ☐Benign ☐Malignant

BENIGN LESIONS

☐ Complex sclerosing lesion/radial scar   ☐ Multiple papilloma
☐ Periductal mastitis/duct ectasia   ☐ Solitary papilloma
☐ Fibroadenoma   ☐ Sclerosing adenosis
☐ Fibrocystic change   ☐ Solitary cyst
☐ Other (please specify)   ☐ Not present

EPITHELIAL PROLIFERATION

☐ Not present   ☐ Present with atypia (ductal)
☐ Present without atypia   ☐ Present with atypia (lobular)

MALIGNANT LESIONS
IN SITU CARCINOMA

☐ Not present   ☐ Ductal, intermediate nulear grade
☐ Ductal high nuclear grade   ☐ Ductal low nuclear grade
         Growth patterns......................................
☐ Lobular   ☐Paget's disease present   SIZE (ductal only)..........................mm

MICROINVASIVE CARCINOMA (<1mm)   Not present   Present   Possible

INVASIVE TUMOUR
☐ Not present   ☐ Mucinous carcinoma
☐ 'Ductal' carcinoma - no specific type (NST) ☐ Tubular carcinoma
☐ Lobular carcinoma   ☐ Mixed (Please tick component types present)
☐ Medullary carcinoma   ☐ Not assessable

Other primary carcinoma (please specify)..
Other malignant tumour (please specify)..

GRADE   ☐I   ☐II   ☐ III   ☐Not assessable
VASCULAR INVASION (blood or lymphatic)   ☐Present   ☐ Not seen
MAXIMUM DIAMETER OF INVASIVE TUMOUR......................................mm
WHOLE SIZE OF TUMOUR (to include DCIS extending >1mm beyond invasive area).....................mm

DISEASE EXTENT   ☐Localised   ☐Multiple   ☐Not assessable
EXCISION MARGINS   ☐Reaches margin ☐Uncertain   ☐ Does not reach margin (nearest.............mm)
OESTROGEN RECEPTOR STATUS   ☐Not done   ☐Negative   ☐ Positive (% cells positive)
AXILLARY NODES PRESENT ☐Yes   ☐No   Number positive......................Total number...................
OTHER NODES PRESENT   ☐Yes   ☐No   Number positive......................Total number...................
                                                  Site of other nodes..

COMMENTS/ADDITIONAL INFORMATION

HISTOLOGICAL DIAGNOSIS ☐ NORMAL ☐ BENIGN ☐MALIGNANT ☐ MALIGNANT BUT
                                                        CURRENT SPECIMEN BENIGN

2.9 Standard proforma including the minimum data set. DCIS = ductal carcinoma *in situ*.

stimuli for introducing quality assurance (QA) measures into breast pathology. A QA programme was set up in the UK in association with the national screening programme, and a similar initiative has been developed on the European mainland. Four major outcome objectives were identified:

1. to improve the identification and pathological characterisation of lesions producing mammographic abnormalities;
2. to improve the consistency of diagnoses made by pathologists;
3. to improve the quality of prognostic information in pathological reports;

4. to minimize the number of unnecessary surgical operations.

The first objective was addressed by defining standards of macroscopic examination as described earlier in this chapter. The second and third were approached by devising a standard reporting form, which ensured that a standard set of data was collected from each patient, using the same terminology. Inconsistency could, however, still arise through the use of different diagnostic criteria, and so guidelines were produced in which, *inter alia*, these criteria were defined. The fourth objective was concerned with improving the standard of non-operative diagnosis and consequently involved defining standards for fine needle aspiration cytology and needle core biopsy (see Chapter 4). Standards of clinical and radiological diagnosis are also, of course, important in reducing unnecessary surgery.

Having taken the initiative to improve diagnostic consistency, a mechanism for monitoring it was required so that the quality of the data collected could be evaluated and corrective action taken if necessary. Such action could include teaching and training, improving guidelines, changing grading or classification systems or even not recording data if there was little or no prospect of achieving an acceptable level of consistency. An external quality assessment (EQA) scheme of the 'consensus' variety was, therefore, set up.

In consensus schemes, there is no prejudgement about the correct diagnosis, which is generally accepted to be that made by the majority of participants unless there is clear evidence to the contrary. In addition to evaluating diagnostic consistency, they have educational value by allowing participants regularly to compare and discuss their diagnoses with other participants. Furthermore, some rare and difficult lesions can be included because cases unsuitable for assessing performance are simply identified by a low level of agreement among the participants. The substandard performance of individuals can be defined as those falling repeatedly into a small subgroup whose diagnoses deviate significantly from those of the majority. These features contrast with the so-called proficiency testing schemes in which the correct diagnoses are determined in advance by the organizers, who thus function similarly to examiners conducting an examination. Although these schemes are effective at identifying substandard performance, they have little educational value as most participants will inevitably be of the required standard, and there is little or no opportunity to discuss the slides. Furthermore, they are able to test neither the performance of pathologists collectively nor the robustness of the diagnostic and classification systems they use.

The following account of EQA in breast histopathology is based on two similar schemes run in association with the UK National Breast Screening Programme and the breast screening programmes within the European Union funded by the Europe Against Cancer Programme. The former is much larger, having more than 400 participants in each circulation, of whom about 25 are members of the National Co-ordinating Group. The latter currently involves about 30 pathologists representing almost all the member states of the EU. Where similar analyses have been performed, the UK and European Working Groups achieve very similar results. In both schemes, cases are selected randomly within certain diagnostic categories. They are not selected because they are thought to be particularly difficult or interesting examples (except where specifically used for educational purposes) as this would make unfair demands on participants and confound the consistency analyses. Participants report the sections using a standard reporting form such as that in Fig. 2.9 above but modified by excluding data that cannot be supplied by examining histological sections alone. The findings are presented to the participants in a number of different ways.

Table 2.1 shows the results obtained for six selected cases from one of the circulations of the EC Working Group, in which 23 pathologists participated. The diagnoses have been divided into four major categories: benign, atypical hyperplasia, *in situ*/microinvasive

TABLE 2.1 Distribution of overall diagnoses

Slide	Overall diagnosis				Majority diagnosis	% readers
	Benign	AH	ISC/Micro	Invasive		
184	0	0	22	0	ISC/micro	100
187	0	0	0	22	Invasive	100
200	13	5	4	9	Benign	59
417	0	0	22	0	ISC/micro	100
419	0	2	20	0	ISC/micro	91
425	0	0	0	22	Invasive	100
κ^1	0.76	0.25	0.81	0.94	Overall κ	0.75
κ^2	0.74	0.27	0.87	0.94	Overall κ	0.84
κ^3	0.70	0.17	0.70	0.83	Overall κ	0.64
κ^4	0.79	0.18	0.75	0.88	Overall κ	0.77

κ^1 23 UK pathologists examining 72 cases (Sloane *et al.*, 1994).

κ^2 23 European pathologists examining 107 cases (Sloane *et al.*, 1999).

κ^3 250 UK pathologists examining 72 cases (Sloane *et al.*, 1994).

κ^4 450 UK pathologists examining 216 cases (Sloane *et al.*, 2000).

AH = atypical hyperplasia; ISC/Micro = *in situ* or microinvasive carcinoma.

carcinoma and invasive carcinoma. In the left-hand column are listed the slide numbers, and in the right-hand column the majority opinions. In four cases (numbers 184, 187, 417 and 425), there is complete agreement. In case 200, there was intraluminal proliferation interpreted as non-atypical hyperplasia by the majority but as atypical hyperplasia or even DCIS by others. In case 419, a substantial majority was in favour of DCIS, but two participants felt that the appearance fell short of this diagnosis and preferred atypical hyperplasia. This form of analysis allows cases that are associated with particular difficulties in interpretation to be identified and discussed. Such cases can be very useful in teaching and training, and in refining diagnostic criteria. The analysis also gives participants the opportunity to assess the spread of opinions in relation to their own diagnoses.

At the foot of the table are summarized the levels of consistency achieved in these four categories in four studies undertaken by UK and European pathologists. The cases and pathologists are different, but the methods of case selection and consistency analysis are identical. Kappa (κ) statistics have been used to measure diagnostic consistency. Values of κ range from zero for chance agreement only to +1 for perfect agreement, a negative value implying systematic disagreement. Landis and Koch (1977) suggest the following interpretation of different ranges of κ: 0–0.20 slight, 0.21–0.40 fair, 0.41–0.60 moderate, 0.61–0.80 substantial and 0.81–1.00 almost perfect.

One disadvantage of κ statistics is their dependence on the prevalence of cases in each category; this will in particular influence comparisons between different circulations. The level of agreement that can reasonably be expected of a large group of pathologists varies with the histological feature being assessed. For a basic diagnosis of invasive carcinoma, near-perfect agreement would be expected with a κ value in excess of 0.9. The reporting of prognostic features is inherently more subjective, and acceptable values are more difficult to define. In general, however, those in excess of 0.5 would be regarded as acceptable and 0.7 as desirable. Not surprisingly,

Table 2.1 shows that, of the major diagnostic categories, only atypical hyperplasia is associated with unacceptably low diagnostic consistency. Indeed, the relatively low κ value for the benign category results largely from cases in which some diagnoses of atypical hyperplasia were made.

The consistency achieved by the UK National Co-ordinating Group of 23 pathologists (κ^1) and the EC Working Group of 23 pathologists (κ^2) 5 years later is very similar. There is some improvement in consistency except in diagnosing atypical hyperplasia (AH), which was very low in both studies, and invasive carcinoma, which was very high in both. The values κ^3 and κ^4 were obtained by all participants in the UK National EQA scheme after 6 and 18 circulations, respectively, and show an improvement in all categories except AH.

Table 2.2 shows κ statistics obtained by the same groups of pathologists for some of the prognostic features of *in situ* and invasive carcinomas included in the reporting form. Again, the results obtained by the UK and EC working groups of 23 pathologists are very similar, the participants in the UK EQA scheme showing an improvement in grading invasive carcinomas between 6 and 18 circulations. This improvement was not gradual but occurred rapidly after the publication of revised guidelines in 1995 giving more explicit, illustrated guidance on grading. Table 2.2 shows that subtyping invasive carcinomas is generally performed satisfactorily but that the consistency of reporting vascular invasion is low and that some method of improving consistency is needed. The consistency of grading DCIS represents a significant improvement on that previously achieved using an architecture-based system, but there is still room for improvement.

Table 2.3 shows the major diagnostic categories, but this time the pathologists are listed in the left-hand column. It can be seen that each pathologist has a code number known only to him- or herself (the numbers being fictitious in the table). No one knows anyone else's code number, so the scheme is anonymous. Participants can read across the major categories and identify in the last column their overall agreement with the majority for that particular circulation. In order to make allowance for the clinical significance of any disagreement, a score is given to each pathologist for each case as follows:

TABLE 2.2. Consistency of reporting histological features of breast carcinomas expressed as κ statistics

Histological feature	Kappa			
Nuclear grade of ductal carcinoma in situ (×3)				
High	0.43[1]	0.44[2]		
Intermediate	0.17[1]	0.19[2]		
Low	0.49[1]	0.32[2]		
Overall	0.35[1]	0.32[2]		
Nuclear grade of ductal carcinoma in situ (×2)				
High versus other	0.46[1]	0.44[2]		
Subtype of invasive carcinoma				
No special type	0.50[2]	0.51[3]		
Lobular	0.70[2]	0.76[3]		
Medullary	0.48[2]	0.56[3]		
Tubular	0.55[2]	0.61[3]		
Mucinous	0.89[2]	0.92[3]		
Overall	0.56[2]	0.58[3]		
Grade of invasive carcinoma				
Grade 1	0.36[5]	0.46[2]	0.58[4]	0.56[3]
Grade 2	0.18[5]	0.29[2]	0.40[4]	0.35[3]
Grade 3	0.21[5]	0.66[2]	0.38[4]	0.70[3]
Overall	0.26[5]	0.47[2]	0.46[4]	0.53[3]
Vascular invasion				
Present, not seen, overall	0.30[2]	0.38[3] (κ is identical as there are only two groups)		

(1) 23 European pathologists examining 33 cases (Sloane *et al.*, 1998).
(2) 450 UK pathologists after 18 circulations of the UK national external quality assessment (EQA) scheme (Sloane *et al.*, 2000).
(3) 23 European pathologists examining 107 cases (Sloane *et al.*, 1999).
(4) 23 UK pathologists examining 72 cases (Sloane *et al.*, 1994).
(5) 250 UK pathologists after 6 circulations of the UK national EQA scheme (Sloane *et al.*, 1994).

TABLE 2.3. Individual diagnoses and measure of agreement

Pathologist	Benign	Atypical hyperplasia	*In situ*/ microinvasive	Invasive	Measure of agreement (%)	No. readings outside +/− 3 mm of median
1	3	0	2	7	100	1
2	1	0	4	7	100	0
3	1	0	4	7	100	0
4	2	1	3	6	97	0
5	1	1	2	8	90	0
6	2	1	2	7	100	0
7	1	1	3	7	100	0
8	2	0	3	7	100	1
9	1	1	3	7	100	0
10	3	0	2	7	100	0
11	1	1	3	7	100	0
12	1	2	2	7	100	0
13	1	2	2	7	100	0
14	1	1	3	7	100	0

- 3 – the diagnosis accords with the majority opinion;
- 2 – the diagnosis deviates by one group;
- 1 – the diagnosis deviates by 2 groups;
- 0 – the diagnosis deviates by 3 groups.

Thus, for a majority diagnosis of invasive carcinoma, scores of 3, 2, 1 and 0 would be given for diagnoses of invasive carcinoma, *in situ* carcinoma, AH and benign, respectively. Participants' scores are then added up and expressed as a percentage, which in Table 2.3 is calculated on only 10 of the 12 cases where there was at least 80% agreement among all participants. This explains why some participants achieve 100% agreement despite having a different number of cases in each of the four categories. Cases in which the majority diagnosis is made by fewer than 80% of the participants are not regarded as being suitable for assessing performance, although they can be highly educational. Scores falling below a predetermined level in two consecutive rounds are regarded as substandard and would stimulate an investigation of the possible reason for this. The last column provides an assessment of the participants' ability to measure tumour size by showing the number of cases where their measurements deviated by more than 3 mm from the median value for all participants.

EQA schemes are, of necessity, to some extent artificial. The amount of tissue examined is usually limited, and there is usually less clinical and macroscopic information. Participants are obliged to report specific categories without the opportunity to express any uncertainty. As the sections are not cut and stained in the participants' own laboratories, they may exhibit appearances somewhat different from those to which they are accustomed. Finally, participants may not devote the same attention to EQA cases as to those forming part of their surgical workload. Care should therefore be exercised in assessing substandard performance from consensus schemes, and a number of safeguards are necessary.

First, an adequate number of participants is needed for the consensus diagnosis to have any validity. Second, it is inappropriate to assess performance on cases in which there is a significant level of disagreement; in the UK scheme, a case is not regarded as being suitable for assessing performance unless the majority diagnosis has been made by at least 80% of the participants (see above). Third, any diagnosis that deviates from the consensus should have clinical significance. Fourth, there should be no evidence, for example from follow-up information, that the majority diagnosis is wrong. Finally, deviation from the majority diagnosis should occur persistently before action is taken.

An important question is whether consensus schemes actually improve performance. Sloane *et al.* (1994, 2000) reported overall κ values for new and previous participants in the UK scheme. Kappa was always higher for experienced participants than for those who were taking part for the first time. Tables 2.2 and 2.3 show that participants in this scheme are achieving greater consistency after 18 circulations than they did after 6 in many diagnostic categories (κ^3 versus κ^4 in Table 3.1 and (5) versus (2) in Table 3.2 above). Further evidence is provided by comparing the results

of this scheme with those obtained in a previous study funded by the Medical Research Council in the UK in association with the Trial of Early Detection of Breast Cancer (TEDBC) (Swanson Beck *et al.*, 1985). Higher κ statistics were obtained for all diagnostic categories. This achievement is all the more significant given that only nine pathologists participated in the TEDBC scheme and that the same slides were examined by all participants. It thus appears that efforts over several years to improve diagnostic consistency in breast pathology have met with some success, although it is clear that improvement cannot continue indefinitely, and there is evidence that a series of plateaux are being reached for the various histological features of clinical importance, the height of each plateau being determined by the robustness of the histological criteria. In the case of AH no progress has been made in improving diagnostic consistency.

REFERENCES

Ashikari R., Huvos A.G., Snyder R.E. (1977) Prospective study of non-infiltrating carcinoma of the breast. *Cancer*, **39**, 435–9.

Bauermeister D.E., Hall M.H. (1973) Specimen radiography – a mandatory adjunct to mammography. *Am. J. Clin. Pathol.*, **59**, 782–9.

Champ C.S., Mason C.H., Coghill S.B., Robinson M. (1989) A perspex grid for localization of non-palpable mammographic lesions in breast biopsies. *Histopathology*, **14**: 311–15.

Cross S.S., Angel C.A. (1997a) Five audit cycles of the informational content of histopathological reports of bladder carcinoma. *J Pathol.*, **181**, 7A.

Cross S.S., Angel C.A. (1997b) Four audit cycles of the informational content of histopathological reports of resected colorectal carcinomas. *Gut* **40**, A65.

Cserni G. (1999) Metastases in axillary sentinel lymph nodes in breast cancer as detected by intensive histopathological work up. *J. Clin. Pathol.*, **52**, 922–4.

Davies J.D. Roberts, G., Richardson P.J. (1973) A serial whole-organ slicing technique for examining surgically resected breasts. *J. Clin. Pathol.*, **26**, 891–2.

Davies J.D., Sharp S., Chinyama C.N. *et al.* (1997) 3-D histo-radiographic comparison of surgical clearances of microcalcified lesions in breast localization biopsies. *J. Pathol.*, **182**, 45–53.

Dey P., Woodman C.B.J., Gibbs A., Coyne J. (1997) Completeness of reporting on prognostic factors for breast cancer: a regional survey. *J. Clin. Pathol.*, **50**, 829–31.

European Commission (1996) *European Guidelines for Quality Assurance in Mammography Screening*, 2nd edn. Office for Official Publications of the European Communities.

Frappart L., Boudeulle M., Boumendil J. *et al.* (1984) Structure and composition of microcalcifications in benign and malignant lesions of the breast: study by light microscopy, transmission and scanning electron microscopy, microprobe analysis and X-ray diffraction. *Hum. Pathol.*, **15**, 880–9.

Gauvin G.P., Shortsleeve M.J., Ostheimer J.T. (1990) A rapid technique for accurately localizing microcalcifications in breast biopsy specimens. *Am. J. Clin. Pathol.*, **93**: 557–60.

Gonzalez J.E.G., Caldwell R.G., Valaitis J. (1991) Calcium oxalate crystals in the breast: pathology and significance. *Am. J. Surg. Pathol.*, **15**, 586–91.

Graham R.A., Homer M.J., Sigler C.J. *et al.* (1994) The efficacy of specimen radiography in evaluating the surgical margins of impalpable breast carcinoma. *Am. J. Roent.*, **162**, 33–6.

Homer M.J., Safail H., Smith T.J., Marchant T.J. (1989) The relationship of mammographic microcalcification to histologic malignancy: radiologic-pathologic correlation. *Am. J. Roentgenol.*, **153**, 1187–9.

Landis J.R., Koch G.G. (1977) The measurement of observer agreement for categorical data. *Biometrics*, **33**, 159–74.

Manton S.L., Ferguson D.J.P., Anderson T.J. (1981) An automated technique for the rapid processing of breast tissue for subgross examination. *J. Clin. Pathol.*, **34**, 1189–91.

Marcum R.G, Wellings S.R. (1969) Subgross pathology of the human breast: method and initial observations. *J. Natl Cancer Inst.*, **42**, 115–21.

National Coordinating Group for Breast Screening Pathology (1995) *Pathology Reporting in Breast Cancer Screening*. NHSBSP Publication No.3.

Rosen P.P. (1978) Frozen section diagnosis of breast lesions: recent experience with 556 consecutive biopsies. *Ann. Surg.*, **187**, 17–19.

Rosen P., Snyder R.E., Foote F.W., Wallace T. (1970) Detection of occult carcinoma in the apparently benign breast biopsy through specimen radiography. *Cancer*, **26**, 944–52.

Schnitt S.J., Wang H.H. (1989) Histologic sampling of grossly benign breast biopsies. How much is enough? *Am. J. Surg. Pathol.*, **13**, 505–12.

Schnitt S.J., Wang H.H., Owings D.V., Hann L. (1989) Sampling grossly benign breast biopsy specimens. *Lancet*, **ii**, 1038.

Sloane J.P., Ellman R., Anderson T.J. *et al.* (1994) Consistency of histopathological reporting of breast lesions detected by screening: findings of the UK National EQA Scheme. *Eur. J. Cancer*, **30A**, 1414–19.

Sloane J.P., Amendoeira I., Apostolikas N. *et al.*(1998) Consistency achieved by 23 European pathologists in categorising ductal carcinoma *in situ of* the breast using 5 classifications. *Hum Pathol.*, **29**, 1056–62.

Sloane J.P., Amendoeira I., Apostolikas N. *et al.* (1999) Consistency achieved by 23 European pathologists from 12 countries in diagnosing breast disease and reporting prognostic features of carcinomas *Virchows Archiv.*, **434**, 3–10.

Sloane J.P. *et al.* (2000) Impact of the national EQA scheme on breast pathology in the United Kingdom (in preparation).

Swanson Beck J. and members of the Medical Research Council Breast Tumour Pathology Panel (1985) Observer variability in reporting of breast lesions. *J. Clin. Pathol.*, **38**, 1358–65.

Symonds D.A. (1990) Use of the von Kossa stain in identifying occult calcifications in breast biopsies. *Am. J. Clin. Pathol.*, **94**, 44–8.

Turner R.R., Ollila D.W., Stern S., Giuliano A.E. (1999) Optimal histopathologic examination of the sentinel lymph node for breast carcinoma staging. *Am. J. Surg. Pathol.*, **23**, 263–7.

Van Diest P.J. (1999) Histopathological work up of sentinel lymph nodes: how much is enough? *J. Clin. Pathol.*, **52**, 871–3.

Walker T.M., Horton L.W.L., Menai Williams R. (1992) Impalpable breast lesions: marking of surgical specimens for pathology. *Clin. Radiol.*, **45**, 179–80.

3 Histochemical and molecular pathological methods of examining the breast

HISTOCHEMICAL STAINS

Mucin

The commonly employed alcian blue–periodic-acid–Schiff stain (AB-PAS) at pH 2.5 reveals the presence of both neutral and acidic mucins in normal and neoplastic breast epithelium. The acid mucin is usually sialidase susceptible and hyaluronidase resistant (Spicer *et al.*, 1962). In some breast carcinomas, mucin may be demonstrated in the form of intracytoplasmic globules (Gad and Azzopardi, 1975). The larger globules may exhibit an alcianophilic rim and a central PAS-positive dot, producing a bull's-eye appearance (Fig. 3.1). Such vacuoles are most frequently found in *in situ* and infiltrating lobular carcinomas and have been shown by electron microscopy to be lined by microvilli (Spriggs and Jerrome, 1975). They thus seem to be forms of intracytoplasmic lumina (see below). Although bull's-eye vacuoles have been reported in carcinomas of other organs such as the stomach and lung, they may have limited value in establishing that a carcinoma in the breast is of local origin in the absence of an *in situ* component.

Patterns of mucin staining may also assist in the diagnosis of the less common variants of breast carcinoma (see Chapter 11). In mucinous carcinoma, the lakes of mucin are

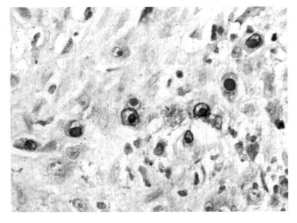

3.1 Alcian blue–periodic-acid–Schiff (AB-PAS) stain at pH 2.5 of an infiltrating lobular carcinoma. The cells contain large intracytoplasmic globules that displace the nucleus to one side of the cell. The central dots are PAS positive and the peripheral rims alcianophilic.

hyaluronidase resistant and sialidase susceptible. In the rare adenoid cystic carcinoma, there is a biphasic appearance in which the stromal 'cysts' are positive for AB only whereas the true ductal structures usually stain with PAS.

Elastin

The major ducts of the normal breast are surrounded by a cuff of fibrillary elastic tissue that is absent from the terminal ducts and acini. Larger ducts have more elastin than smaller ones, and the material tends to diminish on involution.

Increase in elastic tissue (elastosis) has been reported in up to 86% of breast carcinomas (Azzopardi and Laurini, 1974), mostly around

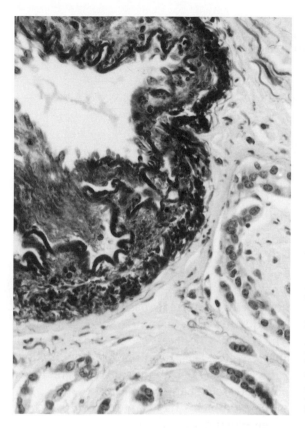

3.2 Breast carcinoma stained for elastin by the Weigert method. At the top left is a blood vessel showing a very marked increase in elastin. At the bottom and right are nests of infiltrating ductal (no special type) carcinoma.

ducts and blood vessels (Fig. 3.2) but sometimes diffusely in the stroma. It is much less prominent in medullary and mucinous carcinomas.

Elastosis is not specific for carcinoma and may also occur in certain benign proliferative lesions of the breast, particularly radial scars and complex sclerosing lesions (see Chapter 6). It is, however, very rarely associated with carcinomas metastatic to the breast and elastin stains may thus be of value in deciding whether a tumour is primary or secondary. Elastosis is uncommon in metastatic deposits of breast carcinoma to other organs.

Silver stains

Some breast carcinomas are argyrophilic and contain classic double membrane neuro-secretory granules on electron microscopy. Some exhibit cytological and architectural features of neuroendocrine tumours (*see* p. 191), some are mucinous carcinomas (*see* p. 178) and a minority have a non-specific appearance. Grimelius is the most sensitive and convenient stain for identifying these granules. Papotti *et al.* (1989) found that only

3 out of 43 carcinomas exhibiting evidence of neuroendocrine differentiation were Grimelius negative. Furthermore, on ultrastructural examination, Grimelius positivity was localized to double membrane-bound dense-core granules. The proportion of breast carcinomas exhibiting argyrophilia appears to be slightly less than 5% (Partenen and Syrjanen, 1981; Azzopardi *et al.*, 1982). Several polypeptide products have been demonstrated in these tumours but no associated clinical syndromes have yet been recorded.

Argentaffin positivity of breast carcinomas, due to colonization by melanocytes, has also been reported (Azzopardi and Eusebi, 1977) and appears to be a relatively common phenomenon in tumours that infiltrate the skin. As pigment may be present in the carcinoma cells as well as the melanocytes, confusion with malignant melanoma may arise. However, the mixture of tumour cells and dendritic melanocytes, as well as restriction of pigmentation to tumour in the upper dermis, should make the distinction clear.

IMMUNOHISTOCHEMICAL STAINS

Steroid receptors

Oestrogen receptor

The human *oestrogen receptor (ERα)* is a steroid-dependent, 65 kDa, DNA-binding protein with a 'zinc finger' binding motif. The gene has been mapped to chromosome 6q25.1. It belongs to a superfamily of nuclear receptors that includes those for thyroid hormone and the hormonal forms of vitamins A and D, as well as receptors for other steroid hormones. It is synthesized in the cytoplasm but translocates to the nucleus and thereafter shuttles between nucleus and cytoplasm. It is divided into several structural/functional domains:

- The *A/B domain* has a cell- and promoter-specific, ligand-independent, *trans*-activating function.
- The *C domain* contains two zinc finger motifs that are responsible for the specific DNA-binding activity of the protein.

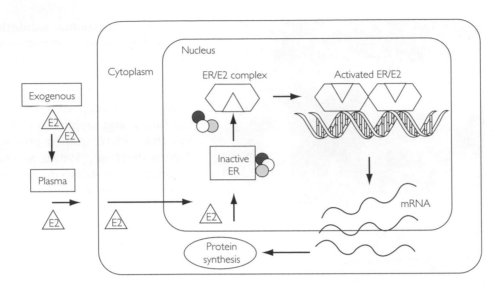

3.3 Oestrogen receptor (ER) action. (Illustration kindly supplied by Dr Balvinder Shoker).

- The *D domain* is a flexible 'hinge' region that may have a role in nuclear localization and DNA binding.
- The *E domain* contains the ligand-binding site and ligand-dependent dimerization activity, and a ligand-dependent *trans*-activation function.
- The *F domain* is thought to have a specific modulatory function on transcriptional responses to oestrogens and anti-oestrogens.

Prior to binding oestrogen, the receptor is in its inactive oligomeric form, associated with other proteins, including heat shock proteins (hsp) 90, 70 and 56, and p23, p50 and p54. On hormone binding, the receptor/hsp complex dissociates and the oestrogen/ER complex becomes activated, binding to DNA at oestrogen-responsive elements (ERE) as a homodimer. The binding results in the transcription and subsequent synthesis of proteins that are often collectively known as oestrogen-inducible proteins (*see* Fig. 3.3 above). These include progesterone receptor, cathepsin D and pS2 (see below).

For many years, ER expression was determined by ligand-binding assays, but they are time consuming and suffer from sampling problems; thus, not only is it sometimes difficult to define the extent of a tumour macroscopically, but the cellularity and degree of necrosis may also vary greatly. Furthermore, an increasing number of small carcinomas is now being detected, particularly since the introduction of mammographic screening, which makes it necessary to utilize all available tissue for histological examination, particularly if all prognostic data are to be provided (see Chapter 12).

These problems have largely been overcome by employing immunohistochemistry, which can be used to demonstrate ERs in formalin-fixed, paraffin-embedded sections. Only nuclear staining is assessed, cytoplasmic positivity being disregarded (Fig. 3.4). The results correlate well with those obtained by ligand-binding assays, and the technique has actually been found to be superior to the latter in predicting the response to adjuvant endocrine therapy (Harvey *et al.*, 1999). Furthermore, it has allowed ERs to be demonstrated in normal breast, benign breast changes and *in situ* carcinomas, although this currently has no clinical relevance. Other advantages of immunohistochemistry are that it can detect receptors occupied by high levels of oestrogen, as occurs in premenopausal women, and it can be applied to cytological samples. A major disadvantage, however, is that the technique gives no information about the functional state of the receptor. At the time of writing, the most common method employs the monoclonal antibody 1D5, which is applied to conventional formalin-fixed paraffin-embedded sections after microwave antigen retrieval (Goulding *et al.*, 1995).

3.4 (a) Immunostaining of a formalin-fixed, paraffin-embedded section of premenopausal breast for oestrogen receptors (ERs) using the 1D5 monoclonal antibody after microwave antigen retrieval. On the left is a normal lobule exhibiting a nuclear positivity of scattered epithelial cells. On the right is an invasive ductal (nst, that is, no special type) carcinoma showing a strong positivity of nearly all the cells. (b) Grade 3 invasive ductal (nst) carcinoma showing ER positivity restricted to the cytoplasm. This tumour should be regarded as negative.

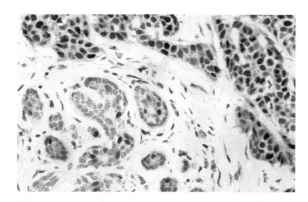

(a)

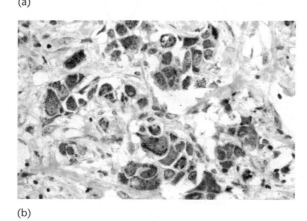

(b)

Histopathologists providing ER services should be aware of the problem of interlaboratory discrepancy resulting from variations in technical quality and inconsistent interpretation by pathologists. It is thus essential for any laboratory providing an immunohistochemistry-based ER service to participate in an external quality assessment scheme. The UK National External Quality Assessment Scheme for Immunohistochemistry has found that, overall, 70% of participating laboratories produce acceptable staining of ERs on slides provided by the scheme organizers and 97% on their own material (Barnes et al., 1998). These figures fall dramatically, however, when performance is assessed on tumours expressing a low level of ER, for which there is a false-negative rate of 30–60%. This lack of sensitivity appears to be caused by minor differences in methodology that may be rectified by a fine adjustment of the overall technique (Rhodes et al., 2000). It is especially important to include a weakly positive control.

The most elaborate scoring method is the so-called H score, which takes into account the percentage of positive cells and their staining intensity. The latter is graded as 0 (negative), 1 (weakly positive), 2 (moderately positive) or 3 (strongly positive). The score is then calculated as follows:

(% weakly positive cells × 1) + (% moderately positive cells × 2) + (% strongly positive cells × 3).

The maximum score is thus 300 and the minimum 0.

This system is, however, very time consuming and impracticable for most laboratories. The 'Quick' score method is simpler and has been shown to possess clinical validity (Reiner et al., 1990; Barnes et al., 1996). It involves assessing staining intensity as 0 (negative), 1 (weak), 2 (moderate) or 3 (strong) and the proportion of positive cells as 0 (no positive cells), 1 (1–25% positive), 2 (26–50%), 3 (51–75%) or 4 (76–100%). The intensity and proportion scores are *added* together, giving a range of 0–7. A similar system has been reported by Harvey et al. (1999), in which the proportion of positive cells is scored as follows: 0 (none), 1 (<1%), 2 (1–10%), 3 (10–33%), 4 (33–67%), 5 (>67%). To this is added the intensity score: 0 (none), 1 (weak), 2 (intermediate) or 3 (strong). This gives scores of 0–8 (without a score of 1), which correlate well with the probability of response to endocrine therapy.

Many laboratories, including the author's own, simply report the percentage of positive cells to the nearest 10%. It has been shown that intensity and evenness of staining are reported inconsistently by histopathologists even on identically stained sections (EC Working Group on Breast Screening Pathology, in preparation). Greater consistency is achieved in reporting the percentage of positive cells, the level increasing inversely with the number of groups. There is, at the time of writing, a lack of consensus over the level of precision required for reporting ER status for clinical purposes. Given that response to hormone therapy is related to the amount of ER (Elledge and Osborne, 1997), laboratories should give a value rather than simply report positive or negative.

In the normal premenopausal breast, ER is demonstrable on about 5–15% of epithelial cells, which are dispersed singly and rather unevenly in the ducts and lobules (*see* Fig. 3.4a above). Interestingly, these cells do not express the proliferation marker Ki67 or take up [³H] thymidine, indicating that the dividing cells in the normal breast are separate from those expressing ER. The same is true for the progesterone receptor (see below) (Clarke *et al.*, 1997). There is evidence that the number of ER-positive cells is lower in the second half of the menstrual cycle than the first and that a reduced number is seen for up to 5 years following a pregnancy and in women taking oral contraceptives. (Williams *et al.*, 1991, Battersby *et al.*, 1992). The percentage of ER-positive cells changes with age, being lowest during reproductive life. A larger proportion is seen in prepubertal girls and postmenopausal women as well as in normal males of all ages. These observations suggest an inverse relationship between the number of ER-positive cells and the plasma oestrogen and progesterone levels.

In involuting lobules, immunostaining may be seen on contiguous cells, sometimes occupying a whole lobule (Fig. 3.5). Increased expression, often on contiguous cells, may also be seen in a variety of benign changes including fibroadenoma, sclerosing adenosis, radial scar, papilloma and ductal and lobular hyperplasias, even in premenopausal women (Shoker *et al.*, 1999a, 1999b). Furthermore, the cells in these lesions, like those of carcinomas, frequently co-express Ki67.

The *oestrogen receptor-beta (ERβ)* shares similar structural and functional features with ERα and activates the transcription of target genes through EREs. The human *ERβ* gene is located on chromosome 14q22–q24 (Enmark *et al.*, 1997) and is much shorter than the alpha gene. The DNA-binding domain shows 97% homology with ERα, the ligand-binding domain 59%, the hinge domain 30%, the A/B domain 17.5% and the F domain 17.9% (Enmark *et al.*, 1997). Overall, ERβ shows approximately 47% identity with ERα. ERβ is

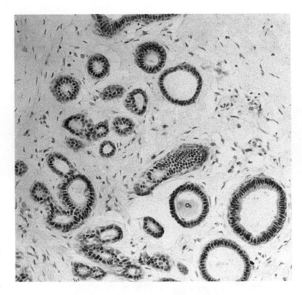

3.5 An involuting lobule from a postmenopausal woman stained for oestrogen receptors by the same method used in Fig. 3.4. There is a strong positivity of all the epithelial cells.

present in a variety of tissues, including kidney, intestine, lungs, thymus, spleen, bone marrow, blood leucocytes, pituitary gland, testis, uterus, ovaries and mammary glands. The tissue distribution is not identical to that of ERα but shows a considerable overlap.

The heterodimerization of ERα and ERβ has been demonstrated and suggests that crosstalk of the two signalling pathways can occur. Oestradiol action in a given tissue may thus depend on the relative expression of the two receptors. In breast cancers, it has been shown that the ratio of ERα to ERβ is higher in ER-positive tumours than in normal breast tissue (Leygue *et al.* 1998). The increased ratio is mainly due to an increased expression of ERα. Furthermore, the ratio of differently-sized ERβ transcripts has been shown to change with increasing tumour inflammation and grade, suggesting that the relative changes may be important during tumorigenesis and tumour progression (Leygue *et al.* 1998). ERβ has also been detected in ER-negative tumours, as determined by ligand-binding assay, and the possibility that ERβ may be involved in endocrine therapy responsiveness has been suggested (Dotzlaw *et al.* 1999).

The antibodies currently used to demonstrate ER for clinical purposes recognize the alpha variant.

Progesterone receptor

The progesterone receptor (PR) has been mapped to chromosome 1 and is regulated by ERs. PRs can also be demonstrated by immunohistochemistry in formalin-fixed, paraffin-embedded sections and is seen on virtually the same cells as ERs. Clarke *et al.* (1997) found that, in the normal breast, 96% of steroid receptor-positive cells synthesize both ER and PR. Contiguous PR-positive cells may be seen in older women, sometimes occupying a whole involuting lobule. The number of PR-positive cells appears to be reduced for up to 5 years after pregnancy (Battersby *et al.*, 1992), but, in contrast to ERs, the number of cells expressing PRs does not appear to vary throughout the normal menstrual cycle. There is, however, a steady increase throughout the cycle in women taking oral contraceptives (Williams *et al.*, 1991, Battersby *et al.*, 1992).

Most tumours that are positive for PR are also ER positive, although there are rare exceptions. The expression of PR is a predictor of response to endocrine therapy and has been shown to improve prediction when combined with ER determination. Thus ER+/PR+ tumours respond more frequently than those which are ER+/PR–, which in turn respond more frequently than the small number that are ER–/PR+ (NIH Consensus Development Conference, 1980). At the time of writing, however, few histopathology laboratories provide PR services as modern endocrine therapy is generally given on the strength of ER status alone. Furthermore, an external quality assessment scheme for PR determination is currently not available. Given the problems encountered by a significant number of laboratories in detecting a low level of ER (see above), it is the view of the author that they should first be able to deliver a reliable ER service before attempting one for PRs. The scope of PR services varies. At one extreme, some laboratories determine PR status on all tumours routinely whereas others investigate only ER-negative tumours for which endocrine therapy may be considered. The scope of a PR service should be determined by pathologists in consultation with clinicians and based on the current management protocols of the breast unit.

Oestrogen-regulated proteins

Various oestrogen-regulated proteins have been identified, mainly by stimulating ER-positive cell lines with oestrogen and then studying the cell supernatant for secreted protein or cell extracts for cDNA.

The *cathepsin D* gene is located on the short arm of chromosome 11, close to the c-Ha-*ras* gene, although no mutation, rearrangement or amplification has been found in breast carcinomas. The protein is a lysosomal enzyme that can digest extracellular matrix directly or indirectly by initiating the proteolytic cascade responsible for the breakdown of basement membranes (Rochefort, 1992). It is expressed in many breast carcinomas and could thus play a role in invasion. Studies of the relationship between cathepsin D and prognosis in invasive breast carcinomas are summarized on p. 229. A new cathepsin, *cathepsin K*, has recently been found to be expressed in breast epithelial cells and carcinomas, although it is not yet known whether this protein is under oestrogenic control (Littlewood-Evans *et al.*, 1997).

The *pS2* gene was identified in cDNA extracted from an ER-positive cell line stimulated with oestrogen (Masiakowski *et al.*, 1982) and encodes a cysteine-rich trefoil protein having similarities with insulin-like growth factor-1 (IGF-1). It is thought to have a role in cell growth, but its precise function is not clear. An increased expression of pS2 and another trefoil protein, *intestinal trefoil factor*, has been found in most benign and malignant breast lesions (Poulsom *et al.*, 1997). The expression of pS2 by breast cancers is further discussed on p. 229.

The *insulin-like growth factor receptor-1* (IGFR-1) is a tetrameric glycoprotein with an extracellular ligand-binding domain and an intracellular domain with tyrosine kinase activity. It is structurally similar to the insulin receptor. IGFR has been demonstrated in 50–93% of breast carcinomas (Pekonen *et al.*, 1988; Peyrat *et al.*, 1988), its level relating to the amount of ER and PR. Amplification of the *IGFR* gene in breast carcinomas has been reported but is very rare (Berns *et al.*, 1992). In an immunohistochemical study using frozen sections fixed in acetone, Happerfield *et al.* (1997) found that epithelial and myoepithelial cells of the normal breast showed cytoplasmic and membrane positivity, the latter often in a basolateral distribution. Endothelial cells were often weakly or moderately positive. Ninety per cent of carcinomas were also positive, invasive lobular carcinomas showing less reactivity than the ductal (nst, that is, no special type) type. A strong correlation with oestrogen and progesterone receptor positivity was observed.

Type 1 growth factor receptors and their ligands

Type 1 growth factor receptors are a group of transmembrane glycoproteins characterized by an extracellular ligand-binding domain, a transmembrane spanning sequence and an intracellular domain with tyrosine kinase activity. Two (epidermal growth factor and c-erbB-2) have been studied extensively in *in situ* and invasive breast cancer in recent years, another (c-erbB-3) being investigated to a much lesser degree.

The *epidermal growth factor receptor* (EGFR, c-erbB-1) is a 170 kDa glycoprotein so called because it was first detected in epidermoid carcinoma cells (Krupp et al., 1982). The gene is located on chromosome 7p13–p12. It can be activated by its ligand, epidermal growth factor (EGF), or by transforming growth factor-α (TGFα). Dimerization of the receptor follows ligand binding, and it is this that initiates the tyrosine kinase activation. The frequency with which EGFR positivity has been found on immunohistochemical examination has varied with the choice of antibody, fixative and staining method. With currently available antibodies, EGFR can be demonstrated on the majority of epithelial and myoepithelial cells in the normal breast in formalin-fixed, paraffin-embedded sections. EGF has been found in human breast cancer and breast cancer cell lines, suggesting that an autocrine loop could occur. EGF secretion by tumour-associated macrophages has been

reported (O'Sullivan et al., 1993). The expression of EGFR on breast carcinomas and its possible prognostic significance are discussed on p. 229.

C-erbB-2 is also known as *neu* and *Her2*, the former because it was first identified as a transforming gene in rat neuroblastomas (Bargmann *et al.*, 1986). It encodes a transmembrane protein of 185 kDa that has extensive homology with EGFR. The gene is located on chromosome 17q11.2–q12. Like the other members of this family of molecules, it exhibits intracellular tyrosine kinase and extracellular ligand-binding-like domains. There is cross-communication between c-erbB-2 and EGFR, and heterodimerization has been observed between the two following ligand binding to EGFR. At the time of writing, the major role of c-erbB-2 appears to be to form heterodimers with c-erbB-1, 3 and 4 to produce high-affinity receptors. Gene amplification, from two- to greater than 20-fold, accompanied by an overexpression of the mRNA and protein, is found in about 30% of human breast carcinomas (Slamon *et al.*, 1987). There is general agreement on this figure, but it should be noted that different antibodies and fixatives profoundly affect the incidence of immunopositivity (Penault-Llorca *et al.*, 1994). Tsutsumi *et al.* (1990) found that positivity could be obtained in epithelial cells in frozen sections of normal breast post-fixed in acetone. In the majority of cases, there is a good correlation between gene amplification and membrane staining as detected by immunohistochemistry of formalin-fixed, paraffin-embedded sections, but this is not always the case, particularly if sensitive staining methods are used. Furthermore, King *et al.*, (1989) found that a significant overexpression of c-erbB-2 mRNA could occur in the absence of gene abnormalities.

The demonstration of an increased expression of c-erbB-2 by immunohistochemistry or of gene amplification by *in situ* hybridization (in which an increased number of copies of the gene are observed as multiple signals in individual nuclei) has become very important in selecting patients for treatment with the humanized anti-c-erbB-2 antibody, Herceptin (*see* p. 230). For a discussion of the relationship between c-erbB-2 expression and prognosis, see p. 229.

C-erbB-2 immunopositivity is seen less frequently in invasive carcinomas than in ductal carcinomas *in situ*, of which 40–70% of cases are positive. It is positive in virtually all DCIS associated with Paget's disease (*see* Chapter 8). The reasons for this are not clearly understood but could simply be due to the higher proportion of detected cases of ductal carcinoma *in situ* that are of high nuclear grade.

The *c-erbB-3* gene encodes a 180 kDa protein that binds the ligand, heregulin (Carraway *et al.*, 1994). The gene is located on chromosome 12q13. Binding of the ligand to the c-erbB-3 receptor alone results in little tyrosine kinase activity, whereas in the presence of c-erbB-2 a high-affinity binding site is formed by dimerization, which results in greater activity in the presence of heregulin (Sliwkowski *et al.*, 1994). The relationship between c-erbB-3 and prognosis in carcinoma is discussed on p. 230.

c-erbB-4 is the most recently described member of the family. It has a molecular weight of 180 kDa. Heregulin and β-cellulin can stimulate the tyrosine phosphorylation of c-erbB-4 alone or in combination with EGFR, c-erbB-2 or c-erbB-3. The expression of c-erbB-4 by breast carcinomas has been found to be greater than normal in a minority of cases and less than normal in the majority (Srinivasan *et al.*, 1998). At the time of writing, there is no evidence that detecting the expression of c-erbB-4 has any clinical value in diagnosing or classifying breast disease.

c-Src is a protein tyrosine kinase involved in the signal transduction pathways activated by several growth factors, including EGFR and c-erbB-2. Its activity is elevated 4–30-fold above normal in breast cancers of various histological types. On immunostaining, the protein is seen mainly around the nucleus in malignant cells and more evenly distributed in the cytoplasm in normal cells (Verbeek *et al.*, 1996). There is no evidence at present, however, that demonstrating the protein has any use in diagnosing or classifying breast disease.

Transforming growth factor-β and its receptors

There are three mammalian isoforms of transforming growth factor-β (TGFβ), which are the products of different genes. Their effects are diverse, including growth suppression and regulation, differentiation and stromal production. They are particularly important in embryogenesis and wound healing. Their receptors fall into two families: type I and type II (TGFβR-I and TGFβR-II), each having small cysteine-rich extracellular regions and intracellular protein kinase domains. Receptor activity is complex. One of the TGFβ isoforms, $TGF\beta_2$, binds TGFβR-II with only a low affinity and requires an accessory receptor, TGFβR-III. It appears that both the homodimerization of type I receptors and the hetero-oligomerization of the type II receptor are needed for TGFβ to have an antimitotic effect. Alterations in TGFβ receptors, particularly TGFβR-II, can result in a loss of the growth inhibitory effect of TGFβ. Mutations in the extracellular or kinase domains of TGFβR-II have been found in colonic, gastric and endometrial cancers but not breast cancer, even though a loss of expression of TGFβR-II has been found in some carcinomas and hyperplasias (see p. 230). A family of genes known as *smads* mediates downstream signalling. The role of TGFβ may be very complex, and there is evidence that it acts in a biphasic manner, acting as an antipromoter in normal breast and early lesions but as a promoter in invasive cancers. The relative level of the different TGFβ receptors may be important in determining these different effects (for a review, see Walker, 2000).

p53

p53 is the protein product of the *TP53* gene. It is a nuclear phosophoprotein that was first identified as a co-immunoprecipitant with the large T antigen in cells infected with the SV40 virus (Lane and Crawford, 1979). It binds DNA and regulates transcriptional activity, eventually leading to growth arrest or apoptosis in cells with DNA damage (Lane, 1992). Abnormalities in p53 are probably the most common molecular change in human cancer.

Mutations are frequent in breast cancer and may be somatic or rarely germline (Malkin *et al.*, 1990). They are often associated with cell transformation, and, perhaps not surprisingly, most that are encountered in tumours occur in the central region of the gene that codes for the DNA-binding domain. Mutation usually results in a protein with a much longer half-life than the normal, wild-type protein. Consequently, mutants are usually demonstrable by immunohistochemistry, in contrast to the wild type, which is generally undetectable.

It should be noted that while positive immunostaining for p53 is usually associated with a gene mutation, this is not always the case. In some cases, the immunopositivity results from an overexpression of the wild-type protein, which may have become stabilized. Possible mechanisms include binding to viral or cellular proteins such as the SV40 large T antigen or the product of the *mdm2* gene (for a review, see Hall and Lane, 1994). Another possibility is that an immunopositive cell may be responding normally to a genotoxic or other stressful insult. Furthermore, the choice of antibody and fixation method influence immunostaining (Fisher *et al.*, 1994). Conversely, not all mutations result in immunopositivity. Negative immunostaining may be observed when normal p53 function is lost as a consequence of genetic deletion (Chen *et al.*, 1995).

Somatic mutations and/or immunostaining have been studied extensively in *in situ* and invasive breast cancer and are associated with high histological or nuclear grade (*see* p. 231).

p21 is the protein product of the *WAF1/Cip1* gene, which contains a p53 response element. It is thought to prevent cyclin/cyclin-dependent kinase complex activity and prevent cells from passing from the G1 to the S phase of the cell cycle. It thus appears to be an important part of the p53 growth arrest pathway but can also be regulated by p53-independent mechanisms. It has been studied in breast cancer, where it has been found to have some prognostic significance (McClelland *et al.*, 1999) (*see* p. 231).

bcl-2

The *bcl-2* gene is located on chromosome 18q21.3 and has been defined by molecular cloning of the translocation t(14;18)–(q32.3;q21.3) found in the majority of follicular lymphomas. It encodes a 26 kDa protein located on the mitochondrial membrane that appears to protect cells from apoptosis (Hockenbery *et al.*, 1990). Immunostaining reveals the positivity of normal breast epithelial cells. The expression of bcl-2 has been studied in both *in situ* and invasive breast carcinomas (*see* p. 231).

nm23/NDP-kinase

The *nm23* gene was identified by Steeg *et al.* (1988), who found that the metastatic potential of murine melanoma cell lines was inversely related to the level of *nm23* RNA. It was therefore proposed that *nm23* is a tumour-suppresser gene with reference to metastasis. It has since been found that the sequences of *nm23* and NDP-kinase (NDP-K) are identical. Studies of human breast cancer have been undertaken using *in situ* hybridization for *nm23* mRNA and antibodies to NDP-K to determine whether the expression of this gene is related to prognosis (*see* p. 231).

Cell cycle proteins

The *cyclin D1* gene is located on chromosome 11q13. It is amplified in about 20% of human breast cancers (Buckley *et al.* 1993) and is overexpressed at the protein level in about 40–80%. It can form activated complexes with cyclin-dependent kinases 4 and 6 to permit transit through the G1 to the S phase of the cell cycle (Fig. 3.6). It may also play an important role in differentiation. The activated complexes phosphorylate the retinoblastoma protein and can be inhibited by p16 and the p53-inducible protein p21/WAF1(see above) (Kamb *et al.*, 1994, Waldman *et al.*, 1996). Cyclin D1 levels may increase in response to oestrogen (Musgrove *et al.*, 1993). That cyclin D1 may be involved in the pathogenesis of breast cancer is evidenced by the occurrence of hyperplasias and breast cancer in transgenic mice engineered to overexpress it in mammary epithelium (Wang *et al.*, 1994).

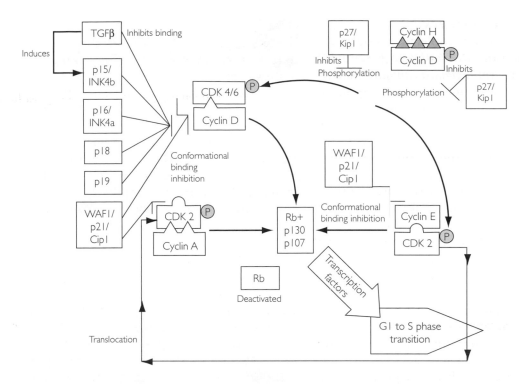

3.6 Cyclin D1 and its interactions during the cell cycle. (Illustration reproduced with permission from Novocastra.) TGFβ = transforming growth factor-β; CDK = Cyclin-dependent kinase; Rb = retinoblastoma.

Cyclin D1 knockout mice develop normally but do not display marked proliferation in pregnancy and consequently do not lactate despite normal hormone levels (Sicinski *et al.*, 1995). For studies of cyclin D1 in atypical hyperplasia and ductal carcinoma *in situ* see p. 109, and in invasive carcinoma see p. 232.

The monoclonal antibodies Ki67 and MIB-1 have been used to stain sections of breast and bind to a protein expressed throughout the cell cycle except for early G1 (for a review, see Brown and Gatter, 1990). Positive cells are thus found in normal breast, benign lesions and carcinomas. The proliferative activity of breast carcinomas provides important prognostic information, and the MIB-I labelling index correlates with histological features and clinical outcome. Perhaps surprisingly, assessing proliferative index by counting Ki67-positive cells has been shown to be associated with low interobserver consistency. This and the additional cost of immunohistochemistry in time and money mean that counting mitotic figures still remains the method of assessing proliferation in routine diagnostic practice, particularly in grading invasive carcinomas (for a review, see Pinder *et al.*, 1996).

Neuroendocrine markers

The antibodies most frequently used to demonstrate neuroendocrine differentiation in breast carcinomas are those against chromogranins A and B, synaptophysin and neurone-specific enolase. The last of these, however, lacks specificity and has been demonstrated in as many as 30% of breast carcinomas. The chromogranins are a specific component of the matrix of neurosecretory granules and have been shown, on electron microscopy using the immuno-gold technique, to localize to double membrane-bound dense-core granules (Papotti *et al.*, 1989). Synaptophysin, on the other hand, localizes to the membranes of a population of small clear vesicles with a size range similar to that of synaptic vesicles (Navone *et al.*, 1986). Synaptophysin and the chromogranins thus exhibit a different intracellular localization. In the study of Papotti *et al.* (1989), 30 of 43 of carcinomas showing neuroendocrine differentiation were positive for one or both of the chromogranins, 34 were positive for synaptophysin, and all 43 were positive for at least one of the three markers. The proportion of positive cells varied from 10% to 95%.

Epithelial cell markers

Antibodies against low molecular weight or a broad spectrum of *cytokeratins* (e.g. Cam 5.2, MNF116) and *epithelial membrane antigen* (EMA) (Fig. 3.7) give immunopositivity in the vast majority of breast carcinomas. Consequently, they are useful in distinguishing carcinomas from non-epithelial tumours such as sarcomas and lymphomas (see Chapter 14). The detection of minute metastatic deposits of breast carcinoma in tissues that do not normally express the markers, such as lymph node, liver and bone marrow, is also facilitated (Fig. 3.8) (Sloane *et al.* 1980, 1983; Dearnaley *et al.*, 1983; Redding *et al.*, 1983). EMA is useful for demonstrating intracytoplasmic lumina in lobular carcinomas.

Antibodies against different *isoforms of keratin* may be useful in distinguishing epithelial from myoepithelial cells. Cytokeratins 5/6 identify two types of cells: myoepithelial cells, which co-express smooth muscle actin, and luminal cells, which lack other differentiation antigens and are often known as basal keratin cells. In contrast, epithelial cells express keratins 15, 16, 18 and 19. Hyperplasia of the usual type usually comprises both types of cell, whereas *in situ* carcinomas usually express the luminal epithelial-type keratins only (Boecker *et al.*, 1992). Some workers have used antibodies to an apocrine cyst fluid protein, GCDFP-15, to identify apocrine differentiation in *in situ* and invasive carcinomas and to distinguish primary from metastatic carcinomas in the breast (Eusebi *et al.*, 1986; Kaufmann *et al.*, 1996).

An account of appropriate markers for diagnosing *non-epithelial tumours*, such as lymphomas and sarcomas, is beyond the scope of this book. It should, however, be noted that immunopositivity for *vimentin* may be encountered in both benign and malignant breast epithelial cells and is thus not a reliable indicator of mesenchymal differentiation (Heatley *et al.*, 1993).

Myoepithelial cell markers

The immunohistochemical demonstration of myoepithelial cells is mainly of value in distinguishing pseudo-infiltrative disorders and *in situ* carcinomas from invasive carcinomas as the latter are almost invariably devoid of a myoepithelial layer. Myoepithelial cells contain a high concentration of contractile proteins and are demonstrable using antibodies to these components. Anti-smooth muscle

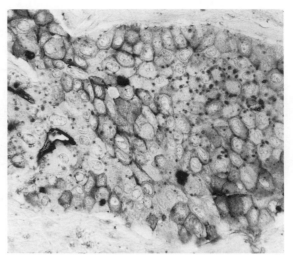

3.7 Formalin-fixed, paraffin-embedded section of an infiltrating breast carcinoma immunostained for epithelial membrane antigen. There is strong staining of cell membranes, luminal membranes (left) and numerous small intracytoplasmic lumina.

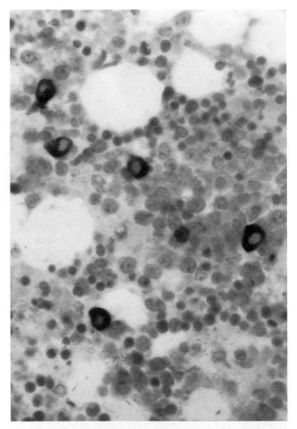

3.8 Dispersed epithelial membrane antigen-positive metastatic breast carcinoma cells in a paraffin-embedded section of a bone marrow aspirate. This specimen was thought to be free of tumour on H&E-stained sections.

3.9 Formalin-fixed, paraffin-embedded section of normal breast immunostained with an antibody to smooth muscle actin. The myoepithelial cells are positive and form a layer around all the acini of this lobule. Note the staining of the pericytes of the small blood vessel in the upper part of the picture.

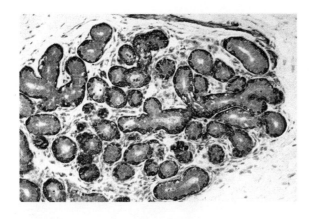

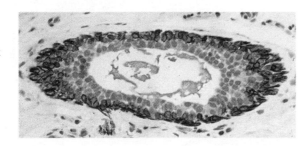

3.10 An interlobular duct immunostained with the antibody LLOO2 against cytokeratin 14. The myoepithelial layer is strongly stained.

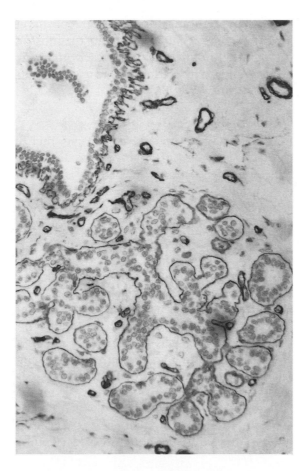

3.11 Methacarn-fixed, paraffin-embedded section of normal breast stained immunohistochemically with a monoclonal antibody to type IV collagen. Basement membrane staining is seen around acini, blood vessels and an interlobular duct (top left).

actin antibodies are the most frequently used (Fig. 3.9). A major problem, however, is that actin is also strongly expressed on stromal myofibroblasts, which may be closely applied to the periphery of invasive tumour cell masses, giving the false impression of a myoepithelial layer. Actin antibodies are therefore best used in combination with those against non-smooth muscle components such as cytokeratin 14 (Fig. 3.10), although this keratin is less consistently expressed, particularly in pathological processes. Antibodies to smooth muscle myosin, calponin and high molecular weight caldesmon have also been employed to distinguish myoepithelial from epithelial cells. The first two of these also react with stromal myofibroblasts (Lazard *et al.*, 1993) and are thus associated with the same interpretative problems as smooth muscle actin.

A positive immunostaining of myoepithelium can be obtained for S100 and glial fibrillary acidic proteins but, in the author's experience, is usually weak in normal cells and often undetectable in myoepithelial tumours. Furthermore, S100 positivity is often seen in ordinary breast carcinomas (Matsushima *et al.*, 1994). Recent work has, however, shown that S100-β is usually expressed in myoepithelial cells but rarely in epithelial cells, in contrast to S100-α, for which the converse is true (Ichihara *et al.*, 1997). For most practical purposes, immunostaining for smooth muscle actin and cytokeratin 14 is usually sufficient to demonstrate myoepithelium around *in situ* carcinomas and the glandular structures of pseudo-infiltrative lesions, but more extensive panels of antibodies may be required for conclusively demonstrating myoepithelial differentiation in myoepithelial tumours.

Basement membrane components

Intact basement membrane can be visualized around the epithelium of the normal breast (Fig. 3.11) but not of invasive carcinomas (Siegal *et al.*, 1981). Its demonstration thus has the same diagnostic value as identifying myoepithelial cells. In ductal carcinoma *in situ*, however, there may be zones where the staining lacks definition, and in microinvasive foci, fragmentation and focal absence of staining may be seen. Basement membrane is also present around blood vessels, and immunohistochemical staining for type IV collagen has been used to detect vascular invasion by breast carcinoma (Bettelheim *et al*, 1984).

Endothelial markers

The significance of lymphatic and blood vessel invasion by breast carcinomas is discussed in Chapter 12. It is often very difficult to be certain whether small clumps of infiltrating carcinoma are within blood vessels or are merely surrounded by stroma exhibiting retraction artefact. Antibodies to factor VIII-related antigen (*see* Fig. 12.13), CD31, CD34 or thrombomodulin can demonstrate vascular endothelial cells and may be useful in detecting vascular invasion (Bettelheim *et al.*, 1984) or assessing angiogenesis. Although some studies have demonstrated a relationship between microvessel density and prognosis, others have failed to do so (*see* p. 226). Specific immunohistochemical stains for lymphatic endothelium have not been found until recently, when Jussila *et al.* (1998) reported that monoclonal antibodies against the extracellular domain of the vascular endothelial growth factor-C receptor (VEGFR-3) specifically stained the endothelial cells of lymphatic vessels.

Milk proteins

The initial hope that milk proteins would serve as tissue-specific markers for mammary carcinoma or have prognostic significance has not been realized. Bailey *et al.* (1982) demonstrated α-lactalbumin in the normal pregnant and lactating breast as well as in a small proportion of non-pregnant women, either in lobules appearing normal or in lobular lesions known as lactational foci. They were unable to detect the protein in breast carcinomas even when they were removed from pregnant or lactating women (Fig. 3.12). This study did not, however, include all histological types of breast carcinoma, and it has since been found that

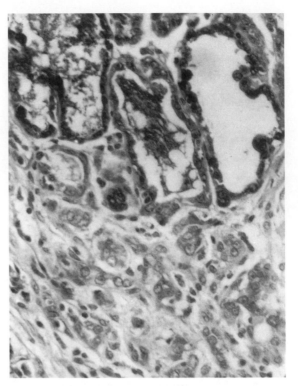

3.12 Immunohistochemical stain for α-lactalbumin on a formalin-fixed, paraffin-embedded section of a carcinoma arising in a lactating breast. The normal lactating epithelium at the top is strongly positive, whereas the tumour at the bottom is negative (× 315). (Illustration reproduced with permission from the *Journal of Pathology*.)

secretory carcinomas are generally positive, a characteristic that is useful in diagnosing these rare tumours. Similar reactions have been found with antibodies to casein (Earl and McIlhinney, 1985).

Adhesion molecules

As invasion and metastasis involve highly complex cascades of changes in adhesion molecule expression, it is perhaps naive to expect that studying any one of them will give valuable pathological or clinical information. Several have, however, received a significant amount of attention in the breast cancer literature.

E-Cadherin and the catenins

E-Cadherin is an epithelium-specific adhesion molecule, the gene for which is located on chromosome 16q. It is a member of a family of transmembrane glycoproteins that mediate calcium-dependent cell–cell adhesion. It complexes with three different cytosolic proteins – α, β and γ catenins – which link E-cadherin to the actin filament network and other transmembrane proteins. The catenins

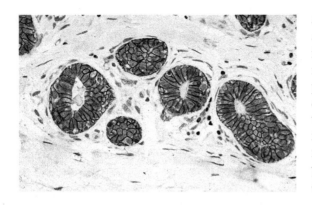

3.13 A normal lobule stained immuno-histochemically for E-cadherin. The basolateral membranes of all the acini are strongly positive.

appear to be necessary for E-cadherin to express its full adhesive function. In the normal breast, immunostaining for E-cadherin and α and β catenin reveals positivity of the basolateral surfaces of the luminal epithelial cells and myoepithelial cells of the interlobular ducts and terminal duct–lobular units (Gamallo *et al.*, 1993; Moll *et al.*, 1993; Oka *et al.*, 1993, Hashizume *et al.*, 1996) (Fig. 3.13). Most *in situ* and invasive ductal carcinomas are positive for E-cadherin and α and β catenin, although staining is often reduced in high-grade tumours. The most significant finding in breast disease is the negativity of most lobular carcinomas (*see* Chapters 9 and 11).

Integrins

The integrins are heterodimeric transmembrane proteins consisting of α and β chains. Variations in the sequence of these chains and the combinations with which they associate give rise to a large family of molecules, mediating cell–stroma and cell–cell interactions. Immunostaining with antibodies to most integrins shows a similar appearance, with strong membrane positivity of the myoepithelial cells and weak-to-moderate staining of the basolateral surfaces of the epithelial cells (Pignatelli *et al.*, 1992).

Downregulation of the α chain of the integrin α2β1 (VLA-2) and a loss of α6β4 have been found in invasive carcinomas, more frequently in high-grade tumours. In contrast, αvβ3 (the vitronectin receptor) has been found to be weak or absent in normal breast epithelium but is present in a minority of invasive ductal (nst) carcinomas and a high proportion of invasive lobular carcinomas. *Carcinoembryonic antigen*

and carcinoembryonic-related antigens function as accessory adhesion molecules and are found in a high proportion of breast carcinomas, mainly in the cytoplasm, although membrane polarization is significantly reduced (Pignatelli *et al.*, 1992). There thus appears to be widespread deregulation of the expression of integrins and their accessory adhesion molecules in breast cancer, but they do not as yet appear to have any value in pathological diagnosis or prognostication.

Metalloproteinases

The matrix metalloproteinases (MMPs) are a family of enzymes capable of modifying and remodelling the extracellular matrix. In certain experimental systems, their activity is required for tumour progression and metastasis. There are many types with different functions. Interstitial and neutrophil *collagenases* and collagenase-3 are capable of degrading interstitial collagens. The two gelatinase enzymes, *MMP-2* and *MMP-9*, are also known as type IV collagenases and degrade basement membrane collagen. *Stromelysin-1 and -2* and *matrilysin* have broad substrate specificity against proteoglycans and glycoproteins such as laminin and fibronectin. *Stromelysin-3*, *metalloelastase* and *membrane-type matrix metalloproteinases* (MTI-MMPs) have more restricted specificity, the latter being a potent activator of the MMP-2 zymogen. Some of the enzymes have been studied in human breast cancer using immunohistochemistry or *in situ* hybridization to detect mRNA. The tissue inhibitors of metalloproteinases, *TIMP-1* and *TIMP-2*, have also been found in tumour and stromal cells. *Gelatinase A* mRNA has been demonstrated in normal myoepithelial cells (Monteagudo *et al.*, 1990). Despite the importance of this family of molecules in cancer, they have not been studied extensively in histological sections of breast carcinoma in relationship to prognosis at the time of writing.

MOLECULAR GENETIC TECHNIQUES

Genetic abnormalities in breast carcinomas may be inherited or acquired. Cancer arising in patients with inherited mutations is discussed on p. 207. Acquired genetic abnormalities are numerous and varied, and include amplifications, deletions, point mutations, structural rearrangements and translocations affecting the function of genes controlling virtually all the major cell functions, including proliferation, apoptosis, DNA repair, genetic stability, differentiation, and their ability adhere to each other and various substrates. There are numerous methods of studying molecular genetic changes in human breast tissue, most of which are beyond the scope of this book. Below are listed a few approaches that have been used to investigate human breast lesions in histopathological material and to which reference is made elsewhere in this book.

Polymerase chain reaction

The value of the PCR technique lies in its ability to amplify minute amounts (theoretically single copies) of DNA to quantities that are sufficiently large to investigate. DNA from specific genes or chromosomal loci can be amplified by choosing synthetic primers of appropriate sequence that span the DNA under investigation. Primers are short specific DNA sequences, generally about 20 nucleotides in length, which are designed to hybridize to complementary sequences in the DNA under investigation and serve as templates for the action of DNA polymerase. The DNA between the hybridization sites of the two primers is thus replicated. Multiple rounds of PCR are performed, the quantity of DNA under investigation theoretically doubling in each of the 30–40 rounds.

There are variations of this technique, including nested PCR, in which the PCR product is subjected to further rounds of amplification using a second pair of primers internal to the first, thus increasing the sensitivity and specificity. Tissue from formalin-fixed, paraffin-embedded sections can be used, but, in the author's experience, it is difficult to amplify sequences greater than 400 base pairs owing to the degradation of DNA that occurs in processing.

When studying histological material, it is usual to employ some method of microdis-section to ensure that only DNA from the cells under investigation is amplified. A variety of techniques can be employed, the degree of sophistication depending on the number and distribution of the cells under study. The simplest method is simply to scrape tissue from the glass slide with a needle or fine scalpel blade, usually under a dissecting microscope. In one method used to study microscopic breast lesions, the sections were mounted on clear, double-sided adhesive tape and stained with methylene blue (Stratton *et al.*, 1995). The advantages of this method are that the cells of interest are easily visualized, and dissection is facilitated by the cohesion of the tissue provided by the tape, which need not be separated from the cells when they are added to the PCR mixture. It is possible to dissect structures as small as 0.5 mm using this method. Further refinement can be achieved using a micromanipulator, which allows structures as small as 0.1 mm to be recovered. At the time of writing, the most sophisticated method is laser capture, which allows single cells to be separated from the surrounding tissue (Emmert-Buck *et al.*, 1996). The amplified DNA can then be studied in a variety of ways.

Mutations can be detected by various methods, including the detection of single-stranded conformational polymorphisms, in which single-stranded DNA is run in non-denaturing gels. Mutations result in changes in the conformation of the DNA, which consequently migrates to a different position in the gel from that of the wild-type DNA. Alternatively, or in addition, direct sequencing can be undertaken.

PCR has been used most frequently on microdissected breast lesions to detect *allelic imbalance* (AI) (loss of heterozygosity) by using primers that span microsatellite nucleotide repeat sequences at specific chromosomal loci. It is necessary to choose subjects who are heterozygous, that is, the sequence of generally 1–4 nucleotides being repeated more times on one chromosome than the other. Consequently, when the PCR products are run in gels, they migrate to different positions and form two bands. The loss of one band cannot confidently be attributed to deletion as the picture could be explained by an overrepresentation of the other allele. Combined analysis with PCR and *in situ* hybridization is useful in these circumstances (see below). Relatively pure cell populations are needed as the imbalance will be masked by a significant contribution of DNA from contaminating normal (or neoplastic) cells not exhibiting it. In order to overcome this problem, PCR analysis can be combined with an appropriate microdissection technique (see above).

AI is a common finding in invasive carcinoma and has been reported at many chromosomal loci using conventional Southern analysis on frozen samples of breast tissue as well as by microdissection and PCR, as described above. The major interest of AI to the molecular biologist is that it may indicate the presence of a tumour-suppressor gene at the locus at which it is found. In most cases, however, the presence of AI merely reflects genomic instability, and it is a relatively non-specific (albeit nevertheless useful) method of detecting tumour-suppressor genes. More recent studies using the microdissection of formalin-fixed, paraffin-embedded sections and PCR have also demonstrated AI at various chromosomal loci in ductal carcinoma *in situ* (Stratton *et al.*, 1995), atypical ductal hyperplasia (Lakhani *et al.*, 1995) and hyperplasia of usual type (Lakhani *et al.*, 1996). Caution has to be exercised in interpreting the significance of AI, however, as it has been found at various chromosomal loci in histologically normal tissue in cancerous breasts and in reduction mammoplasty specimens from patients without cancer. AI involving the wild-type allele of the *BRCA-1* gene in a patient with an inherited *BRCA-1* mutation has even been found in apparently normal cells (Lakhani *et al.*, 1999). The molecular *milieu* of the cells showing AI is clearly of great importance.

A phenomenon related to AI, as detected by the PCR amplification of microsatellites, is *microsatellite instability* (MI), in which the microsatellites are themselves unstable and exhibit random increases or decreases in length. MI is a characteristic feature of the hereditary non-polyposis colorectal cancer syndrome, in which it is associated with inherited mutations of the human homologues of the bacterial mismatch repair genes (Thibodeau *et al.*, 1993; Karran, 1996). When the PCR products are subjected to gel electrophoresis, those from the lesional tissue migrate to different positions in the gel from those of normal tissue, reflecting their change in size. This is in contrast to AI, in which one of the products migrates to the normal position and the other is lost altogether. MI has been described in invasive breast cancer, but its incidence has varied greatly from one study to another. Fewer studies have been undertaken in ductal carcinoma *in situ*, where MI has been found in a significant minority of cases, generally of high nuclear grade and often c-erbB-2 positive (Walsh *et al.*, 1998)

Interphase cytogenetics

This technique has largely replaced conventional cytogenetic analysis in the investigation of breast disease as it is not dependent on obtaining metaphase spreads from dividing cells in culture. Furthermore, it allows a direct correlation of cytogenetic changes with morphology. A limited number of conventional cytogenetic analyses have been undertaken on breast lesions, mostly on invasive carcinomas; they are referred to in the relevant places in this book.

Interphase cytogenetics involves the *in situ* hybridization of specific nucleotide probes to complementary DNA sequences in histological sections or cytological smears. Two main types of probe have been used: centromeric and locus specific.

Centromeric probes hybridize to repeated sequences near the centromeres of chromosomes, and in view of the abundance of the target sequences they are relatively easy to use. Consequently, studies using these probes are more numerous. As the centromeric sequences are chromosome specific, they allow the determination of the number of a particular chromosome in a cell. Alternatively, locus-specific probes can detect a change in the number of specific genes or loci. This is technically more demanding as a signal has to be generated from a single target sequence. Large, heavily labelled probes and sensitive detection systems are therefore required.

In the past, probes were usually labelled with radioactive isotopes, but it is now more common to use fluorochromes or enzyme histochemical techniques (generally peroxidase or alkaline phosphatase), usually in combination with biotin- or digoxigenin-labelled probes. The main advantage of the enzyme histochemical approach, as in immunohistochemistry, is that it is possible simultaneously to see the histological and cytological detail of the tissue under study. The advantage of fluorescence *in situ* hybridization (FISH), however, is that it is easier to use multiple probes. Images can be superimposed and processed so that changes in multiple genes and chromosomes can be visualized in the same cell. Changes in gene copy number can also be related to the number of copies of the particular chromosome on which the gene is located by the combined use of locus and centromeric probes. It is also easier to combine FISH with immunohistochemistry so that genotype and phenotype can be compared in the same cell.

Interphase cytogenetics thus gives quantitative information on the number copies of genes, specific chromosomal loci or whole chromosomes in individual cells and can therefore overcome the significant problem of tumour heterogeneity. It thus provides information complementary to that obtained from AI analysis. It will not reveal mutations in genes, but translocations may be seen where two normally separate signals are seen side by side, or when two adjacent loci become separated by translocation. Most studies using probes for specific chromosomal loci have been undertaken on cytological preparations. Studies of histological sections, particularly formalin-fixed, paraffin-embedded sections, have generally employed centromeric probes. Problems arise in interpreting signals from sections because of the truncation of nuclei, which inevitably occurs on sectioning. Correction factors can, however, be applied to overcome this problem (Southern and Herrington, 1996), but it may still be difficult to identify small subpopulations of abnormal cells with confidence.

Interphase cytogenetic studies on formalin-fixed, paraffin-embedded sections using pericentromeric probes have shown abnormal chromosome numbers in invasive and *in situ* carcinoma and hyperplasia (Micale *et al.*, 1994).

Comparative genomic hybridization

This technique involves the hybridization of differently labelled genomic DNA (usually with fluorescein and rhodamine) from tumour and normal cells simultaneously to normal metaphase spreads. The ratio of intensity of hybridized tumour and normal DNA is then determined by digital imaging microscopy. If DNA at a particular chromosomal locus is overrepresented in the tumour, this will be reflected in a greater intensity of the fluorescence from the fluorochrome used to label the tumour DNA at that locus in the metaphase spread. The reverse is true if the DNA is underrepresented. This method can thus be used to determine changes in gene copy number over the whole genome in one investigation, but it is limited in its sensitivity to changes that involve more than about 10 megabases of DNA or very high-level amplification of smaller regions (Gray *et al.*, 1994). Another limitation is that the observed changes represent the summation of all those in the tissue and take no account of tumour heterogeneity or of contamination by non-neoplastic cells, which, if significant, could mask any changes in the tumour. This problem has, however, been minimized by analysing DNA from cells that have been microdissected from histological sections.

FLOW CYTOMETRY

There is a significant body of evidence supporting an association between a high S-phase fraction, and to a lesser extent aneuploidy, and the increased risk of recurrence and death for patients with breast cancer. This appears to be independent of tumour size, nodal involvement and steroid hormone receptor status but not tumour grade. Although flow cytometry is more objective than histological grading, it is more

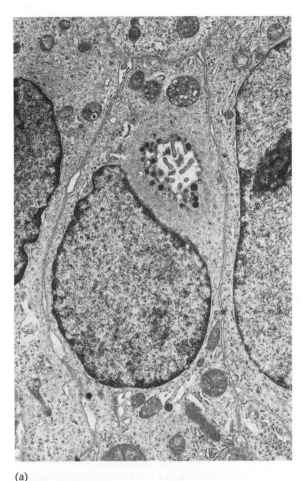

(a)

(b)

3.14 (a) Electron micrograph of an infiltrating breast carcinoma cell containing an intracytoplasmic lumen lined by microvilli in the upper central part of the picture (× 15 714). (b) Part of the cytoplasm of another tumour showing double membrane-bound, dense-core granules, indicative of neuroendocrine differentiation (same magnification).

and Ellis, 1991) if grading criteria are adhered to (Sloane *et al.*, 1999).

ELECTRON MICROSCOPY

There have been several extensive reviews of the ultrastructure of the normal and disordered human breast (Ozello, 1971; Fisher, 1976; Ahmed, 1980). Although electron microscopy almost invariably increases the understanding of the morphology of the normal and diseased breast, it rarely enables a diagnosis of a breast disorder to be made that cannot be established by light microscopy.

Breast carcinomas differ from normal cells ultrastructurally by showing a marked variation in the prominence and distribution of their organelles. Cytoplasmic filaments may be found, some of which resemble those seen in non-neoplastic epithelial cells, while others are thick and irregularly clustered in groups. Sometimes filaments may be arranged in thick, wavy bundles. Filaments with the characteristics of those seen in myoepithelial cells are not usually observed. Intracytoplasmic lumina may be seen that consist of small, membrane-bound lumina lined by microvilli within the cytoplasm (Fig. 3.14). They appear to represent invaginations of the plasma membrane. A small proportion of breast carcinomas exhibit intracytoplasmic double membrane-bound dense-core granules or small, clear, synaptic-like vesicles indicative of neuroendocrine differentiation (Fig 3.14). In intraduct carcinomas, electron microscopy frequently shows breaks in the basal lamina through which epithelial cells may protrude, possibly indicating areas of early invasion. None of these features is, however, specific for malignancy, and all may occasionally be seen in non-neoplastic states.

Ahmed (1980) found that electron microscopy may be of value in distinguishing sclerosing adenosis from tubular carcinoma by identifying the myoepithelial layer in the former. This feature may be impossible to ascertain by conventional light microscopy but can usually be demonstrated by immunohistochemistry (see above). The electron microscope may be useful, as in any organ, in distinguishing epithelial from

expensive and time consuming, and little has been done to standardize methods of flow cytometric analysis in different laboratories (for a review, see O'Reilly and Richards, 1992). Intratumour heterogeneity has been found to be a problem in flow cytometric determinations (Bergers *et al.*, 1996). Furthermore, it has been shown that pathologists can achieve at least a moderate level of agreement on tumour grade using the Nottingham method (Elston non-epithelial lesions, in particular densely cellular carcinomas from malignant lymphomas, and spindle cell carcinomas from sarcomas. All these problems, however, may also be solved by immunohistochemical techniques, which are cheaper and suffer less from sampling problems.

SCANNING ELECTRON MICROSCOPY

Although it is possible to examine only the surfaces of tissues with this technique, it allows a rapid observation of a large number of cells and often provides an appreciation of surface morphology that cannot be inferred from conventional transmission electron microscopy.

There have been few scanning electron microscopy studies of the breast, and although some interesting observations have been made, there is little to suggest that it has a significant role to play in diagnosing breast disease.

REFERENCES

Ahmed A. (1980) Ultrastructural aspects of human breast lesions. *Pathol. Ann.*, **15**, 411–43.

Azzopardi J.G., Eusebi V. (1977) Melanocyte colonization and pigmentation of breast carcinoma. *Histopathology*, **1**, 21–30.

Azzopardi J.G. and Laurini R.N. (1974) Elastosis in breast cancer. *Cancer*, **33**, 174–83.

Azzopardi J.G., Muretto P., Goddeeris P., Eusebi V., Lauweryns J.M. (1982) 'Carcinoid' tumours of the breast: the morphological spectrum of argyrophil carcinomas. *Histopathology*, **6**, 549–69.

Bailey A.J., Sloane J.P., Trickey B.S., Ormerod M.G. (1982) An immunocytochemical study of a-lactalbumin in human breast tissue. *J. Pathol.*, **137**, 13–23.

Bargmann C.I., Hung M.C., Weinberg R.A. (1986) The neu oncogene encodes an epidermal growth factor receptor-related protein. *Nature*, **319**, 226–30.

Barnes D.M., Harris W.H., Smith P., Millis R.R., Rubens R.D. (1996) Immunohistochemical determination of oestrogen receptor: comparison of different methods of assessment of staining and correlation with clinical outcome of breast cancer patients. *Br J Cancer*, **74**, 1445–51

Barnes D.M., Millis R.R., Beex L.V.A.M., Thorpe S.M., Leake R.E. (1998) Increased use of immunohistochemistry for oestrogen receptor measurement in mammary carcinoma: the need for quality assurance. *Eur. J. Cancer*, **34**, 1677–82.

Battersby S., Robertson B.J., Anderson T.J., King R.J.B., McPherson K. (1992) Influence of menstrual cycle, parity and oral contraceptive use on steroid receptors in normal breast. *Br. J. Cancer*, **65**, 601–7.

Bergers E., van Diest P.J., Baak J.P.A. (1996) Tumour heterogeneity of DNA cell cycle variables in breast cancer measured by flow cytometry. *J. Clin. Pathol.*, **49**, 931–7.

Berns E.M.J.J., Klijn J.G.M., van Staveren I.L., Portengen H., Foekens J.A. (1992) Sporadic amplification of the insulin-like growth factor 1 receptor gene in human breast tumours. *Cancer Res.*, **52**, 1036–9.

Bettelheim R., Mitchell D., Gusterson B.A. (1984) Immunocytochemistry in the identification of vascular invasion in breast cancer. *J. Clin. Pathol.*, **37**, 364–6.

Boecker W., Bier B., Freytag G. *et al.* (1992) An immunohistochemical study of the breast using antibodies to basal and luminal keratins, α smooth muscle actin, vimentin, collagen IV and laminin. *Virchows Archiv. A Pathol. Anat.*, **421**, 323–30.

Brown D.C., Gatter K.C. (1990) Monoclonal antibody Ki-67: its use in histopathology. *Histopathology*, **17**, 489–503.

Buckley, M.F., Sweeney, K.J.E., Hamilton, J.A. *et al.* (1993) Expression and amplification of cyclin genes in human breast cancer. *Oncogene*, **8**, 2127–33.

Carraway K.L., Sliwkowski M.X., Akita R. *et al.* (1994) The c-erbB-3 gene product is a receptor for heregulin. *J. Biol. Chem.*, **269**, 14303–6.

Chen Y.H., Li C-D., Yap E.P.H., McGee J.O'D. (1995) Detection of loss of heterozygosity of p53 gene in paraffin embedded breast cancers by non-isotopic PCR-SSCP. *J. Pathol.*, **177**, 129–34.

Clark, G.M., Harvey, J.M., Osborne, C.K., Allred, D.C. (1997) Estrogen receptor status determined by immunohistochemistry is superior to biological ligand-binding assay for evaluating breast cancer patients. *Proc. Am. Soc. Clin. Oncol.*, **16**, 129.

Clarke R.B., Howell A., Potten C.S., Anderson E. (1997) Dissociation between steroid receptor expression and cell proliferation in the human breast. *Cancer Res.*, **57**, 4987–91.

Dearnaley D.P., Ormerod M.G., Sloane J.P. *et al.* (1983) Detection of isolated mammary carcinoma cells in the marrow of patients with primary breast cancer. *J. Roy. Soc. Med.*, **76**, 359–64.

Dotzlaw H., Leygue E., Watson P.H., Murphy L.C. (1999) Estrogen receptor-beta messenger RNA expression in human breast tumor biopsies: relationship to steroid receptor status and regulation by progestins. *Cancer Res.*, **59**, 529–32.

Earl H.M., McIlhinney R.A.J. (1985) Monoclonal antibodies to human casein. *Mol. Immunol.*, **22**, 981–91.

Elledge R.M., Osborne C.K. (1997) Oestrogen receptors and breast cancer. It is time for idivdualised treatment based on oestrogen receptor status. *Br. Med. J.*, **314**, 1843–4.

Elston C.W., Ellis. (1991) Pathological prognostic factors in breast cancer. I. The value of histological grade in breast cancer: experience from a large study with long term follow up. *Histopathlogy*, **19**, 403–10.

Emmert-Buck M.R., Bonner R.F., Smith P.D. *et al.* (1996) Laser capture microdissection. *Science*, **274**, 998–1001.

Enmark E., Pelto-Huikko M., Grandien K. *et al.* (1997) Human estrogen receptor beta-gene structure, chromosomal localization, and expression pattern. *J. Clin. Endocrinol. Metab.*, **82**, 4258–65.

Eusebi V., Millis R.R., Cattini M.G., Bussolati G., Azzopardi, J.G. (1986) Apocrine carcinoma of the breast . Amorphological and immunocytological study. *Am. J. Pathol.*, **123**, 532–41.

Fisher C.J., Gillett C.E., Vojtesek B., Barnes D.M., Millis R.R. (1994) Problems with p53 immunohistochemical staining: the effect of fixation and variation in the methods of evaluation. *Br. J. Cancer.*, **69**, 26–31.

Fisher E.R. (1976) Ultrastructure of the human breast and its disorders. *Am. J. Clin. Pathol.*, **66**, 291–374.

Gad A., and Azzopardi J.G. (1975) Lobular carcinoma of the breast: a special variant of mucin-secreting carcinoma. *J. Clin. Pathol.*, **28**, 711–16.

Gamallo C., Palacios J., Suarez A. *et al.* (1993) Correlation of E-cadherin expression with differentiation grade and histological type in breast carcinoma. *Am. J. Pathol.*, **142**, 987–93.

Goulding H., Pinder S., Cannon P. *et al.* (1995) A new immunohistochemical antibody for the assessment of estrogen receptor status on routine formalin-fixed tissue samples. *Hum. Pathol.*, **26**, 291–4.

Gray J.W., Collins C., Henderson I.C. *et al.* (1994) Molecular cytogenetics of human breast cancer. *Cold Spring Harbor Symposia on Quantitative Biology*, **LIX**, 645–52.

Hall P.A., Lane D.P., (1994) p53 in tumour pathology: can we trust immunohistochemistry? – revisited! *J. Pathol.*, **172**, 1–4.

Happerfield L.C., Miles D.W., Barnes D.M., Thomsen L.E., Smith P., Hanby A.M. (1997) The localisation of the insulin-like growth factor receptor (IGFR-1) in benign and malignant breast tissue. *J. Pathol.*, **183**, 412–17.

Harvey J.M., Clark G.M., Osborne C.K., Allred D.C. (1999) Estrogen receptor status by immunohistochemistry is superior to the ligand binding assay for predicting response to adjuvant endocrine therapy in breast cancer. *J. Clin. Oncol.*, **17**, 1474–81.

Hashizumi R., Koizumi H., Ihara A., Ohta T., Uchikoshi T. (1996) Expression of β catenin in normal breast tissue and breast carcinoma: a comparative study with epithelial cadherin and α-catenin. *Histopathology*, **29**, 139–46.

Heatley M., Whiteside C., Maxwell P., Toner P. (1993) Vimentin expression in benign and malignant breast epithelium. *J. Clin. Pathol.*, **46**, 441–5.

Hockenbery D., Nunez G., Milliman C., Schreiber R.D., Korsmeyer S.J. (1990). Bcl-2 is an inner mitochondrial protein that blocks programmed cell death. *Nature*, **348**, 334–6.

Ichihara S., Koshikawa T., Nakamura S., Yatabe Y. and Kato K. (1997) Epithelial hyperplasia of usual type expresses both S100-α and S100-β in a heterogeneous pattern but ductal carcinoma *in situ* can express only S100-α in a monotonous pattern. *Histopathology*, **30**, 533–41.

Jussila L., Valtola R., Partanen T.A. *et al.* (1998) Lymphatic endothelium and Kaposi's sarcoma spindle cells detected by antibodies against the vascular endothelial growth factor receptor-3. *Cancer Res.*, **58**, 1599–604.

Kamb A., Gruis N.A., Weaver-Feldhaus J. *et al.* (1994) A cell cycle regulator potentially involved in the genesis of many tumour types. *Science*, **264**, 436–40.

Karran P. (1996) Microsatellite instability and DNA mismatch repair in human cancer. *Semin. Cancer Biol.*, **7**, 15–24.

Kaufmann O., Deidesheimer T., Muehlenberg M., Deicke P., Dietel M. (1996) Immunohistochemical differentiation of metastatic breast carcinomas from metastatic adenocarcinomas of other common primary sites. *Histopathology*, **29**, 233–40.

King R.C., Swain S.M., Porter L., Sreinberg S.M., Lippman M.E., Gelman E.P. (1989) Heterogeneous expression of c-erbB-2 messenger mRNA in human breast cancer. *Cancer Res.*, **49**, 4185–91.

Krupp M.N., Connolly D.T., Lane M.D. (1982). Synthesis, turnover and down-regulation of epidermal growth factor receptors in human A431 epidermoid carcinoma cells and skin fibroblasts. *J. Biochem.*, **257**, 11489–96.

Lakhani S.R., Collins N., Stratton M.R., Sloane J.P. (1995) Atypical ductal hyperplasia of the breast: a clonal proliferation with loss of heterozygosity on chromosomes 16q and 17p. *J. Clin. Pathol.*, **48**, 611–15.

Lakhani S.R., Slack D.N., Hamoudi R.A., Collins N., Stratton M.R., Sloane J.P. (1996) Detection of allelic imbalance indicates that a proportion of mammary hyperplasia of usual type are clonal, neoplastic proliferations. *Lab. Invest.*, **74**, 129–35.

Lakhani S.R., Chaggar R., Davies S. *et al.* (1999) Genetic alterations in 'normal' luminal and myoepithelial cells of the breast. *J Pathol.*, **189**, 496–503.

Lane D.P. (1992) Cancer. p53, guardian of the genome. *Nature (London)*, **258**, 15–16.

Lane D.P., Crawford L.V. (1979). T antigen is bound to host protein in SV-transformed cells. *Nature*, **278**, 261–3.

Lazard D., Sastre X., Frid M.G., Glukhova M.A., Thiery J.P., Koteliansky V.E. (1993) Expression of smooth muscle-specific proteins in myoepithelium and stromal myofibroblasts of normal and malignant human breast tissue. *Proc. Natl Acad. Sci. USA*, **90**, 999–1003.

Leygue E., Dotzlaw H., Watson P.H., Murphy L.C. (1998) Altered estrogen receptor alpha and beta messenger RNA expression during human breast tumorigenesis. *Cancer Res.*, **58**, 3197–201.

Littlewood-Evans A.J., Bilbe G., Bowler W. *et al.* (1997) The osteoclast associated protease Cathepsin K is expressed in human breast carcinoma. *Cancer Res.*, **57**, 5386–90.

Malkin D., Li F.P., Strong L.C. *et al.* (1990) Germ line p53 mutations in a familial syndrome of breast cancer, sarcomas and other neoplasms. *Science*, **250**, 1233–8.

Masiakowski P., Breathnach R., Bloch J. *et al.* (1982). Cloning of cDNA sequences of hormone-regulated genes from the MCF-7 human breast cancer cell line. *Nucl. Acids Res.*, **10**, 7895–902.

Matsushima S., Mori M., Adachi Y., Matsukuma A., Sugimachi K. (1994) S100 protein positive breast carcinomas: an immunohistochemical study. *J. Surg. Oncol.*, **55**, 108–13.

McClelland R.A., Gee J.M.W., O'Sullivan L. *et al.* (1999) p21WAF1 expression and endocrine response in breast cancer. *J Pathol.*, **188**, 126–32.

Micale M.A., Visscher D.W., Gulino S.E., Wolman S.R. (1994) Chromosomal aneuploidy in proliferative breast disease. *Hum. Pathol.*, **25**, 29–35.

Moll R., Mitze M., Frixen U.H., Birchmeier W. (1993) Differential loss of E-cadherin expression in infiltrating ductal and lobular breast carcinomas. *Am. J. Pathol.*, **143**, 1731–42.

Monteagudo C., Merino M.J., San-Juan J., Liotta L.A., Stetler-Stevenson W.G. (1990) Immunohistochemical distribution of type INVASIVE collagenase in normal, benign, and malignant breast tissue. *Am. J. Pathol.*, **136**, 585–92.

Musgrove E.A., Hamilton J.A., Lee C.S., Sweeney K.J., Watts C.K., Sutherland R.L. (1993) Growth factor, steroid and steroid antagonist regulation of cyclin gene expression associated with changes in T-47D human breast cancer cell cycle progression. *Mol. Cell Biol.*, **13**, 3577–87.

Navone F., Jahn R., Di Gioia C., Stukenbrok H., Greengard P., De Camilli P. (1986) An integral membrane protein specific for small clear vesicles of neurones and neuroendocrine cells. *J. Cell Biol.*, **103**, 2511–27.

NIH Consensus Development Conference on Steroid Receptors in Breast Cancer (1980). *Cancer*, **46**, 2759–963.

Oka H., Shiozaki H., Kobayashi K. *et al.* (1993) Expression of E-cadherin cell adhesion molecules in human breast cancer tissues and its relationship to metastasis. *Cancer Res.*, **53**, 1696–701.

O'Reilly S.M., Richards M.A. (1992) Is DNA flow cytometry a useful investigation in breast cancer? *Eur. J. Cancer*, **28**, 504–7.

O'Sullivan C.O., Lewis C.E., Harris A.L., McGee J.O'D. (1993) Secretion of epidermal growth factor by macrophages associated with breast carcinoma. *Lancet*, **342**, 148–9.

Ozzello L. (1971) Ultrastructure of the human mammary gland. *Pathol. Ann.*, **6**, 1–59.

Papotti M., Macri L., Finzi G., Capella G., Eusebi V., Bussolati G. (1989) Neuroendocrine differentiation in carcinomas of the breast: a study of 51 cases. *Semin. Diagn. Pathol.*, **6**, 174–88.

Partanen S., Syrjanen K. (1981) Argyrophilic cells in carcinoma of the female breast. *Virchows Arch., Pathol. Anat.*, **391**, 45–51.

Pekonen F., Paitanen S., Makinen T., Rutanen E.M. (1988). Receptors for epidermal growth factor and insulin-like growth factor 1 and their relation to steroid receptors in human breast cancer. *Cancer Research*, **48**, 1343–7.

Penault-Llorca F., Adelaide J., Houvenaeghel G., Hassoun J., Birnbaum D., Jacquemier J. (1994) Optimization of immunohistochemical detection of ERBB2 in human breast cancer: impact of fixation. *J. Pathol.* **173**, 65–75.

Peyrat J.P., Bonneterre J., Beauscart R., Dijiane J., Demaille A. (1988) Insulin-like growth factor I receptors in human breast cancer and their relationship to estradiol and progesterone receptors. *Cancer Res.*, **48**, 6429–33.

Pignatelli M., Cardillo M.R., Hanby A., Stamp G.W.H. (1992) Integrins and their accessory adhesion molecules in mammary carcinomas: loss of polarisation in poorly differentiated tumors. *Hum. Pathol.*, **23**, 1159–66.

Pinder S.E., Elsto C.W., Ellis I.O. (1996). Proliferative activity in invasive breast carcinoma. *J. Clin. Pathol.*, **49**, 868–9.

Poulsom R., Hanby A.M., Lalani E-N., Hauser F., Hoffmann W., Stamp G.H. (1997) Intestinal trefoil factor (TFF3) and pS2 (TFF1) but not spasmolytic polypeptide (TFF2) are co-expressed in normal, hyperplastic and neoplastic human breast epithelium. *J. Pathol.*, **183**, 30–8.

Redding W.H., Monaghan P., Imrie S.F. *et al.* (1983) Detection of micrometastases in patients with primary breast cancer. *Lancet*, **ii**, 1271–4.

Reiner A., Neumeister B., Spona J., Reiner G., Schemper M., Jakesz R. (1990) Immunocytochemical localization of estrogen and progesterone receptor and prognosis in human primary breast cancer. *Cancer Res.*, **50**, 7057–61

Rhodes A., Jasani B., Barnes D.M., Bobrow L.G., Miller K.D. (2000) Reliability of immunohistochemical demonstration of oestrogen receptors in routine practice: interlaboratory variance in the sensitivity of detection and evaluation of scoring systems. *J. Clin. Pathol.*, **53**, 125–30.

Rochefort H. (1992) Biological and clinical significance of cathepsin D in breast cancer. *Acta Oncol.*, **31**, 125–30.

Shoker B.S., Jarvis C., Sibson R., Walker C., Sloane J.P. (1999a) Oestrogen receptor expression in the normal and pre-cancerous breast. *J. Pathol.*, **188**, 127–244.

Shoker B.S., Jarvis C., Clarke R.B. *et al.* (1999b) Estrogen receptor positive proliferating cells in the normal and precancerous breast. *Am. J. Pathol.* **155**, 1811–15.

Sicinski P., Donaher J.L., Parker S.B. *et al.* (1995) Cyclin D1 provides a link between development and oncongenesis in the retina and breast. *Cell*, **82**, 621–30.

Siegal G.P., Barsky S.H., Terranova V.P., Liotta L.A. (1981) Stages of neoplastic transformation of human breast tissue as monitored by dissolution of basement membrane components: an immunoperoxidase study. *Invest. Metast.*, **1**, 54–70.

Slamon D.J., Clark G.M., Wong S.G., Levin W.J., Ullrich A., McGuire W.L. (1987) Human breast cancer: correlation of relapse and survival with amplification of the HER-2/neu oncogene. *Science*, **235**, 177–82.

Sliwkowski M.X., Schaefer G., Akita R.W. *et al.* (1994) Coexpression of erbB-2 and erbB-3 proteins reconstitutes a high affinity receptor for heregulin. *J. Biol. Chem.*, **269**, 14661–5.

Sloane J.P., Ormerod M.G., Imrie S.F., Coombes R.C. (1980) The use of antisera to epithelial membrane antigen in detecting micrometastases in histological sections. *Br. J. Cancer*, **42**, 392–8.

Sloane J.P., Hughes F., Ormerod M.G. (1983) An assessment of the value of epithelial membrane antigen and other epithelial markers in solving diagnostic problems in tumour histopathology. *Histochem. J.*, **15**, 645–54.

Sloane J.P. Amendoeira I., Apostolikas N. *et al.* (1999) Consistency achieved by 23 European pathologists from 12 countries in diagnosing breast disease and reporting prognostic features of carcinomas *Virchows Archiv.*, **434**, 3–10.

Southern S.A., Herrington C.S. (1996) Assessment of intra-tumoural karyotypic heterogeneity by interphase cytogenetics in paraffin wax sections. *J. Clin. Pathol. Mol. Pathol.*, **49**, M1–M7.

Spicer S.S., Neubecker R.D., Warren L., Henson J.G. (1962) Epithelial mucins in lesions of the human breast. *J. Natl Cancer Inst.*, **29**, 963–75.

Spriggs A.I., Jerrome D.W. (1975) Intracellular mucous inclusions: a feature of malignant cells in effusions in the serous cavities, particularly due to carcinoma of the breast. *J. Clin. Pathol.*, **28**, 929–36.

Srinivasan R., Poulsom R., Hurst H.C., Gullick W.J. (1998). Expression of the c-erbB-4/HER4 protein and mRNA in normal human fetal and adult tissues and in a survey of nine solid tumour types. *J. Pathol.*, **185**, 236–45.

Steeg P.S., Bevilacqua G., Kopper L. *et al.* (1988) Evidence for a novel gene associated with low tumour metastatic potential. *J. Natl Cancer Inst.*, **80**, 200–4.

Stratton M.R., Collins N., Lakhani S.R., Sloane J.P. (1995) Loss of heterozygosity in ductal carcinoma in situ of the breast. *J. Pathol.*, **175**, 195–201.

Thibodeau S.N., Bren G., Schaid D. (1993) Microsatellite instability in cancer of the proximal colon. *Science*, **260**, 816–19.

Tsutsumi Y., Naber S., DeLellis R.A. *et al.* (1990) *neu* oncogene protein and epidermal growth factor receptor are independently expressed in benign and malignant breast tissues. *Hum. Pathol.*, **21**, 750–8.

Verbeek B.S., Vroom T.M., Adriaansen-Slot S.S. *et al.* (1996) c-Src protein expression is increased in human breast cancer. An immunohistochemical and biochemical analysis. *J. Pathol.*, **180**, 383–8.

Waldman T., Lengauer C., Kinzler K.W., Vogelstein B. (1996) Uncoupling of S phase and mitosis induced by anticancer agents in cells lacking p21. *Nature*, **381**, 713.

Walker R.A. (2000) Transforming growth factor beta and its receptors: their role in breast cancer. *Histopathology*, **36**, 178–80.

Walsh T., Chappell S.A., Shaw J.A., Walker R.A. (1998) Microsatellite instability in ductal carcinoma *in situ* of the breast. *J. Pathol.*, **185**, 18–24.

Wang T.C., Cardiff R.D., Zukerberg L., Lees E., Arnold A., Schmidt E.V. (1994) Mammary hyperplasia and carcinoma in MMTV-cyclin D1 transgenic mice. *Nature*, **369**, 669–71.

Williams G., Anderson E., Howell A. *et al.* (1991) Oral contraceptive (OCP) use increases proliferation and decreases oestrogen receptor content of epithelial cells in the normal breast. *Int. J. Cancer*, **48**, 206–210.

4 Non-operative diagnosis

P.A. Trott and J.P. Sloane

INTRODUCTION

Current evidence indicates that the use of fine needle aspiration cytology (FNAC) and/or needle core biopsy (NCB) can substantially reduce the number of unnecessary surgical operations performed for both benign and malignant disease, with a consequent reduction in discomfort and inconvenience to the patient as well as financial savings. Decisions concerning whether and how to operate on patients can be decided preoperatively by the 'triple assessment' of mammography, clinical examination and cytology/needle biopsy (Thomas et al., 1978, Di Pietro et al., 1987, Dixon et al., 1984), thus avoiding the need for intraoperative frozen sections. Other forms of imaging such as ultrasound may be used in addition to mammography.

The correlation of clinical and radiological data and the findings from needle specimens is best achieved in multidisciplinary meetings where the clinician, radiologist and pathologist discuss the findings and reach a consensus on diagnosis and on the appropriate management of each patient following predefined protocols. The accuracy of this method of assessment is particularly important in those patients in whom a diagnosis of malignancy will lead directly to treatment, such as primary medical therapy (Trott and Nasiri, 1997) or definitive surgery, rather than open biopsy.

If the needle sample is negative in the face of strong clinical or radiological evidence of malignancy, it can be repeated; if it is still negative, an open biopsy should be undertaken. The detection of carcinoma in needle specimens depends not only on the ability of the pathologist to identify malignancy, but also on the skill with which the operator can localize the lesion with the needle and obtain a representative sample of adequate size and quality, free from artefact. The failure to detect malignancy by needling in a patient with cancer may thus be caused by factors beyond the pathologist's direct control. Adequate multidisciplinary discussion and a unit audit of performance parameters can lead to the identification of problems and allow appropriate corrective measures to be taken. Consequently, reporting forms have been devised for use in European Breast Screening Programmes, which allow sensitivity, specificity and other measures of performance to be calculated and monitored (see below).

Until recently, needle aspiration was the more widely used technique, but core biopsy is increasingly being used (Britton, 1999). A major factor is the introduction of the biopsy gun, which relies on a 'firing' action and is less painful than the Tru-cut needle. There has been much discussion concerning the relative merits and disadvantages of FNAC and NCB (Britton and McCann, 1999) (Table 4.1). The latter has several advantages. It is possible to

TABLE 4.1 Relative merits and disadvantages of needle core biopsy (NCB) and fine needle aspiration cytology (FNAC) in diagnosing breast diseases

	NCB	FNAC
Distinguishing *in situ* from invasive carcinoma	Usually possible	Not possible
Diagnosing low-grade invasive carcinomas	Usually possible	Occasionally possible
Benign samples	A specific diagnosis can usually be made	Usually only a general diagnosis of benignity is possible (C2)
Specimen radiography	Possible	Not possible
Reporting prognostic features	More reliable	Less reliable
Immunohistochemistry for oestrogen receptors and other markers	Good correlation with findings on excision specimens	Correlation with excision specimens less predictable. Currently no external quality assessment schemes for reporting oestrogen receptors
Speed of operation	Slower – needs local anaesthetic	Fast – allows definitive preoperative diagnoses to be made in 'one-stop' clinics
Multiple passes	More difficult	Easier
Localization of small and impalpable lesions	More difficult	Easier
Skill and experience of operator	Essential	Essential

distinguish *in situ* from invasive carcinomas, although the technique has greater positive than negative predictive value as the invasive component of a tumour may not always be included in the biopsy. It is easier to recognize as malignant those carcinomas with low-grade cytological features (e.g. tubular, cribriform and lobular carcinomas), which are difficult to diagnose without architectural interpretation. Specific benign diagnoses can be made, and this allows a better correlation of clinical, radiological and histological features.

A major advantage of needle biopsies is that they can be subjected to specimen radiography to ensure that the mammographic abnormality has been sampled. If the relevant calcification is included in the biopsy and is clearly associated with a benign process, an unnecessary operation is avoided. It is important, however, to ensure that calcification seen histologically corresponds to that on the specimen radiograph. Dahlstrom *et al.* (1966) reported that calcification of less than 100 μm is not visible on core biopsy radiographs. The radiological detection of numerous smaller foci could, however, occur by summation.

Although reporting the histological features of carcinomas associated with prognosis is best left to the subsequent open biopsies, tumour type (if pure) and grade can be given with a reasonable degree of accuracy if open surgery cannot be performed. Vascular invasion is sometimes identifiable in core specimens. Immunohistochemical staining for oestrogen receptors and other markers can also be undertaken on needle core biopsies, the results showing a very high level of concordance with those obtained on excision specimens (Jacobs *et al.*, 1998). Distinguishing ductal carcinoma *in situ* from atypical ductal hyperplasia, although theoretically possible, is very difficult, and in Dahlstrom *et al.*'s (1998) study, most patients with the latter diagnosis on stereotactic core biopsy were found to have ductal carcinoma *in situ* at open biopsy. Finding atypical hyperplasia in a core biopsy is thus a clear indication to perform an excision biopsy.

FNAC, on the other hand, is quicker and cheaper than needle biopsy. It is easier to perform, does not require local anaesthetic and consequently uses less clinic time. Multiple passes with the needle increase diagnostic accuracy with both techniques but are easier with FNAC. Small and impalpable lesions are also easier to localize, particularly if image localization is used. As FNAC is a quicker technique, cytopathologists can provide diagnoses during assessment clinics so that the triple assessment process, on which the decision to operate will be made, can be completed in a single visit (see below). Furthermore, if unequivocally malignant cells are identified on FNAC, it is possible to make a confident diagnosis of invasive carcinoma (as opposed to ductal carcinoma *in situ*) if the radiological and clinical appearances are typical. Most pathologists, however, find it easier to interpret needle biopsy specimens, the standard of interpretation being generally higher except in the major cytopathology centres. Owing to differences in preparation and processing, the immunohistochemical staining of cytological smears for oestrogen receptors and other markers may not be comparable to that obtained on excision specimens, and the provenance of all the positive cells may not be certain. Furthermore, at the time of writing, there are no external quality assessment schemes for reporting receptor status on cytological specimens.

It is thus clear that FNAC and NCB are complementary methods of arriving at a preoperative diagnosis and that the choice of technique should depend on the clinical circumstances. In one centre, the frequency with which preoperative diagnoses could be made on screen-detected lesions increased from 72% using FNAC alone to 90% using the two techniques in combination (Pinder *et al.*, 1996). The same centre found that one or the other investigation was positive in 97% of patients who were elderly or had locally advanced breast cancer and who were being considered for primary medical therapy (Poole *et al.*, 1996). As stated previously, however, the efficacy of both methods is heavily dependent on the skill and experience of the operator, who is usually not a pathologist.

The findings from FNAC or NCB are particularly important when investigating solid breast masses in younger patients, particularly those under 35 years. Mammography is often unsatisfactory at this age because of the denseness of the breast, and the clinician is often inclined to discount a diagnosis of cancer in view of its rarity. The most common cause of a solid lump in a young person is a fibroadenoma, which can be conclusively diagnosed by FNAC or NCB, as of course can the unexpected carcinoma. In a review (Yelland *et al.*, 1991) of 150 women with breast cancer aged less than 35 years undergoing FNAC, aspiration cytodiagnosis was more effective in diagnosing carcinoma than was clinical examination and mammography.

PERFORMING FINE NEEDLE ASPIRATION

There have been many advances in breast FNAC since the first edition of this book, but the purpose of the technique remains the detection of malignant disease with the maximal sensitivity, specificity and positive predictive value possible. The investigation is comparatively painless, and a result can be available within a few minutes.

Aspiration technique for palpable lesions

The simplest method is to insert a hypodermic needle into a lesion, apply suction with the syringe and then squirt the aspirated material onto a slide. A syringe holder has been used widely in Scandinavia, and there are other devices available, mostly designed by surgeons, to enable them to aspirate more conveniently.

The syringe holder requires dexterity to use it properly, but once this has been mastered, it is useful in increasing the yield and presumably the accuracy of the technique. Many practitioners, however, consider that simply using a 10 ml syringe held in the hand with a green (20 gauge) or blue (22 gauge) hypodermic needle is equally suitable. Good results can also be obtained using a 27 gauge needle, and an evaluation of the use of this narrower, and consequently less traumatic, needle is being undertaken (Querci della Rovere, personal communication, 1999).

The recommended method using a hand-held syringe is as follows:

1. Clean the skin and fix the breast lump between the finger and thumb or between the fingers, preferably with the patient supine.
2. Draw up 2 ml air into the syringe, and ensure that the needle is firmly fixed into the barrel of the syringe to avoid air leakage.
3. Insert the needle tip into the centre of the lesion in an 'angled' (as opposed to 'vertical') direction in order to reduce the chance of puncturing the pleural cavity.
4. Aspirate with much negative pressure in the syringe, up to the 9 or 10 ml graduation, while moving the needle tip within the tumour, which should be kept fixed. This is the critical part of the operation. Some large tumours may be necrotic in their centres, so it is wise to aspirate round the periphery if this can be identified. It is also important to aspirate in many directions so that samples from different areas of the tumour are aspirated. Such wide sampling is not possible when performing a needle biopsy for histopathological diagnosis (see above).
5. It is extremely important to release the negative pressure in the syringe before extracting the needle from the tumour. If this is not done, air will rush in as the needle is pulled through the skin, and the contents of the needle will be sucked into the barrel of the syringe and thus be difficult to extract.
6. Make blobs at the ends of several slides and smear appropriately, remembering that those destined for Papanicolaou staining should be rather thick and those for Giemsa staining thin.
7. The syringe and needle contents are now rinsed into buffered saline or culture medium for centrifuging for special stains or research purposes.

The procedure should be undertaken in a confident manner in order to reassure the patient, with a good light and with an assistant nearby.

Preparation and staining

The Papanicolaou (equivalent to H&E) and Giemsa techniques are the most commonly used staining methods, each requiring a different preparatory procedure. In order to achieve perfect Papanicolaou stained smears, for example, the material has to be fixed before it dries, using the universal gynaecological spray-fix, whereas smears destined to be stained with Giemsa must dry instantaneously, a hair dryer being provided in some laboratories for the purpose. The consequence of this is that smears destined for Papanicolaou staining that dry before they are fixed give poor results, and smears destined for Giemsa that do not dry quickly enough also provide poor preparations. In practice, smears earmarked for Papanicolaou staining should be smeared rather more thickly on the slide than those destined for Giemsa staining.

The aspirator

There is controversy over whether it is better for the clinician (surgeon or physician) or the pathologist to perform FNAC (Stanley, 1990). In favour of the former is that aspiration can be an important part of clinical assessment, giving the operator additional physical signs that enhance clinical diagnosis. Aspirating breast cysts in clinics is often diagnostic and may even be curative. The consistency of a tumour can be revealed by fine needle aspiration. Lumps that are rubbery and 'grip' the needle are more often benign. Carcinomas, on the other hand, often feel 'gritty'.

The pathologist who subsequently undertakes the microscopic interpretation is also concerned with clinical features, which should always be taken into account when making a pathological diagnosis. Moreover, the pathologist is more knowledgeable about preparation techniques and the effect they have on microscopic appearances (see above) and is better able to recognize an inadequate smear so that aspiration can be repeated immediately rather than at the patient's next clinic visit. Consequently, smears are likely to be of higher quality when pathologists undertake the aspiration.

Cytology clinics

In Sweden, under a scheme pioneered at the Karolinska Hospital in Stockholm (Franzen and Zajicek 1968), all patients requiring FNAC, including that of the breast, are referred to the Cytology Clinic. This practice is the major factor contributing to the quality of aspiration cytology services in this region, where a consistently high level of specificity and sensitivity is achieved. The Cytology Clinic is an autonomous unit staffed by nurses and secretaries as well as pathologists, to whom the patient is referred. General practitioners as well as hospital clinicians are able to refer patients to these clinics, the reports being sent out appropriately. Pathologists can make use of their clinical training and may not only take full histories and even examine X-rays, but also palpate masses and perform other appropriate investigations where necessary. In this way, the pathologist is able accurately to assess clinical, radiological and other data in making a cytological diagnosis.

In the UK, many pathologists appreciate the advantages of this arrangement, which has also been welcomed by clinicians. The cost of the tests is much reduced, not only because unsatisfactory specimens are extremely rare, but also because definitive diagnoses can more frequently be achieved. Notable examples of this approach in the UK are found in Northampton (Brown and Coghill, 1992), University College Hospital, London (Kocjan, 1991) and several other centres. Similar clinics have been established in the USA, including one in San Francisco, which is designed along Scandinavian lines and has reported excellent results (Abele and Miller, 1993). Over a 7-year period, there had been a 20-fold increase in the number of patients referred for investigation. Specimens consist mainly of breast aspirates but also include samples of thyroid, prostate, salivary gland and subcutaneous soft tissue tumours.

As many clinicians are reluctant to lose the extra clinical data they obtain from aspirating tumours themselves, a compromise has been reached in many centres. The pathologist attends the clinic to ensure that the specimens are prepared to the highest standard and reports them before the patient leaves (Kocjan, 1991). These 'one-stop' clinics have the advantage of speed and thereby convenience for the patient, who will discover during the same clinic visit her diagnosis and what her management will be. This immediate reporting does not require such radical reorganization as does the establishment of autonomous cytology clinics and has therefore become established in many hospitals in the UK. Gui et al. (1995) considered that such a scheme maximizes outpatient resources. Harcourt et al. (1998), in a report of an evaluation of a one-stop breast lump clinic, reported that anxiety was reduced in women found to have benign lesions, but some doubt was raised over the value of such clinics for women found to have carcinoma.

Complications of FNAC

The most frequent complication of aspiration cytodiagnosis is local haematoma, which can largely be prevented by firm pressure for about 2 minutes after withdrawing the needle. Pneumothorax is rare but was reported in one review (Gateley et al., 1991) to have occurred in seven patients, with an incidence of 4% of aspirates. Not all workers have experienced this high rate, and indeed in a recent review of 49 Italian Institutions (Catania et al., 1993), involving over 200 000 needle aspirates, an incidence of 0.01 per cent was reported. It must be admitted, however, that many such punctures may go undetected. In their review, Christie and Bates (1999) suggested that it is not necessary to warn patients of this potential complication.

Tumour seeding along the needle tract is of mainly theoretical interest as most carcinomas will be at least excised or given other forms of treatment.

NIPPLE SMEARS

The examination of smears can be of diagnostic value in local and systemic disease. Nipple discharge can, however, be physiological in girls at puberty and when lactation continues after breast-feeding has ceased. Furthermore, mechanical factors such as compression of the breast at mammography may induce nipple secretion, which may not necessarily be pathological. Radiographers are well placed to observe any nipple secretion during mammography and can be instructed to collect smears for cytological assessment. Nipple discharge sometimes occurs as a side-effect of drug therapy, notably with phenothiazines or oral contraceptives.

Bilateral serous nipple discharge may be symptomatic of a pituitary tumour, especially where patients have amenorrhoea and a raised prolactin level. Unilateral nipple discharge usually relates to local disease, and evidence of origin from a single lactiferous duct should be obtained by careful inspection. Blood-stained or discoloured fluid is associated with an underlying tumour, but not all bloody discharges indicate a neoplasm, and clear fluid should not be discounted as an innocent event. The presence of blood can be confirmed by Hemastix testing. In an analysis of 176 patients undergoing microdochectomy for blood-stained or persistent discharge, 15 (9 per cent) had a carcinoma 78 (44 per cent) an intraduct papilloma and the rest a range of abnormalities including duct ectasia, fibrocystic change, inflammation and hyperplasia. The percentage with bloody discharge was only slightly higher (59%) in the neoplastic groups than in the remainder (56 per cent) (Fung *et al.*, 1990).

Samples can be collected onto a glass slide by touching the nipple in the region of the discharge, which may need to be encouraged by gentle palpation, and then smearing the fluid along the slide. Another method of obtaining smears is by using a breast pump or suction device. This consists of an airtight chamber connected to a syringe or pump, which is used to create a vacuum. The microscopic examination of the aspirate shows a few epithelial cells but the sample will consist mainly of macrophages (Mitchell *et al.*, in press) in a proteinaceous fluid, in which fat is present in the form of small vacuoles (Fig. 4.1). In air-dried samples, the fat can be demonstrated using Oil Red O, but in wet fixed smears it is dissolved by the alcohol. The macrophages have finely vacuolated cytoplasm and indistinct cell borders. Some of the epithelial cells may exhibit a similar appearance.

Intraduct papilloma

The nipple smear from a papilloma often contains both fresh and altered blood, with many foamy macrophages. When altered blood (indicative of previous haemorrhage into the affected duct) is present, there may be many siderophages that stain dark blue in air-dried smears. The hallmark of a duct papilloma is the presence of papillary clusters of small cohesive benign ductal cells (Fig. 4.2). The clusters themselves are usually small and the cells may be cytologically bland or slightly enlarged with visible nucleoli. Apocrine cells may be seen infrequently.

In cases of Paget's disease, gentle scraping of the affected nipple (Fig. 4.3) will usually produce sufficient material for diagnostic

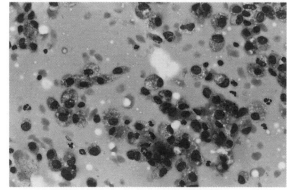

4.1 Cells in a nipple aspirate sample consisting mainly of foamy macrophages with scattered non-specific inflammatory cells and some red blood cells.

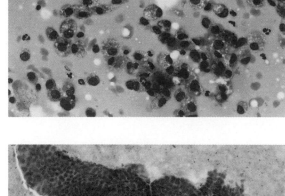

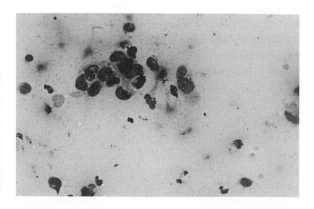

4.2 (Left) Papillary clusters of monomorphic epithelial cells characteristic of a benign papilloma.

4.3 (Right) Cells obtained after scraping a nipple showing Paget's disease. Note clusters and single large irregular cells with pleomorphic nuclei. They generally show squamoid appearance.

purposes (Lucarotti *et al.*, 1994), but better samples are obtained after wetting the nipple with a warm, saline-soaked gauze pad for a few minutes. This prevents the air-drying artefact often seen in wet-fixed scrapes of the nipple (Masukawa *et al.*, 1973).

CYTOLOGY OF BENIGN LESIONS

Cysts

The aspiration of fluid from a cyst, suspected clinically to be malignant, brings relief to the clinician and joy to the patient, who is cured of the lump and reassured. A review of a large number of cases of breast cyst aspiration by Ciatto *et al.* (1987) indicated that the routine cytological examination of cyst fluid is unnecessary and certainly not cost-effective. These authors reviewed 6782 cyst fluid specimens from 4105 patients. One incidental case of occult lobular carcinoma *in situ* was detected. Five clinically and radiologically inapparent intracystic papillomas were detected, but all had produced blood-stained fluid; cytology was negative in two of these cases. Otherwise all the cancers detected had been suspected on physical examination and/or mammography. This study supports the general recommendation (Haggensen, 1971) that fluid aspirated from a breast cyst should be examined cytologically only when it is discoloured or blood stained, or when the lump persists after aspiration. To this may be added cysts that have internal echoes on ultrasound examination. Medullary carcinoma occasionally produces blood-stained fluid (Howell and Kline, 1990).

In cytological smears, cysts contain granular debris, foam cells and often apocrine cells, polymorphonuclear leucocytes and altered blood (Fig. 4.4). Although they have features of histiocytes, the foam cells may sometimes be epithelial cells that have been shed into the cyst lumen. They have rounded or bean-shaped nuclei with sharp margins, a noticeable nucleolus and foamy, finely vacuolated cytoplasm. In the wet-fixed, Papanicolaou-stained smear, intracytoplasmic inclusion bodies may be observed. These are believed to be large lysosomes that develop as a result of phagocytic activity (Nagy *et al.*, 1989).

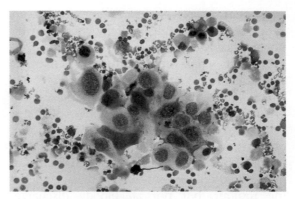

4.4 Clusters of cells aspirated from a benign cyst. Although having large pleomorphic nuclei, the cells still resemble histiocytes and should not be mistaken for carcinoma. Note the small granules in the background which are thought to originate from apocrine cells.

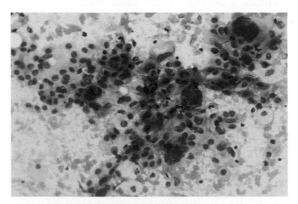

(a)

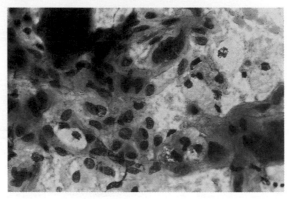

(b)

4.5 Atypical but benign cells aspirated from a cyst. (a) At low power, squamous cells and histiocytes are present. (b) At high power, the benign nature of the nuclei is evident.

Occasionally, cellular atypia is seen, in the form of nuclear enlargement and degenerative changes such as blurring of nuclear outlines and cytoplasmic vacuolation. This atypia should not be mistaken for malignancy (Fig. 4.5).

Sheets of apocrine cells are frequently seen. These are large cells with abundant cytoplasm, eccentric nuclei, prominent nucleoli and cytoplasmic granules that show up clearly on

4.6 (Left) Cytology – fibroadenoma. Ductal sheets with blunt, club-shaped branches are another feature often seen in fibroadenomas. Note the bare nuclei in the background.

4.7 (Right) Stroma aspirated from a fibroadenoma which stains pink with Giemsa.

4.8 (Left) Cytology – fibroadenoma. A high-power view of benign ductal cells shows their smooth rounded nuclear outlines, vesicular chromatin pattern and visible nulceoli (Pap).

4.9 (Right) Cytology – atypical fibroadenoma. On the left note the orderly arrangement of small uniform ductal cells. On the right the cells are pleomorphic and appear to be dissociating. This is a pitfall which can be avoided by searching for bare nuclei and noting that in areas some of the pleomorphic cells are attached to sheets of benign ductal cells (Pap).

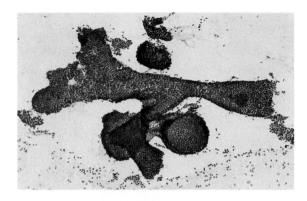

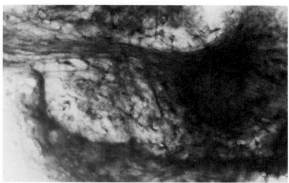

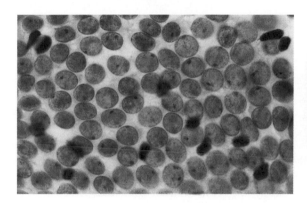

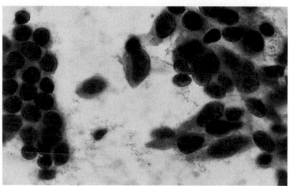

the air-dried smear stained with Giemsa. Although much debris resembling the granular material of apocrine cell cytoplasm is seen in cyst fluid smears, necrotic cellular debris is never seen in benign cysts and if present should always prompt a thorough search for malignant cells from an encysted ductal carcinoma *in situ*.

Fibroadenoma

Aspirates of fibroadenomas, especially those from young women, are usually very cellular and contain large flat sheets of small uniform benign epithelial cells showing an 'antler-horn' branching effect (Fig. 4.6). The margins of the sheets are usually smooth and the cells cohesive. Scattered between the epithelial clusters are a large number of small hyperchromatic cells, which can occur singly or in pairs and are generally thought to be myoepithelial cells. The third characteristic feature is the presence of fragments of metachromatic-staining connective tissue stroma. These vary in cellularity, showing

spindle-shaped fibroblasts in a myxoid-type matrix that stains bright pink with Giemsa (Fig. 4.7). The epithelial cells in the sheets often have conspicuous nucleoli indicative of active growth, and mitotic figures may be seen. The chromatin pattern, however, is vesicular and the nuclear outlines smooth and rounded (Fig. 4.8). Apocrine cells and foamy macrophages are occasionally seen. It is not possible to tell from the cytology whether a fibroadenoma is of the pericanalicular or intracanalicular type.

Proliferation of the epithelial component of a fibroadenoma may be so extensive as to produce a highly cellular aspirate with epithelial cells showing pleomorphism (Fig. 4.9) that has been mistaken for carcinoma. This mistake can, however, be avoided by identifying the pairs and single myoepithelial cells that are always present in large numbers. Fibroadenomas may show lactational changes (*see* p. 238) (Tavassoli and Yeh, 1987). The cells aspirated from such lesions show cytoplasmic vacuolation, prominent nucleoli and some cell disassociation. Here again, the presence of bipolar nuclei is helpful in arriving at the correct diagnosis. Deen *et al.* (1999) analysed in detail the cytological features of 39 fibroepithelial lesions that included phyllodes tumours. High-grade phyllodes tumours could be separated from the benign variant and fibroadenomas by the appearances of the stromal spindle cells.

Acute mastitis

Acute mastitis is obvious clinically by pain, redness, swelling and tenderness over the affected area of the breast, and it is not usually aspirated. A course of antibiotics clears the condition, but a non-tender mass occasionally remains in the breast and may arouse suspicions of carcinoma. An FNAC sample from such an area will be cellular and contain many foamy macrophages, histiocytes, polymorphonuclear leucocytes and background debris (Fig. 4.10). Clusters of benign epithelial cells are seen that may show some reactive atypia. Reaspiration for microbiological investigation may be necessary. Fibrinous streaks are also reported.

Granulomatous mastitis

Granulomatous mastitis may be mistaken clinically for carcinoma as it exhibits a defined hard mass that may have skin tethering. In Western countries it is usually non-specific, but in the Indian subcontinent a high proportion of inflammatory breast lesions have a specific cause, including tuberculosis and histoplasmosis. In typical cases, aspiration cytology shows foamy macrophages, footprint-shaped epithelioid histiocytes, proliferative blood vessels and multinucleated giant histiocytes (Figs 4.11 and 4.12). The atypical nature of the histiocytes may lead to a mistaken diagnosis of carcinoma by the unwary. If sufficient material is available, fungal and tuberculous infections may be detected using special stains such as periodic acid–Schiff and Ziehl–Neilsen. Sarcoidosis may produce a similar cytological picture, while in silicone granuloma vacuoles of various sizes are seen within histiocytes (Dodd *et al.*, 1993).

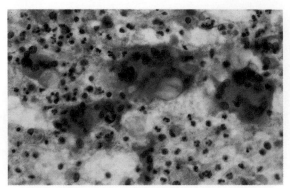

4.10 Cytology – subareolar abscess. The cytological appearances are similar to those seen in mastitis, with multinucleated giant cells, histiocytes and polymorphs. However, note the pale orange anucleate squames in the background (Pap).

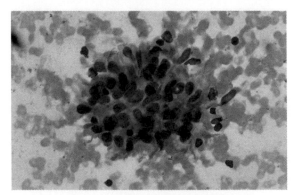

4.11 Cytology – granulomatous mastitis. This is a collection of epithelioid histiocytes with elongated footprint-shaped nuclei, associated with granulomatous mastitis. A scattering of lymphocytes is also present (MGG).

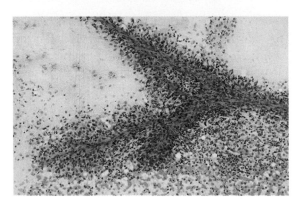

4.12 Cytology – granulomatous mastitis. This low-power field shows the proliferating capillaries often observed in aspirates from granulomatous mastitis (Pap).

Fat necrosis

FNAC is very useful in this condition, which often presents as a hard irregular mass. A history of trauma may be elicited on careful questioning, but there is sometimes quite a long interval between the trauma and the development of symptoms, the injury being forgotten. Mammography is helpful in excluding carcinoma. Aspirates from fat necrosis show variable degrees of cellularity. Degenerate fat cells are present that often

4.13 Cytology – fat necrosis. Degenerate fat cells and foamy macrophages are illustrated here, suggesting a diagnosis of fat necrosis (MGG).

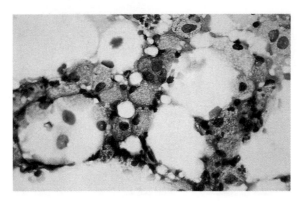

resemble foamy macrophages (Fig. 4.13). Inflammatory cells, including polymorphs, lymphocytes, histiocytes and multinucleated histiocytes, are seen. Usually no epithelial cells are evident (Orell *et al.*, 1992). Differential diagnosis from granulomatous mastitis is difficult, but, with a helpful history, precise diagnosis is possible.

Other benign lesions

Within this large range of histological changes, there are proliferative lesions in which the cells may mimic carcinoma. Cells aspirated from benign lesions generally show good cohesion and form flat, single-layered sheets of cells, which may show branching. The borders of the clusters are usually circumscribed. The cells themselves may show a 'honeycombing' effect, within which smaller more pyknotic nuclei are present that may represent myoepithelial cells, although this is an unreliable sign of a benign tumour. Occasionally, intact lobules are aspirated,

4.14 Benign epithelial cells showing lactational change. Note the rather loose appearance of the cluster and the finely vacuolated cytoplasm. The nuclei are enlarged.

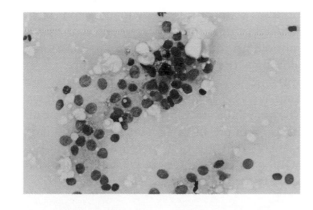

which appear three-dimensional. In addition, the background will contain single and pairs of benign nuclei as well as a variety of other cells that may include foam cells and apocrine cells, suggesting a cystic component to the lesion. There may also be a mixture of non-specific inflammatory cells.

There have been several attempts to correlate appearances suspicious of carcinoma with the atypical ductal or lobular hyperplasias described histologically (Stanley *et al.*, 1993). This has not been successful, and atypical cytology is most often caused by either frank carcinoma, perhaps of the low-grade variety, or common benign lesions. Aspirates and nipple smears from patients with duct ectasia generally show sheets of degenerate epithelial and inflammatory cells as well as epithelial, foam and occasionally apocrine cells. The inflammatory component may be prominent.

Lactational changes

During pregnancy and lactation, the epithelial cells have a large amount of vacuolated cytoplasm (Fig. 4.14). Furthermore, the nuclei are enlarged and may have one or two prominent nucleoli. This latter feature can be misinterpreted as malignancy, and it is important that the clinician informs the pathologist that the patient is pregnant or lactating. Focal lactational changes have been reported in the breasts of non-pregnant, non-lactating women, sometimes associated with the use of hormone therapy, antipsychotic drugs or hypertensive therapy (Tavassoli and Yeh, 1987). Fibroadenomas may also show lactational changes during pregnancy.

A galactocoele is the accumulation of milk in ducts deep to the nipple after the termination of lactation, causing cyst formation. It may be a palpable lump, the squeezing of which may induce a clear nipple secretion. The specimen is generally poorly cellular with scattered macrophages and epithelial cells. Simple cysts deep to the nipple can also present with a serous discharge. In these samples, a few scattered foam cells will be seen against a background of thin proteinaceous fluid.

Uncommon benign lesions

The cytopathologist should be aware of the range and variety of breast pathology, which includes uncommon lesions that may cause especial difficulty when aspirated. Although it is sufficient to identify the benign lesions as being only benign, the ability to suggest a rare diagnosis without perhaps being too dogmatic provides zest to the report and may impress clinicians.

In *juvenile papillomatosis* (*see* p. 114), aspirates may show an alarming degree of epithelial cell atypia. The cellularity is dense, and three-dimensional clusters may sometimes be present. Although benign bipolar nuclei may be seen, there is a danger of overdiagnosis, which should be avoided, particularly in young women.

Aspirates from cases of *gynaecomastia* in the early phase of the lesion can be very cellular and have been mistaken for carcinoma (Chang, 1990). Large sheets of epithelial cells are sometimes seen, as well as occasional mitotic figures. As with all benign lesions, it is usually possible to identify benign epithelial cells and benign pairs of myoepithelial cells, which should be diligently sought.

Collagenous spherulosis (Tyler and Coghill, 1991) can mimic adenoid cystic carcinoma, both histologically (*see* p. 87) and in needle aspirates. The cytological features of aspirates reflect the histopathological changes and show rings of epithelial cells surrounding amorphous collagenous material. Adenoid cystic carcinoma can be quite similar, but no benign cells are identified, and the carcinoma cells, although small, are atypical.

Low-grade phyllodes tumours are usually misdiagnosed as fibroadenomas in cytological smears, but it is usually possible retrospectively to identify sheets of hypercellular stroma within the needle aspirate sample.

Granular cell tumours may well be mistaken for carcinoma as the cells are large and may have pleomorphic nuclei. The granules may not be evident in the smears, but the diagnosis can be made when the histiocytic nature of the cells is appreciated. This tumour has rarely been diagnosed preoperatively by

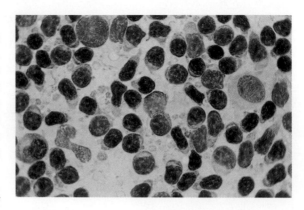

4.15 This shows a range of normal lymphoid cells.

aspiration cytodiagnosis (Simm *et al.*, 1988; Lowhagen and Rubio, 1977).

Aspirates containing lymphoid cells are comparatively common (Fig 4.15) and may result from an *intramammary lymph node*. Lymph nodes are quite common within the breast, especially in the upper outer quadrant, and can be palpated as well as seen mammographically (Pettinato *et al.*, 1991). The smears show a variety of lymphoid cells, including mature and immature forms as well as histiocytes and tingible body macrophages.

CYTOLOGY OF MALIGNANT LESIONS

Criteria of malignancy

Several authors have formulated definitions of the criteria of malignancy. Oertel and Galbum (1986) considered the most important criterion to be the cellularity of the specimen and nuclear atypia. Kline *et al.* (1985) published a useful table in which the frequency of features is listed in various types of malignant breast tumour stained by the Papanicolaou technique. Cellularity, poor cohesion and monomorphism are important features, although the degree of abnormality varies with the carcinoma subtype. Linsk and Franzen (1983) also give useful guidelines. They include the presence of single cells having round or irregular large nuclei and nucleoli that are best seen in Papanicolaou-stained slides. In addition, clusters and bipolar nuclei should be absent.

TABLE 4.2 Cytological criteria of malignancy

Obvious	Large size
	Nuclear border irregularity
	Large nucleoli
	Lack of cohesion
	Cellular pleomorphism
Less obvious	Intranuclear vacuoles
	Monomorphism
	Mitoses
	Single cells with much cytoplasm
	Absence of benign pairs

In Table 4.2, the criteria of malignancy have been divided into those which are 'obvious' and those which are 'less obvious'. This list is an attempt to provide a consensus of criteria gleaned from the literature as well as from personal experience. The 'obvious' criteria are those generally applied to the identification of malignant cells in all cytological samples, lack of cohesion perhaps being particularly relevant to breast aspiration specimens. It is important also to emphasize nuclear border irregularity as this feature occasionally tips the balance towards a malignant diagnosis. The 'less obvious' criteria are worth examining in detail. Intranuclear vacuoles may be the counterpart of the intracellular lumina that can be identified by electron microscopy in carcinoma cells, although they are usually identified in the cytoplasm (Fisher, 1976). This may in some cases be an important observation in the diagnosis of malignancy, although it is certainly also seen in some benign specimens. Vacuoles are seen far more easily in Giemsa than in wet-fixed Papanicolaou-stained preparations, being identified as punched-out, clear areas about the size of a red blood cell or smaller (Fig. 4.16).

Monomorphism (Fig. 4.17) refers to the number of types of cell rather than to the degree of variability when comparing one cell with another. In smears suspicious of harbouring malignancy, the identification of two types of cell – epithelial and myoepithelial – indicates a benign nature. A diagnosis of carcinoma should be considered in smears where the cells are all of the same type, even when they are regular and small, although carcinoma is more easily diagnosed when the cells show individual pleomorphism.

Mitoses (Fig 4.18) are infrequently seen in aspirates from carcinomas. This is curious because they can be common in histological sections, and their number is indeed an important component of histological grading. Their absence in breast aspirates may be the consequence of a lower cell number, as the cells are fresh when smeared and it is unlikely that mitoses would complete after the sample had been taken. Their presence is nevertheless a strong indicator of malignancy, although they are known to occur in some benign lesions, notably fibroadenomas.

The presence of single cells with much cytoplasm has been identified by Linsk and

4.16 (Left) High-power view of a cluster of breast carcinoma cells stained with MGG. Many nuclei show vacuoles of various kinds. The one on the left is 'punched out', others less defined.

4.17 (Right) In this low-power photomicrograph the cells are evenly spread and all one type, although they vary in size. This is monomorphism.

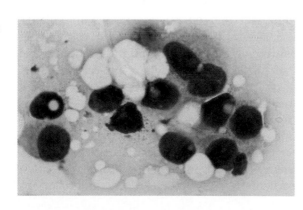

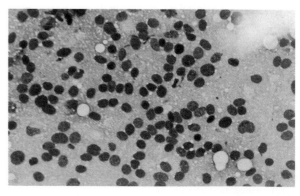

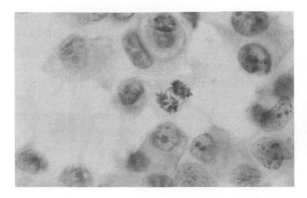

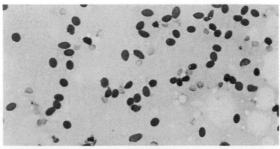

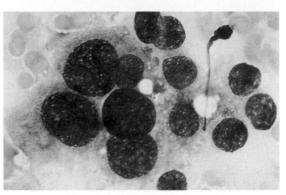

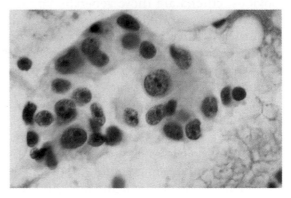

4.18 (Left) High-power field of a metaphase mitosis stained by the Papanicolaou technique.

4.19 (Right) Cytology – bare nuclei. Many myoepithelial cell nuclei, some apparently in groups of two or three. The nuclei are plump and oval, as opposed to spindle-shaped stromal nuclei (MGG).

4.20 High-power photomicrograph showing large polygonal cells with a small nuclear cytoplasmic ratio. Nucleoli are often multiple and there is marked pleomorphism. At the right of the picture an acinus can be identified.

4.21 High-power view of carcinoma cells stained by Papanicolaou, showing prominent nucleoli.

Franzen (1983) as a criterion of malignancy and is often found in malignant aspirates. Their presence should raise the alarm, and other evidence of malignancy should be diligently sought.

The absence of 'benign pairs' is an observation complementary to monomorphism. It is not clear why myoepithelial cells commonly group together in pairs or sometimes in clusters of three or even four nuclei (Fig. 4.19). Zajicek (1974) recognized single 'sentinel' nuclei and claimed them to be of myoepithelial origin, maintaining that they are very rarely observed in aspirates from carcinoma. This has been confirmed in an objective study by Sturgis *et al.* (1998). Pairs of myoepithelial nuclei simply representing two adjacent sentinel cells are more easily identified than single nuclei. It is a convenient rule of thumb, when confronted with an equivocal smear, to hunt for benign pairs of myoepithelial cells and permit a diagnosis of carcinoma only when they are either absent or the atypical cells themselves are large, pleomorphic and irregular, that is, unequivocally malignant. The observance of this rule will prevent the confusion of carcinoma with fibroadenoma where large atypical epithelial cells, which may even be in mitosis, are present but where myoepithelial cells, singly and in pairs, are abundant.

Infiltrating ductal carcinoma

Although there is a wide range of appearances, aspirates from infiltrating ductal carcinomas are usually composed of cells that are large and polygonal with a low nuclear-to-cytoplasmic ratio and marked nuclear border irregularity (Fig. 4.20). In this type of tumour, nucleoli are easily identified and often multiple. The Papanicolaou-stained cells show this well (Fig. 4.21). In other tumours, the aspirated cells are medium sized and grouped in loose aggregates in which the monomorphic appearance of the nuclei is striking (Fig. 4.22). It is these tumours which will often have single cells that satisfy the criteria of malignancy. In many cases, particularly high-grade tumours, the diagnosis

4.22 (Left) Carcinoma cells showing monomorphic nuclei. In a benign cluster, epithelial and myoepithelial nuclei would be identified.

4.23 (Right) High-power view of carcinoma cell showing pink-staining mucin in the cytoplasm.

4.24 (Left) Many cells show basophilic granules in the cytoplasm. These are certainly epithelial cells and the granules probably indicate neuroendocrine differentiation. This is common in breast cancer, and in aspiration cytology of the breast their presence may help in establishing a diagnosis of carcinoma.

4.25 (Right) Two cells are seen centrally with vacuoles in their cytoplasm in which a small blob of mucus is present. These appearances have been described in aspirates from infiltrating lobular carcinoma, although (as in this case) the histological appearances were more in favour of a ductal lesion.

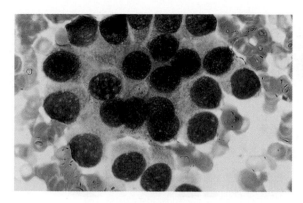

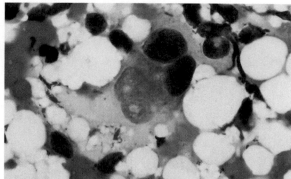

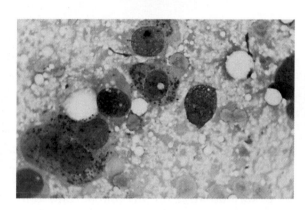

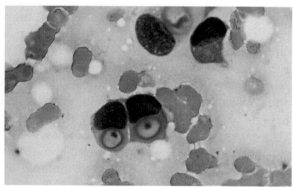

of carcinoma is straightforward, the aspirate revealing loose sheets and single, large, pleomorphic irregular cells obviously fulfilling the criteria of malignancy (*see* Table 4.2 above). Occasional blobs of intracellular mucin (Fig. 4.23) may be seen, and in some tumours there are cells containing neuroendocrine granules (Fig. 4.24). The finding of granules may sometimes confirm suspicions of malignancy and allow a positive diagnosis to be made.

Lobular carcinoma

Antoniades and Spector (1987) studied nine cases of lobular carcinoma in which they compared imprints with thick and thin histological sections. A range of cell sizes was seen, from that just larger than a lymphocyte with a small round-to-oval nucleus, to a signet-ring form with a nuclear size of up to 11.8 μm and large cytoplasmic vacuoles containing mucin (Fig. 4.25). The typical cell was small, with a

round-to-oval nucleus with finely dispersed chromatin and a small distinct nucleolus, and cytoplasm with punched-out vacuoles. Leach and Howell (1992) found, that in needle aspirates of lobular carcinoma, the classic variety (*see* p. 174) was the most likely to result in a false-negative cytodiagnosis. The importance of cytoplasmic vacuoles is again emphasized. However, a few cases of the alveolar variant had large cells and were diagnosed as ductal carcinoma.

Two kinds of cell have generally been described in aspirates from lobular carcinomas: first, loosely dispersed sheets of small cells, seen particularly in postmenopausal women, and second, tight clusters of pleomorphic cells seen in three-dimensional groups. The small cells are often only slightly larger than red blood cells and may be mistaken for lymphocytes from an intramammary lymph node or even malignant lymphoma. The diagnosis is often suspected on low-power microscopy when diffuse sheets of cells are

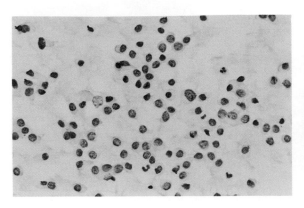

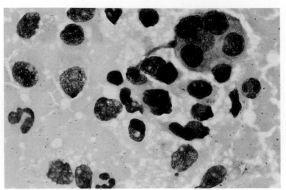

4.26 (Left) Low-power photomicrograph showing a loose sheet of dissociated cells from a small cell carcinoma.

4.27 (Right) High-power view showing the pleomorphic nature of the nuclei and the epithelial clustering. Note that the nuclei are only slightly larger than the polymorph nucleus (left field).

seen (Fig. 4.26), and a prolonged hunt at high power usually reveals one or two cells with a fair amount of cytoplasm and others in which epithelial clustering is apparent (Fig. 4.27). This pattern was recognized by Zajicek (1974) and called 'carcinoma, small cell type'. Experience is required to identify these cases. Those cases that present in aspirates with clusters can also be difficult to recognize. However there is usually nuclear moulding as well as irregular nuclear outlines towards the periphery of the clusters, and in these smears there may also be loose groups of rather larger irregular cells that support the diagnosis, although these may be few and far between.

Medullary carcinoma

The histopathology of these tumours is described on p. 181. In FNAC samples the cells are very large and disaggregated, with prominent nucleoli. The lymphoid stroma is easily identified, and plasma cells are numerous. Despite sampling difficulties in a tumour that must conform to specific histopathological criteria to warrant a good prognosis, it is nevertheless possible to suggest that a tumour may be a medullary carcinoma, by FNAC, particularly when the characteristic mammographic appearance of a circumscribed mass is also seen. Some medullary carcinomas produce cystic fluid when aspirated (Howell and Kline, 1990). In three cases of this kind studied at the Royal Marsden Hospital, the fluid was up to 2 ml in volume and only slightly blood-stained.

Mucinous (mucoid) carcinoma

In this carcinoma, clusters of malignant cells are surrounded by extracellular mucin. The appearances are very characteristic on FNAC (Duane *et al.*, 1987), especially in Giemsa preparations. The mucus appears as pink or purple bands throughout the smear, and the carcinoma cells often appear lined up alongside it (Fig. 4.28). The cells themselves are usually quite small and uniform. The

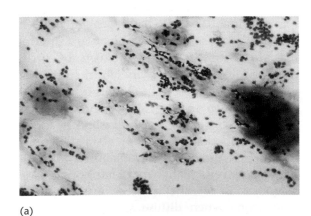

(a)

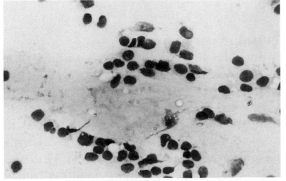

(b)

4.28 (a) Low-power photomicrograph of a needle aspirate showing the characteristic features of a mucinous carcinoma. Broad streaks of pink-staining mucin are present, with loose aggregates and single intervening cells. (b) At high power the cells are small but monomorphic and appear to be lined up along the edge of the mucin. The Giemsa stain is particularly useful in the diagnosis of this type of carcinoma. In the Papanicolaou-stained smears mucin is almost invisible.

4.29 (a) Clusters of monomorphic cells aspirated from a circumscribed lesion in an elderly woman. The groups of cells show a papillary pattern, particularly the clusters to the left of the photomicrograph, in which there is nuclear palisading. (b) Counterpart histology showing a papillary carcinoma.

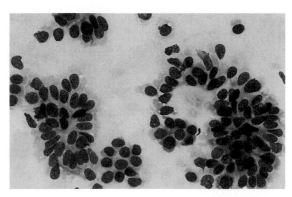

(a)

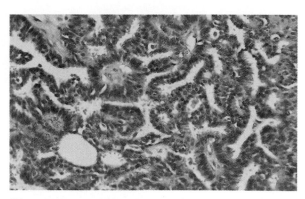

(b)

diagnosis may be difficult when the mucus is either scanty or poorly stained, and as the cells are small and relatively monomorphic, a diagnosis of malignancy may be overlooked in these circumstances. Stanley *et al.* (1989) investigated the cytological appearances of pure mucinous carcinoma and mixed infiltrating ductal and mucinous carcinoma. They identified features indicative of pure mucinous carcinoma consisting of abundant mucin in all smears, with little pleomorphism and no necrosis.

Papillary carcinoma

These tumours may be *in situ* or invasive and may be diagnosed in aspirates or nipple smears if they involve the major ducts. Needle aspirates often include much cystic fluid, which may be contaminated by blood. The cells are usually less pleomorphic than in ductal carcinoma and may occur in papillary clusters (Fig. 4.29). The distinction between papillary carcinoma and papilloma relies on cytological features indicating malignancy that include a high nuclear-to-cytoplasmic ratio, nuclear atypia and large cell size. Myoepithelial cells forming pairs of nuclei are absent. Interpretation in practice is usually difficult, and the pathologist can quite often only be suspicious of malignancy. In these circumstances, an equivocal diagnosis is the safest. The problem is compounded by the presence of papillary patterns in some examples of complex sclerosing lesions, but in aspirates from such lesions a mixture of papillary clusters, benign pairs and single 'naked' nuclei is seen.

In situ carcinoma

Although there have been reports that cells aspirated from pure *in situ* lesions have characteristic appearances (Sneige *et al.*, 1989), there is no certain criterion that will differentiate *in situ* from infiltrating carcinoma. The diagnosis is a histopathological one and depends on the architectural feature of invasion. In lobular carcinomas *in situ*, the cells are small and round, but in ductal carcinoma *in situ*, they are very variable and may be very large and contain prominent nucleoli.

It may be possible with the aid of mammography to conclude that individual lesions are more likely to be ductal carcinoma *in situ* than invasive carcinoma. The cytopathological criteria, however, are too imprecise to indicate this diagnosis with confidence.

Paget's disease

Paget's disease of the nipple is named after Sir James Paget, who first described it in 1874 (*see* p. 138). It is usually identified in nipple smears, which show many squames, debris and large carcinoma cells with abundant cytoplasm. They have hyperchromatic, irregular nuclei and may be binucleate.

Sarcoma

Those sarcomas with epithelium are usually high-grade phyllodes tumours (*see* p. 247). Sarcomas without an epithelial component are less common and are usually fibrosarcomas (*see* p. 260). Heterologous elements such as osteoid, cartilage, muscle and fat may be found. The cytodiagnosis of breast sarcoma is difficult, even when good quality samples containing spindle cells typical of sarcoma are obtained (Fig. 4.30). Consequently, the cytodiagnosis of breast sarcoma should be made with circumspection. Sarcoma can, however, be confidently diagnosed in a breast needle aspirate in recurrent cases where the primary tumour has been properly sampled and assessed histopathologically.

Uncommon malignant lesions

Adenoid cystic carcinoma can be quite similar to collagenous spherulosis, but no benign cells are identified and the carcinoma cells, although small, are atypical. Squamous carcinomas are quite distinctive, especially in Papanicolaou preparations, but it should be remembered that most cases of squamous carcinoma are not pure but have a ductal component. High-grade phyllodes tumours may exhibit sheets of frank sarcoma cells. If they are accompanied by numerous pairs of myoepithelial cells and other clusters showing conventional 'antler' sheets of epithelial cells, a specific diagnosis may be possible (Deen *et al.*, 1999). Malignant lymphomas, in contrast to intramammary lymph nodes or reactive infiltrates, exhibit a monomorphic appearance of lymphoid cells, which may show marked pleomorphism and prominent nucleoli, in which case the diagnosis is comparatively straightforward. Giemsa stain is best for identifying these lesions.

Use of needle aspirate samples to assess prognosis

Although taking breast needle aspirates results in little tumour perturbation and carcinoma diagnosis can be achieved, it has been difficult to assess prognosis using this material compared to samples removed for histopathological diagnosis. Such prognostic information is especially important in patients whose treatment will be decided on triple assessment alone (Denley *et al.*, 2001). Such patients include those who will receive neoadjuvant chemotherapy and those who are unfit for surgery.

Despite this, efforts have been made to derive prognostic information from FNAC samples. Gregory (1998) investigated the use

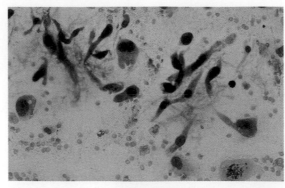

(a)

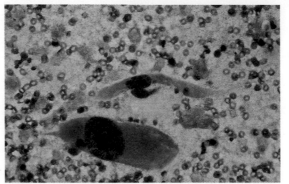

(b)

4.30 (a) Cells aspirated from a soft lump in the inner quadrant of the breast in a 64-year-old woman. Numerous elongated spindle cells are present. (b) One very large bizarrely-shaped cell is seen and another that is elongated. Note that in cytological preparations all the cell is included on the slide, rather than a section through it.

of molecular markers to predict prognosis and response in patients receiving neoadjuvant chemo- or endocrine therapy. A combination of Mib-1 measured in cytospin samples as well as S-phase fraction, and DNA ploidy measured in cell suspensions, provided a means of identifying high and low grade tumours. Furthermore, the expression of c-erbB-2 and P-glycoprotein, together with a high post-treatment apoptotic index, was associated with drug resistance. The use of these markers warrant further investigation in a prospective setting. She also showed that in a trial, c-erbB-2-negative patients who received neoadjuvant chemotherapy had a prolonged disease-free survival compared to those c-erbB-2-negative cases receiving conventional adjuvant therapy. This provided clinical evidence that neoadjuvant chemotherapy may carry a survival benefit. Furthermore, patients with a low apoptotic index following neoadjuvant therapy also had an improved disease-free survival, this also being true of the group of patients who had shown the best response to chemotherapy. Thus, by sampling tumours by FNAC using modern molecular markers, information is beginning to be acquired that may be helpful in guiding therapy and going some way towards tailoring treatment to specific patients.

Following the recognition that histopathological grading has powerful prognostic value, attempts have been made to grade breast carcinoma in needle aspirates. Two of the histopathological features – cellular pleomorphism and mitotic rate – are applicable to cytological material although mitotic figures are unusual in FNAC specimens. However, better nuclear detail (particularly in Papanicolaou-stained slides) allows a range of criteria to be assessed and scored. These include size, uniformity, chromatin patterns and the appearance of the nucleoli and nuclear margins. Cell dissociation can also be assessed.

Although the technology is available for the sophisticated analysis and compilation of parameters using automated image analysis, the expense and time involved currently make it impracticable. The pathologist requires a quick and simple grading scheme that can be undertaken on routinely stained material prepared in a conventional manner. Zajdela et al. (1984) related prognosis to the nuclear diameter of aspirated breast cancer cells measured against red blood cells, reporting a correlation with histopathological grading and prognosis. Hunt et al. (1990) expanded this method by using more parameters, and Robinson et al. (1994), in an analysis of 281 invasive ductal carcinomas, established three cytological grades that matched well with conventional histological grading.

Cytology grading systems are in their infancy and require further development and evaluation, but the demand for them is likely to increase if more patients receive neoadjuvant treatment when a conventional assessment of histological grade, tumour size and lymph node status cannot be made.

The main hope for cytopathological prognostication and the prediction of response to different forms of treatment lies in finding suitable molecular markers that will predict outcome without the need for architectural assessment. Methods being researched currently include flow cytometry (see p. 44) and immunohistochemical staining for specific markers, which are extensively discussed in Chapter 12. Research is also being undertaken using sequential needle aspirates or biopsies in patients receiving primary chemotherapy, in order to assess changes in immunoreactivity that may provide an indication of therapy resistance so that regimens can be altered accordingly (Makris et al.,1997a, b).

REPORTING CYTOLOGY RESULTS

Breast cytopathology reports should be concise (Kline, 1990) and unambiguous. Proforma reporting is now extensively used, the proforma employed by the UK National Breast Screening Programme and the European Breast Screening Network being illustrated in Fig. 4.32. The patient identifiers are given at the top of the form, followed by the anatomical site of the specimen, the type of specimen, the method of localization and the cytological opinion. Any temptation to make a histopathological diagnosis should be avoided, although it is appropriate to consider this in the descriptive section under 'Comment'. A diagnosis such as 'malignant lymphoma', for example, should be reported as C4 or C5 depending on the degree of certainty, but a precise diagnosis may be suggested in the free text. Similarly, an aspirate showing numerous large spindle and bizarrely shaped cells might be considered to contain sarcoma, but spindle cell carcinomas may produce a similar pattern. Unless there is clear immunohistochemical support for mesenchymal origin, the possibility of sarcoma should be discussed in the 'Comment' section but the conclusion should be C4 or C5.

Similarly, when reporting benign changes. The temptation to provide a diagnosis of 'fibrocystic change' should be avoided even though the description of the cells might lead the clinician to conclude such a diagnosis in consultation with the clinical and mammographic appearances. Although the appearances of

Registration Form

BREAST SCREENING CYTOPATHOLOGY

Surname............................ Forenames.. Date of Birth................................

Screening No.................. Hospital No.................. Centre.................. Report No.................

Side ☐ Right ☐ Left

Specimen type ☐ FNA ☐ FNA ☐ Nipple disharge ☐ Nipple or skin scrapings
(solid lesion) (cyst)

Localisation technique ☐ Palpation ☐ X-ray guided ☐ Ultrasound guided

Opinion ☐ 1 Unsatisfactory
☐ 2 Benign
☐ 3 Atypia probably benign
☐ 4 Suspicious of malignancy
☐ 5 Malignant

PATHOLOGIST NAME OF ASPIRATOR DATE

4.31 Cytopathology screening form used in European breast screening programmes. FNA = fine-needle aspiration.

fibroadenoma in needle aspirates are well described and tested prospectively (Bottles *et al.*, 1988), the report should simply provide the appropriate 'C' category. It is appropriate, however, to state in the description section that the appearances are compatible with a fibroadenoma. It is certainly important to diagnose fibroadenomas as, in consultation with the patient, a surgeon might adopt a policy of observation rather than excision. Indeed, these lesions usually disappear later in life.

The macroscopic appearance of the specimen is also important, and the aspirator should inform the cytopathologist of the nature of the sample. The presence of fluid in the syringe indicates a cyst, although the deposit may be acellular. An appropriate report in this situation might read: 'six millilitres of clear fluid aspirated. No cells present. No evidence of malignancy.' When the aspirator is the pathologist, such potential difficulties are eliminated, but if specimens are sent to the laboratory by clinicians without clinical information, the report of 'no cells present', indicating an inadequate specimen, would be inappropriate.

Although the aim is to provide a definitive diagnosis of malignancy or a benign lesion, this is not always possible, although the proportion of equivocal reports reduces with experience. Most pathologists have adopted a numerical classification prefixed with the letter 'C' whereby C1 means inadequate, C2 benign and C5 malignant. C3 denotes a degree of atypia but is probably benign, and C4 is suspicious of malignancy. A detailed definition of these categories is given in the guidelines for the UK National Breast Screening Programme and the European Breast Screening Network (EC 1996), British National Health Service Breast Screening Programme handbook *Guidelines for Cytology Procedures and Fine Needle Aspirates of the Breast* (1994), as well as in the European Commission (1996) Guidelines. These are reproduced here, along with the reporting form (*see* Fig. 4.31 above):

- *C1: Unsatisfactory* – indicates a scanty or acellular specimen or a poor preparation. Scanty cellularity is defined as fewer than five clumps of epithelial cells. Preparative artefact includes crushing, excessive blood obscuring the epithelial cells and unsatisfactory drying that occurs when smears for Giemsa staining dry too slowly, being too thick, or when wet fixed smears are allowed to dry before fixation.

- *C2: Benign* – indicates an adequate sample showing no evidence of malignancy, and thus, if representative, warrants a negative report. The specimen should be cellular (at least five clumps of epithelial cells), and the cells should have morphological characteristics of benignity. The possibility of a specific condition should be mentioned, for example fibroadenoma, fat necrosis, inflammation or lymph node, if sufficient features are present.
- *C3: Atypia* – probably benign. These specimens have the characteristics of a benign aspirate but with additional atypical features such as nuclear pleomorphism and loss of cellular cohesion. Aspirates exhibiting nuclear and cytoplasmic changes resulting from hormonal or other treatment may be included in this category.
- *C4: Suspicious of malignancy* – cases in this group are almost certainly malignant, and although the cells are highly abnormal, the pathologist feels unable to provide a categorical diagnosis of malignancy. These reservations fall into three main categories:
  (a) The specimen may be scanty, poorly preserved or poorly prepared.
  (b) It may show some malignant features but not enough to make a clear-cut diagnosis.
  (c) The overall pattern is benign with a large number of characteristic epithelial and myoepithelial cells, singly and in pairs, but an occasional cluster of large irregular cells with definite malignant features is seen.
- *C5: Malignant* – indicates unequivocal malignancy, characteristic of carcinoma or other malignant tumour. The pathologist should feel 'at ease' in making such a diagnosis. Malignancy should not be diagnosed on the basis of a single criterion, but a combination of such features, such as those listed in Table 4.2 above, will be necessary to achieve this diagnosis.

The proportion of samples reported in each of these groups will clearly vary according to clinical practice and the skill and experience of the cytopathologist and aspirator. Although

a wide range of diagnostic performance has been reported in the literature (Giard and Herman, 1992), many papers have shown a positive predictive value for the diagnosis of carcinoma of 100 per cent (Wells *et al.*, 1994), with a range of sensitivity between 65 and 98 per cent. As far as false-positive reports are concerned, Jatoi and Trott (1996) found four misdiagnoses of carcinoma in an analysis of 1104 cases of positive breast aspirates seen consecutively over a 4-year period. This is an incidence of 0.3 per cent and a positive predictive value of 99.6 per cent. The benign conditions that led to a false-positive diagnosis were radiation-induced changes, granulomatous mastitis and fibroadenoma. The standards for FNAC, in which therapy is partially based on it, have been defined for the UK National Breast Screening Programme and the European Breast Screening Network by various parameters, as shown in Table 4.3.

NEEDLE CORE BIOPSIES

NCB reports

For the purposes of data-recording and quality assurance, it has been recommended by the UK National Co-ordinating Group for Breast Screening Pathology (1997) and the European Commission Working Group on Breast Screening Pathology (2000) that NCBs be

TABLE 4.3 Standards for FNAC

	Percentage
Absolute sensitivity	>60
Complete sensitivity	>80
Specificity (including non-biopsied cases)	>60
Positive predictive value	>98
False-negative rate	<5
False-positive rate	<1
Inadequate rate	<25
Inadequate rate in samples taken from carcinomas	<10
Suspicious rate	<20

Registration Form

BREAST SCREENING WIDE BORE NEEDLE BIOPSY

Surname............................ Forenames.. Date of Birth..............................

Screening No................. Hospital No................. Centre................. Report No.................

Side ☐ Right ☐ Left Number of cores.............................

Calcification present on X-Ray? ☐ Yes ☐ No ☐ Radiograph not seen

Histological calcification ☐ Absent ☐ Benign ☐ Malignant ☐ Both

Localisation technique ☐ Palpation ☐ X-ray guided ☐ Ultrasound guided ☐ Stereotaxis

Opinion ☐ B1. Unsatisfactory/Normal tissue only

☐ B2. Benign

☐ B3. Benign but of uncertain malignant potential

☐ B4. Suspicious of malignancy

☐ B5. Malignant ☐ a. In-situ

☐ b. Invasive

☐ c. Uncertain whether in-situ or invasive

PATHOLOGIST............................ Operator taking biopsy................................ Date............................

Comment ....
....

4.32 Form for reporting needle biopsies in European breast screening programmes.

classified on a 5-point scale in a similar fashion to cytological specimens. A standardized reporting form has been devised for this purpose (Fig. 4.32). Some centres may wish to merge categories B3 and B4 as both indicate the need for further action.

It needs to be emphasized, however, that the categories are not the same as the five cytology categories and have different clinical implications. It is essential that the histological appearances in NCBs are compared with the clinical and radiological findings in order to ensure that the biopsy is representative.

Needle biopsy reporting categories

B1: Normal or uninterpretable – may indicate an unsatisfactory biopsy that is:

(a) uninterpretable because of artefact;
(b) composed of stroma only;
(c) composed of normal breast tissue in cases where a normal appearance is felt to be inconsistent with findings on imaging and clinical examination.

B2: Benign – indicates that the sample contains a benign abnormality. The characteristics of the lesion can be described in an accompanying text report. Biopsies exhibiting a normal appearance may be included in this category if they are felt to be consistent with the findings on imaging and clinical examination (e.g. of a hamartoma). Involutionary calcification should be classified as benign.

B3: Benign but of uncertain biological potential – indicates a benign abnormality that is recognized to be associated with an increased risk of developing breast cancer, or is often associated with the presence of *in situ* or invasive carcinoma in the breast. Examples of such lesions include papillomas and radial scars/complex sclerosing lesions.

B4: Suspicious – indicates that changes suggestive of *in situ* or invasive malignancy are present but a categorical diagnosis cannot be made because of artefact or because the appearances are borderline.

B5: Malignant – indicates the presence of an unequivocal malignant process, usually *in situ* or invasive carcinoma. Category (a) indicates that only *in situ* carcinoma is present, (b) that invasive carcinoma is seen, and (c) that it is not certain whether or not the carcinoma is invasive. If invasive malignancy other than a primary carcinoma is suspected, category 5b should be used but a qualifying statement should be entered in the 'comment' section. It is important to remember that a lesion classified as 5a may be found to have an invasive component in later biopsy or resection specimens.

Calcification

Should an NCB be performed for the investigation of suspicious microcalcification, the report should indicate clearly whether microcalcification has been identified in the biopsy and whether it is associated with a specific abnormality. Radiography of the specimen can assist in identifying microcalcification and confirming that its characteristics are the same as those of the mammographic abnormality.

The patient details, report number, side (right or left), localization technique and names of the pathologist and operator taking the biopsy are also included. In assessing performance it is essential to specify whether the performance indicators (e.g. sensitivity, specificity and positive predictive value) relate to the histological report alone or to the diagnosis reached after consideration of the pathological, radiological and clinical findings.

NEEDLE DIAGNOSIS OF IMPALPABLE BREAST LESIONS

The use of mammography as a screening test for cancer and as part of the investigation and follow-up of symptomatic breast disease has markedly increased in recent years.

Benign lesions such as cysts or fibroadenomas are relatively common among impalpable abnormalities, and most can be confidently identified without the need for further investigation. The assessment of impalpable abnormalities is aided by physical examination of the breast by an experienced clinician. Thus the impalpable may become palpable, or palpable and impalpable lesions may co-exist.

The most common significant abnormality seen in mammography is calcification, which may have characteristic features suggesting malignancy or benignity. Calcification without an opacity presents a less compact target for sampling. If radiological assessment suggests malignancy, samples for cellular diagnosis can be obtained under image guidance.

Methods of localizing abnormalities

These are currently radiography and ultrasonography. The early X-ray techniques combined views from several directions with the use of a perforated grid or plate placed on the skin near the lesion, through which the needle could be inserted in the right direction. This technique was cumbersome and often inaccurate, producing poor-quality material, and has been largely superseded by X-ray stereotaxis, in which the calculations to determine the correct angle and distance to which to insert the needle are undertaken automatically following radiographs taken through different co-ordinates.

Two types of machine are available. In one the patient sits upright and the breast is squeezed between plates. Guidance for inserting the needle is provided by computer analysis, and the needle is inserted by the radiologist. Check films are taken to ensure that the needle tip is adjacent to the lesion. In the second type of machine, the patient lies prone with the breast protruding through a port. Similar procedures to identify the position of the lesion are then undertaken, and a sample is obtained. The general experience is that better samples are usually obtained with the prone technique, although the machine is expensive and can be used only for breast stereotaxis. The upright machine can also be used for other radiological procedures and is far cheaper.

If a lesion is visible by ultrasound, it is far easier to use this technique than stereotaxis to obtain samples for diagnosis. The advantage of ultrasonography is that a hand-held device can be used on the outpatient couch to visualize the needle and guide its positioning in the breast during the procedure. Furthermore, there is no danger from radiation, and the needle can be inserted with ultrasound guidance from different directions so that its tip can be seen 'in real time' to be within the lesion. Conventional transducers unfortunately do not identify microcalcification, which is the most common mammographic abnormality likely to be malignant. However, for complex lesions, especially those which are partly cystic, ultrasonography provides an excellent image that then can be directly needled.

Factors affecting diagnostic success in impalpable abnormalities

The skill of the radiologist lies in selecting the abnormalities most likely to be malignant, as well as in technical expertise in obtaining samples from that particular lesion. Although the amount of material aspirated is usually less than that obtained from palpable lumps, a high level of accuracy can be obtained.

In many centres the quality of the material is assessed during the procedure by staining smears rapidly with toluidine blue or a similar rapid vital stain to check that sufficient material has been obtained. Subsequent conventional staining is possible. Details of preparation and staining depend on personal preferences and experience, but a suggested routine is two smears from each pass, one stained using the Papanicolaou technique and the other by the May–Grunwald Giemsa method. Calcified material is occasionally seen and is good evidence that the needle is correctly positioned. The histological grade of the lesion is an important factor in determining specificity and sensitivity. High-grade *in situ* or invasive carcinomas will be more readily diagnosed than low-grade ones.

REFERENCES

Abele J.S., Miller T.R. (1993) Implementation of an outpatient needle aspiration biopsy service and clinic. In Schmit W.A. (ed.), *Cytopathology Annual*. Baltimore, Williams & Wilkins.

Antoniades K., Spector H.B. (1987) Similarities and variations among lobular carcinoma cells. *Diagn. Cytopathol.*, **3**, 55–9.

Bottles K., Chan J.S., Holly E.A. *et al.* (1988) Cytologic criteria for fibroadenoma. *Am. J. Clin. Pathol.* **89**, 707–13.

Britton P.D. (1999) Fine needle aspiration or core biopsy. *Breast*, **8**, 1–4.

Britton P.D., McCann J. (1999) Needle biopsy in the NHS Breast Screening Programme 1996/97: how much and how accurate? *Breast*, **8**, 5–11.

Brown L.A., Coghill S.B. (1992) Cost effectiveness of a fine needle aspirate clinic. *Cytopathology*, **3**, 275–80.

Catania S., Veronesi P., Marassi A. *et al.* (1993) Risk of pneumothorax after fine needle aspiration of the breast: Italian experience of more than 200,000 aspirations. *Breast*, **2**, 246–7.

Chang A.R. (1990) Fine needle aspiration cytology in a case of florid gynaecomastia. *Cytopathology*, **1**, 357–61.

Christie R, Bates T. (1999) Risk of pneumothorax as a complication of diagnostic fine needle aspiration or therapeutic needling of the breast; should the patient be warned? *Breast*, **8**, 98–9.

Ciatto S., Cariaggi P., Bularesi P. (1987) The value of routine cytologic examination of breast cyst fluids. *Acta Cytol.*, **31**, 301–4.

Dahlstrom J.E., Sutton S., Jain S. (1996) Histologic-radiologic correlation of mammographically detected microcalcification in stereotactic core biopsies. *Am. J. Surg. Pathol.*, **22**, 256–9.

Dahlstrom J.E., Sutton S., Jain S. (1998), Histological precision of steretactic core biopsy in diagnosis of malignant and premalignant breast lesions. *Histopathology*, **28**, 537–41.

Deen S.A., McKee G.T., Kissin M.W. (1999) Differential cytologic features of fibroepithelial lesions of the breast. *Diagn. Cytopathol.*, **20**, 53–6.

Denley H., Pinder S.E., Elston C.W. *et al.* (2001) Preoperative assessment of prognostic factors in breast cancer. *J. Clin. Pathol.*, **54**, 20–24.

Di Pietro S., Fariselli G., Bandieramonte G *et al.* (1987) Diagnostic efficacy of the clinical-radiological cytological triplet in solid breast lumps: results of a second prospective study on 631 patients. *Eur. J. Surg. Oncol.*, **13**, 335–50.

Dixon J.M., Anderson T.J., Lamb J. *et al.* (1984) Fine needle aspiration cytology in relationship to clinical examination and mammography in the diagnosis of a solid breast mass. *Br. J. Surg.*, **71**, 593.

Dodd L.G., Sneige N., Reece G.P., Fornage B. (1993) Fine needle aspiration cytology of silicone granulomas in the augmented breast. *Diagn. Cytopathol.*, **9**, 498–502.

Duane G.B., Canter M.H., Branigan T., Chang C. (1987) A morphologic and morphometric study of cells from colloid carcinoma of the breast obtained by fine needle aspiration. *Acta Cytol.*, **31**, 742–50.

European Commission (1996) *European Guidelines for Quality Assurance in Mammography Screening*, 2nd edn. Office for Official Publications of the European Communities.

Fisher E.R. (1976) Ultrastructure of the human breast and its disorders. *Am. J. Clin. Pathol.*, **66**, 291–375.

Franzen S., Zajicek J. (1968) Aspiration biopsy in the diagnosis of palpable lesions of the breast: critical review of 3479 consecutive biopsies. *Acta Radiol. Ther.*, **7**, 241–62.

Fung A., Rayter Z., Fisher C. *et al.* (1990) Preoperative cytology and mammography in patients with single-duct nipple discharge treated by surgery. *Br. J. Surg.*, **77**, 1211–2.

Gateley C.A., Maddox P.R., Mansel R.E. (1991) Pneumothorax: a complication of fine needle aspiration of the breast. *Br. Med. J.*, **30**, 627–8.

Giard R.W.M., Herman J.O. (1992) The value of aspiration cytologic examination of the breast: a statistical review of the medical literature. *Cancer*, **69**, 2104–10.

Gregory K.R. (1998) Use of molecular markers to predict prognosis and response to neoadjuvant chemoendocrine treatment in primary carcinoma of the breast. MD thesis. University of Newcastle Upon Tyne, UK.

Gui G.P.H., Allum W.H., Perry N.M. *et al.* (1995) One-stop diagnosis for symptomatic breast disease. *Ann. Roy. Coll. Surg. Eng.*, **77**, 24–7.

Haggensen C.D. (1971) *Diseases of the Breast*, 2nd edn. Philadelphia, W.B. Saunders.

Harcourt D., Ambler N., Rumsey N., Cawthorn S.J. (1998) Evaluation of a one-stop breast lump clinic: a randomized controlled trial. *Breast*, **7**, 314–19.

Howell L.P., Kline T.S. (1990) Medullary carcinoma of the breast; a rare cytologic finding in cyst fluid aspirates. *Cancer*, **65**, 277–82.

Hunt C.M., Ellis I.O., Elston C.W., Locker A., Pearson D., Blamey R.W. (1990) Cytological grading of breast carcinoma – a feasible proposition? *Cytopathology*, **1**, 287–95.

Jacobs T.W., Siziopikou K.P., Prioleau J.E. *et al.* (1998). Do prognostic marker studies on core needle biopsy specimens of breast carcinoma accurately reflect the marker status of the tumor? *Mod. Pathol.*, **11**, 259–64.

Jatoi I., Trott P.A. (1996) False positive reporting in breast fine needle aspiration cytology: incidence and causes. *Breast*, **5**, 270–3.

Kline T.S. (1990) Communication and aspiration biopsy cytology: clear, concise and to the point (editorial). *Diagn. Cytopathol.*, **6**, 153.

Kline T.S., Kannan V., Kline I.K. (1985) Appraisal and cytomorphologic analysis of common carcinomas of the breast. *Diagn. Cytopathol.*, **1**, 188–93.

Kocjan G. (1991) Evaluation of the cost effectiveness of establishing a fine needle aspiration cytology clinic in a hospital outpatient department. *Cytopathology*, **2**, 13–8.

Leach, C., Howell L.P. (1992) Cytodiagnosis of classic lobular carcinoma and its variants. *Acta Cytol.*, **36**, 199–202.

Linsk J.A., Franzen S. (1983) *Clinical Aspiration Cytology*. Philadelphia, J.B. Lippincott.

Lowhagen T., Rubio C.A. (1977) The cytology of granular cell myoblastoma of the breast. Report of a case. *Acta Cytol.*, **21**, 314–15.

Lucarotti M.E., Dunn J.M., Webb A.J. (1994) Scrape cytology in the diagnosis of Paget's disease of the breast. *Cytopathology*, **5**, 301–5.

Makris A., Allred D.C. Powles T.J. *et al.* (1997a) Cytological evaluation of biological prognostic markers from primary breast carcinomas. *Breast Cancer Res. Treat.*, **44**, 65–74.

Makris A., Powles T.J., Dowsett M. *et al.* (1997b) Prediction of response to neoadjuvant chemoendocrine therapy in primary breast carcinomas. *Clin. Cancer Res.*, **3**, 593–600.

Masukawa T, Kuzma J.F., Straumfjord J.V. (1973) Cytologic detection of early Paget's disease of breasts with improved cellular collection method. *Acta Cytol.*, **19**, 274–8.

Mitchell G., Trott P.A., Morris L. *et al.* (in press 2001) Cellular characteristics of nipple aspiration fluid during the menstrual cycle in healthy premenopausal women. *Cytopathology*.

Nagy G.K., Jacobs J.B., Mason-Savas A. *et al.* (1989) Intracytoplasmic inclusion bodies in breast cyst fluid are eosinophilic giant lysosomes. *Acta Cytol.*, **33**, 99–103.

National Co-ordinating Group for Breast Screening Pathology (1997) *Guidelines for Breast Pathology Services*. NHSBSP Publication No 2. Oertel Y.C., Galbum L.L. (1986) Fine needle aspiration of the breast: diagnostic criteria. *Pathol. Annu.*, **18**, 375–407.

Orell S.R., Sterrett G.E., Walters M.N.L., Whittaker D. (1992) *Manual and Atlas of Fine Needle Aspiration Cytology*, 2nd edn. Edinburgh, Churchill Livingstone.

Pettinato G., Manivel J.C., Petrella G., De Chiara A. (1991) Primary multilobulated T-cell lymphoma of the breast diagnosed by fine needle aspiration cytology and immunocytochemistry. *Acta Cytol.*, **35**, 294–9.

Pinder S.E., Elston C.W., Ellis I.O. (1996) The role of pre-operative diagnosis in breast cancer. *Histopathology*, **28**, 563–6.

Poole G.H., Willsher P.C., Pinder S.E., Robertson J.F.R., Elston C.W., Blamey R.W. (1996) Diagnosis of breast cancer with core-biopsy and fine needle aspiration cytology. *Aust. N. Z. Surg.*, **66**, 592–4.

Robinson I.A., McKee G., Nicholson A. *et al.* (1994) Prognostic value of cytological grading of fine-needle aspirates from breast carcinomas. *Lancet*, **343**, 947–9.

Simm V., Moretti D., Sacconi P *et al.* (1988) Fine needle aspiration cytopathology of phyllodes tumour: differential diagnosis with fibroadenoma. *Acta Cytol.*, **32**, 63–6.

Sneige N., White V.A., Katz R.L., Troncoso P., Libshitz H.I., Hortobagyi G.N. (1989) Ductal carcinoma-in-situ of the breast: fine-needle aspiration cytology of 12 cases. *Diagn. Cytopathol.*, **5**, 371–7.

Stanley M.W. (1990) Who should perform fine needle aspiration biopsies? *Diagn. Cytopathol.*, **6**, 215–7.

Stanley M.W., Henry-Stanley M.J., Zera R. (1993). Atypia in breast fine needle aspiration smears correlates poorly with the presence of a prognostically significant proliferative lesion of ductal epithelium. *Hum. Pathol.*, **24**, 630–5.

Stanley M.W., Tani E.M., Skoog L. (1989) Mucinous breast carcinoma and mixed mucinous infiltrating ductal carcinoma: a comparative cytologic study. *Diagn. Cytopathol.*, **5**, 134–8.

Sturgis C.D., Sethi S., Cajulis R.S., Hidvegi D.E., Yu G.H. (1998) Diagnostic significance of 'benign pairs' and signet ring cells in fine needle aspirates (FNAs) of the breast. *Cytopathology*, **9**, 308–19.

Tavassoli F.A., Yeh I.T. (1987) Lactational and clear cell changes of the breast in non-lactating, non-pregnant women. *Am. J. Clin. Pathol.*, **87**, 23–9.

Thomas J.M., Fitzharris B.M., Redding W.H. *et al.* (1978) Clinical examination, xeromammography and fine needle aspiration cytology in diagnosis of breast lesions. *Br. Med. J.*, **2**, 1139–41.

Trott P.A., Nasiri N (1997) Treatment of breast cancer before surgery will present pathologists with challenges (letter). *Br. Med. J.*, **314**, 755.

Tyler X., Coghill S.B. (1991) Fine needle aspiration cytology of collagenous spherulosis of the breast. *Cytopathology*, **2**, 159–62.

Wells C.A., Ellis I.O., Zakhour H.D., *et al.* (1994) Guidelines for cytology procedures and reporting on fine-needle aspirates of the breast. *Cytopathology*, **5**, 316–34.

Yelland A., Graham M.D., Trott P.A. *et al.* (1991) Diagnosing breast carcinoma in young women. *Br. Med. J.*, **302**, 618–20.

Zajdela A., DeLa Riva L., Ghossein N. (1984) The relation of prognosis to the nuclear diameter of breast cancer cells obtained by cytologic aspirations. *Acta Cytol.*, **23**, 75–80.

Zajicek J. (1974) Aspiration biopsy cytology. I. Cytology of supradiaphragmatic organs. In Weid G.L. (ed.) *Monographs in Clinical Cytology*. Basel, S. Karger.

5 Development and developmental abnormalities

DEVELOPMENT

Development in the embryo and neonate

At about 5 weeks of intrauterine life, a pair of external thickenings develop on the ventral surface of the embryo, extending from the base of the forelimb buds to points medial to the hindlimb buds. These are known as the mammary ridges or lines (milk lines). Their caudal portions later disappear, but the intermediate portions of their cephalic one third thicken to form the mammary primordium. By the end of the first trimester, there is a well-defined bud from which about 15–20 solid epithelial cords extend into the upper dermis, surrounded by mesenchyme that tends to be more cellular in the immediate vicinity of developing epithelium. In the centre of the bud, the cells exhibit microvilli and desmosomes under the electron microscope, but cytoplasmic organelles are poorly developed (Tobon and Salazar, 1974). At the periphery of the bud, the cells maintain some similarity to the epidermal basal and intermediate cells and are surrounded by a single basal lamina continuous with that of the epidermis.

In the second trimester, the cords acquire lumina to become ducts lined by a double layer of cells. These ducts are surrounded by dense connective tissue and extend deeper into the dermis but do not reach the subcutaneous tissue. Epithelial and myoepithelial differentiation is discernible ultrastructurally at this stage. The epithelial cells lining the ducts exhibit microvilli, tight junctions and more prominent organelles with abundant rough endoplasmic reticulum, large mitochondria and many tonofilaments, although the Golgi apparatus remains sparse. Myoepithelial cells are present at the periphery of the ducts in contact with the basal lamina. They contain a large number of intracytoplasmic myofilaments and are connected to adjoining epithelial and myoepithelial cells by desmosomes, as well as to the basal lamina by hemidesmosomes. A further group of cells with electron-lucent cytoplasm and poorly developed organelles is also identifiable.

In the third trimester, there is an increasing number of branching dilated ducts that now contain secretory material and extend into the subcutaneous fat. Towards the end of pregnancy, the epithelial cells have vacuolated cytoplasm due to the presence of lipid droplets and other secretory products. Secretion can usually be obtained from the nipple at birth, and there is generally some clinical enlargement that later subsides. It has been assumed that these secretory changes near term result from the action of maternal hormones. The onset of these changes during the first few weeks of life in some premature infants, however, indicates that the explanation may not be quite as simple as this (McKiernan and Hull, 1981).

The original epidermal downgrowth appears as a crater into which the mammary ducts open, but near term there is a proliferation of mesenchyme, causing its elevation above the surface to form the nipple. Embryological development is similar in both male and female, so that at term the structure of the breast in the two sexes is the same.

Changes in the expression of various molecules in human breast development have been studied by Gusterson and colleagues in an attempt to gain insight into the development of breast disease (Nathan et al., 1994; Osin et al., 1998). Immunostaining for Ki67 reveals a large number of positive epithelial and stromal cells in the developing fetal breast, the former mainly in the neck of the epithelial bud and the latter randomly distributed. The stromal, and to a lesser extent the epithelial, positivity persists for the first few days of infant life, after which virtually no positive cells are seen. Immunopositivity for transforming growth factor-α (TGFα) is present in a minority of epithelial and mesenchymal cells of the fetal and early infant breast but not in the intralobular or periductal stroma. There may be foci of extramedullary haemopoiesis in the stroma of the fetal breast, always in the TGFα-negative areas. TGFβ1 is restricted to the stroma, particularly surrounding the epithelium, and persists for the first 3 months of infant life, after which it becomes weaker.

Tenascin-C is present in the stromal cells around the neck of the breast bud but absent at the tip. In infants, staining intensity for tenascin-C shows two peaks: one immediately post partum and the other at 6–12 weeks. The second peak coincides with an intriguing morphological change in which the infant breast epithelium changes from a secretory to an apocrine type with cystic dilatation. Type IV collagen immunostaining is seen around the developing epithelial bud, more so around

the neck region than the tip. The anti-apoptotic protein bcl-2 is expressed in the basal layer of the developing fetal breast bud and the surrounding mesenchyme. In the infant heterogeneous positivity is seen in luminal epithelial cells but not in myoepithelial cells or fibroblasts. Staining intensity increases after 2 months of age.

Development in childhood and adolescence

The breast enlargement palpable at birth may persist into the second half of the first year of life, after which it subsides. Breast growth in childhood is isometric, that is, proportional to the growth of the body as a whole. During this time the histological appearances are similar in the male and female, showing a rudimentary duct system devoid of lobules. This appearance persists in the male but changes dramatically in the female at puberty.

Pubertal breast development (thelarche) usually begins about a year before the menarche. Breast growth becomes allometric; that is, it is disproportionately greater than that of the rest of the body. Histological studies of this phase of breast development in the human are sparse. There is marked ductal proliferation, budding and canalization to form a much more extensive duct system from which true lobules arise. Vascularity is also markedly increased, and there is an extensive deposition of connective tissue and fat. The proliferation of skin elements leads to an increase in size and proliferation of the areola and nipple.

DEVELOPMENTAL ABNORMALITIES

Accessory breast tissue

Accessory breast tissue usually occurs along the mammary lines, most frequently in the axilla or between the breast and the umbilicus. There are, however, rare reports of its occurrence at sites remote from the milk lines; Camisa (1980), for example, described an accessory breast on the posterior thigh of an elderly man and quoted other reports concerning the back, shoulder and vulva. The incidence of accessory tissue varies in different studies from about 0.2 to 2% of the general population (De Cholnoky, 1939; Mehes, 1979). Supernumerary breast tissue may take many different forms (Kajava, 1915). Sometimes there is a complete breast with glandular tissue, nipple and areola, but in most cases development is incomplete. There may be glandular tissue without the areola and/or nipple. Similarly, the areola or nipple may exist alone or together but without underlying breast tissue. Occasionally, the nipple and areola overlie a pad of fat devoid of glandular epithelium – a condition known as pseudomamma. The accessory tissue may sometimes be represented only by a patch of hair.

The epithelium and stroma are identical to those of the normal breast and are susceptible to the same alterations. Cysts, hyperplasia, fibroadenoma and other benign changes have been observed as well as carcinoma (De Cholnoky, 1951). Normal proliferative and secretory changes may also occur in pregnancy, and it is sometimes the consequent enlargement that first draws attention to the abnormality. Surprisingly, enlargement may not always occur in the first pregnancy (Greer, 1974).

Cases without underlying glandular or fatty tissue are often mistaken clinically for naevi or other benign cutaneous tumours. Histological examination may reveal very little if the pathologist is unaware of the possibility of an accessory breast. Careful examination, however, often shows the presence of a few poorly formed mammary ductal structures in the skin and subcutaneous tissue (Fig. 5.1).

There may occasionally be more than one nipple in an otherwise normal breast (Brightmore, 1972).

Absence or hypoplasia of the breast

This is rare. Wilson *et al.* (1972) described a family in which congenital absence or hypoplasia of one or both breasts occurred as an inherited, dominant disorder. The absence of breasts may also occur in the inherited syndrome of ectodermal dysplasia (Burck and Held, 1981). A hereditary syndrome of rudimentary nipples, lumpy scalp and odd ears has also been reported (Finlay and Marks, 1978). In addition, inverted nipples may occur as a dominantly inherited disorder (Shafir *et al.*, 1979).

Abnormal development at puberty

Failure of the breast to undergo normal development at puberty may occur in association with disorders such as Turner's syndrome (Haagensen, 1971) and congenital adrenal hyperplasia (Jones and Scott, 1958). Precocious development may also occur, sometimes in association with ovarian tumours but usually for inexplicable reasons. The histological appearances of the breast are normal for the stage of development.

Juvenile hypertrophy of the breast usually follows normal puberty but the breasts continue to grow out of proportion, often to a very large size. The condition does not regress and is sometimes asymmetrical. Surgical intervention is often necessary to alleviate the patient's physical and psychological problems. The breasts show no histological abnormality, most of the enlargement apparently resulting from an overgrowth of normal-appearing fibroadipose stroma.

Associated abnormalities

Subjects with accessory breast tissue, congenital hypoplasia or absence of the breast and Turner's syndrome have an increased incidence of developmental abnormalities of the kidney and renal adenocarcinoma (Goeminne, 1972; Mehes, 1979; Goedert *et al.*, 1981).

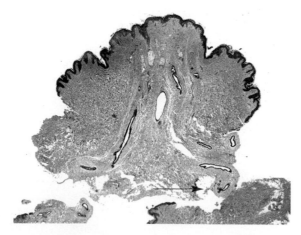

5.1 Accessory breast tissue. The section is of a lesion (thought to be a lipoma) removed from the axilla. The dermis contains several large ducts lined by epithelial and myoepithelial cells. A very small terminal duct–lobular unit is present in the deep aspect of the specimen (arrow) (H&E).

REFERENCES

Brightmore T. (1972) Bilateral double nipples. *Br. J. Surg.*, **59**, 55–7.

Burck U., Held K.R. (1981) Athelia in a female infant – heterozygous for anhidrotic ectodermal dysplasia. *Clin. Genet.*, **19**, 117–21.

Camisa C. (1980) Accessory breast on the posterior thigh of a man. *J. Am. Acad. Dermatol.*, **3**, 467–9.

De Cholnoky T. (1939) Supernumerary breast. *Arch. Surg. (Chicago)*, **39**, 926–41.

De Cholnoky T. (1951) Accessory breast tissue in the axilla. *N.Y. State J. Med.*, **51**, 2245–8.

Finlay A.Y., Marks R. (1978) An hereditary syndrome of lumpy scalp, odd ears and rudimentary nipples. *Br. J. Dermatol.*, **99**, 423–30.

Goedert J.J., McKeen E.A., Fraumeni J.F. (1981) Polymastia and renal adenocarcinoma. *Ann. Intern. Med.*, **95**, 182–4.

Goeminne L. (1972) Synopsis of mammo-renal syndromes. *Humangenetik*, **14**, 170–1.

Greer K.E. (1974) Accessory axillary breast tissue. *Arch. Dermatol.*, **109**, 88–9.

Haagensen C.D. (1971) Abnormalities of breast growth, secretion, and lactation, of physiologic origin. In *Diseases of the Breast*, 2nd edn. London, W.B. Saunders.

Jones H.W., Scott W.W. (1958) *Hermaphroditism, Congenital Abnormalities, and Related Endocrine Disorders*. Baltimore, Williams & Wilkins.

Kajava Y. (1915) *Duodecim*, 31, 143, as quoted by Brightmore T. (1972) *Br. J. Surg.*, **59**, 55–7.

McKiernan J.F., Hull D. (1981) Breast development in the newborn. *Arch. Dis. Child.*, **56**, 525–9.

Mehes K. (1979) Association of supernumerary nipples with other anomalies. *J. Pediatr.*, **95**, 274–5.

Nathan B., Anbazhagan R., Clarkson P., Bartkova J., Gusterson B.A. (1994) Expression of BCL-2 in the developing human fetal and infant breast. *Histopathology*, **24**, 73–6.

Osin P.P., Anbazhagan R., Bartkova J., Nathan B., Gusterson B.A. (1998) Breast development gives insights into breast disease. *Histopathology*, **33**, 275–83.

Shafir R., Bonne-Tamir B., Ashbel S., Tsur H., Goodman R.M. (1979) Genetic studies in a family with inverted nipples (mammillae invertita). *Clin. Genet.*, **15**, 346–50.

Tobon H., Salazar H. (1974) Ultrastructure of the human mammary gland. I. Development of the fetal gland throughout gestation. *J. Clin. Endocrinol. Metab.*, **39**, 443–56.

Wilson M.G., Hall E.B., Ebbin A.J. (1972) Dominant inheritance of absence of the breast. *Humangenetik*, **15**, 268–70.

6 Non-neoplastic epithelial changes

GENERAL REMARKS

The epithelium of the breast may undergo a wide variety of benign alterations that have been grouped together under terms such as fibrocystic mastopathy, cystic hyperplasia, benign breast disease, fibroadenosis and mammary dysplasia.

Although the various lesions that comprise the spectrum are strongly associated with each other (Bartow *et al.*, 1987), the use of these all-embracing diagnoses has many disadvantages. The various changes may not all be present in any one specimen and may occur singly or in any combination. The terms embodied in the general headings (fibrosis, cysts, hyperplasia, adenosis etc.) may thus describe changes that are either not present or form only part of what is observed. Furthermore, there are no clear definitions of precisely what changes should be included.

There is some evidence that the alterations may have an endogenous (Walsh *et al.*, 1984) or exogenous (Berkowitz *et al.*, 1984) hormonal basis, although the effect of hormones may not be the same for all lesions. Cahn *et al.* (1997) reported a higher incidence of sclerosing adenosis and a lower incidence of fibrocystic change and fibroadenoma in women on hormonal replacement therapy.

The changes do not seem to reflect the stage of the menstrual cycle (Bartow *et al.*, 1987). The aetiology is thus very poorly understood, and there is no proof that, in any one patient, all observed changes share the same cause. The implication that many of them actually represent disease is highly questionable in view of the frequency with which they occur in the general population, especially with advancing age.

It is thus preferable to record the individual changes observed without attempting to group them into a single disease entity, or even necessarily to give them pathological significance. This has two major clinical advantages. First, not all have the same implications for the patient's management. There is evidence that some lesions, such as intraductal and intralobular hyperplasias, sclerosing adenosis and papillomas, are associated with an increased risk of developing breast cancer, whereas there is no such evidence of this for changes such as cysts, duct ectasia and lactational foci. Furthermore, the level of risk associated with intraluminal proliferations depends on the degree of atypia.

Second, recording in this way enables histopathological findings to be correlated with clinical and radiological features. Cysts produce rounded fluctuant swellings, whereas zones of fibrosis give rise to hard irregular areas that could be confused with carcinoma. Duct ectasia may produce nipple discharge or retraction, features that may be associated with malignancy. Similarly, radial scars exhibit radiological features like those of invasive carcinomas. It is important for the pathologist to attempt to provide explanations for clinical and radiological findings, especially those which may have serious significance, as an inability to do so may indicate that important pathological changes have not been sampled.

The epithelial alterations described in this chapter exclude intraductal and intralobular proliferations, which are considered later in the book in view of their histological similarity, the extensive literature on their precancerous status and the special problems that they present in diagnosis and risk assessment. Furthermore, intraductal proliferations give rise to particular problems during mammographic screening.

CYSTS (FIBROCYSTIC CHANGE)

Cysts are ovoid or spheroidal structures derived from lobules by the dilatation and coalescence of acini; they are thus generally found in clusters (Fig. 6.1), although they may be solitary, especially if expansion is very marked. Small cysts may represent an involutionary process, as described on p. 7. Others are larger, more numerous and often multi-layered, indicating a proliferative process. Papillary tufting with a fibrovascular core is sometimes seen (Fig. 6.2).

The epithelial lining of cysts frequently exhibits metaplasia, giving rise to cells resembling those of normal apocrine sweat glands (Fig. 6.2). These apocrine cells are large, with rounded nuclei and copious amounts of deeply eosinophilic vacuolated cytoplasm containing periodic acid–Schiff (PAS)-positive, diastase-resistant granules (Fig. 6.3). Ultrastructurally, they exhibit more prominent cytoplasmic organelles than do normal breast epithelial cells and are particularly rich in mitochondria, which vary in size and shape and often exhibit incomplete cristae. There are also bundles of

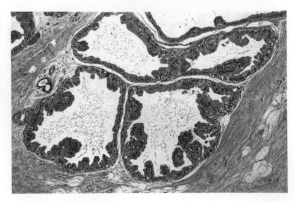

6.1 A cluster of cysts lined by apocrine cells exhibiting papillary hyperplasia (H&E).

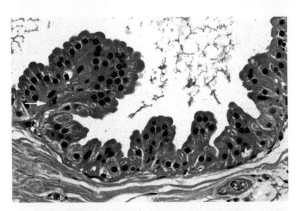

6.2 Higher-power view of Fig. 6.1, showing the papillary tufts with a fibrovascular core on the left (arrow). Although large, the nuclei are regular and normochromic and contain single uniform nucleoli (H&E).

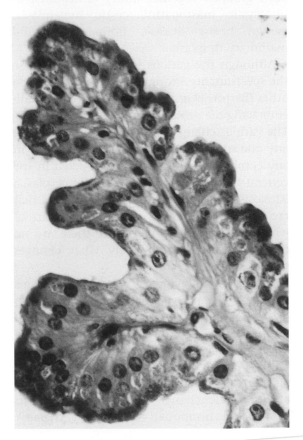

6.3 Wall of an apocrine cyst showing a papillary ingrowth with a fibrovascular core. The section has been stained with periodic acid–Schiff after diastase treatment that reveals numerous small granules between the nuclei and the luminal membranes.

keratin-like filaments, a prominent rough endoplasmic reticulum and well-developed Golgi apparatus (Ahmed, 1975). The cysts are surrounded by elongated myoepithelial cells, which usually contain numerous myofilaments. Ahmed (1975) reported the presence of prominent blood vessels around cysts lying within the epithelial stromal junction, which is normally avascular.

In some cysts the epithelium is attenuated or even absent. These cysts usually contain fluid under pressure and are known as tension cysts. It may be very difficult to distinguish a solitary cyst of this type from a dilated duct. Residual small foci of apocrine cells are very helpful in making the distinction as apocrine metaplasia is hardly ever seen in breast ducts. Even if the epithelium is not recognizably apocrine, the PAS-positive granules may still be demonstrable. Cyst walls usually have no demonstrable elastin, and fibrosis and mononuclear cell infiltration are absent unless a leakage of cyst contents has taken place. Foamy macrophages, often seen in dilated ducts, are usually absent from cysts.

The cyst fluid is complex and comprises a group of proteins often known as gross cystic disease fluid proteins (GCDFPs) (Pearlman *et al.*, 1973). The immunostaining of apocrine cyst epithelium with an antibody against one of them, GCDFP-15, is generally positive and has been used to demonstrate apocrine differentiation in various breast lesions. Immunoglobulins, hormones and electrolytes are also present. Immunostaining apocrine cysts for oestrogen and progesterone receptors is negative, but it is usually positive for androgen receptors (Gatalica, 1997).

Although cysts are commonly responsible for benign breast lumps, they occur with great frequency in the general population. Frantz *et al.* (1951) examined the breasts of 225 autopsies performed on patients with no previous history of breast disease and found cysts in 53%. In 19% the cysts were macroscopically visible, and in half of these subjects there was also some degree of intraductal proliferation (see Chapter 7). There was an externally palpable lump in only one case, however, this being caused by a cyst 20 mm in diameter. The incidence of cysts was much lower below the age of 30. In a forensic autopsy study of 519 women, Bartow *et al.* (1987) found cystic change in up to 65% of all women with no history of breast disease and apocrine metaplasia in up to 50%. Both changes were more common in women of European extraction than in American Indians.

There have been reports of increased breast cancer risk in women with gross cystic disease, particularly in the presence of a family history of breast cancer (Dupont and Page, 1985; Ciatto *et al.*, 1990; Dixon *et al.*, 1999). Most studies have, however, failed to demonstrate an increased risk of developing cancer in women whose cysts are detected histologically (see Chapter 10). Increased surveillance is not justified. Oral contraceptive use has been reported in association with a reduced incidence of cysts (Pastides *et al.*, 1983).

Radiologically, cysts may appear as rounded densities similar to non-calcified fibroadenomas. They occasionally contain calcified material that presents little difficulty on screening mammography (Fig. 6.4). The calcified material may sediment on the floor of the cyst to produce the so-called 'tea-cup' calcification. Wedellite is sometimes detected in cysts (*see* Fig. 2.6).

A *galactocoele* is usually a sub-areolar, solitary, cystic structure distended with milk occurring after an abrupt termination of lactation. Histologically, it is unrelated to the cysts described above and is usually lined by a double layer of epithelial and myoepithelial cells. The former may exhibit active secretion and an abundance of cytoplasmic organelles (Ironside and Guthrie, 1985).

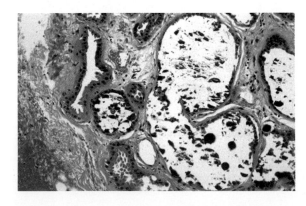

6.4 Collection of apocrine cysts with calcified contents, which were detected by screening mammography (H&E) .

DUCT ECTASIA

A minor degree of dilatation of the interlobular ducts is commonly seen in breast biopsies and is frequently associated with the presence of cysts (Fig. 6.5).

A clinically more important form of duct ectasia is that which involves mainly the major subareolar ducts, which are markedly distended with white or green viscid material that is deeply eosinophilic in histological sections (Fig. 6.6). There is usually a marked periductal infiltration by lymphocytes, plasma cells and histiocytes, together with a significant degree of periductal fibrosis. The process is often called periductal or plasma cell mastitis because of the inflammatory component. A large number of foamy histiocytes is also often present within the lumen, in the periductal zone and within the epithelium itself.

The periductal fibrosis is not always concentric and may take the form of irregular fibrous plaques that can result in considerable ductal distortion (Davies, 1973a). The inflammation may sometimes lead to total ductal obliteration, and in these cases residual ducts may sometimes be identified as solid collagenous plugs surrounded by elastin fibres.

Alterations in periductal elastin may be seen. There is sometimes a fibrous replacement of the elastin, whereas in other cases there may be elastosis similar to that seen in infiltrating breast carcinomas (*see* p. 172). Davies (1973a) found a significant association between elastosis and increasing parity.

The aetiology of the condition is unknown. It has been suggested that the primary process is inflammatory, leading to fibrosis and secondary ductal dilatation. Alternatively, the dilatation may be primary and the inflammation secondary, perhaps related to a leakage of duct contents.

It is important to recognize major duct ectasia as it may be mistaken clinically for carcinoma. The ductal contents may be discharged from the nipple and may rarely be blood-stained. The fibrosis may lead to retraction of the nipple and, together with the ductal dilatation, produce a firm palpable mass. The discharge may occasionally induce

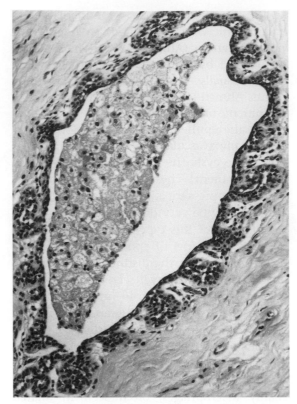

6.5 Interlobular duct showing a minor degree of ectasia. The lumen contains many foamy macrophages, but there is no periductal inflammation or fibrosis (H&E). (Illustration reproduced with permission from Oxford University Press.)

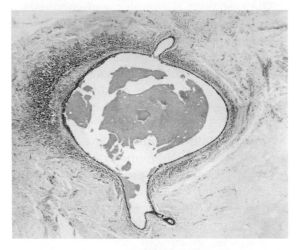

6.6 Major subareolar duct ectasia. The duct is considerably dilated and surrounded by dense chronic inflammation and fibrosis. The lumen is filled with a thick eosinophilic secretion (H&E).

eczema-like changes in the nipple that may be mistaken for Paget's disease.

Calcification may be present within the duct walls, this being seen mammographically in 12 of the 30 patients studied by Rees *et al.* (1977). Even without calcification, however, major duct ectasia could be identified mammographically in all their 30 patients.

Duct ectasia frequently does not give rise to clinical symptoms and is commonly found in mastectomy and autopsy specimens. Frantz *et al.* (1951) noted the presence of 'strikingly dilated nipple ducts containing white or greenish material' at autopsy in 24% of subjects with no history of breast disease. This figure rose to 46% in subjects over 60 years of age.

FIBROSIS

Fibrosis is commonly seen in benign breast biopsies. It may form part of a specific process such as duct ectasia, fat necrosis or diabetic mastopathy. Long-standing fibroadenomas may also consist largely of mature fibrous tissue, but they can usually be recognized by their circumscription and the presence of at least a small amount of residual epithelial tissue. In any fibrous lump in the breast, it is important to exclude the possibility of an infiltrating lobular carcinoma in which the malignant epithelial cells may be very widely dispersed in the fibrous stroma.

A clinically palpable breast lump may sometimes consist of an irregular zone of fibrosis of variable size replacing the epithelial elements of the breast. A hard and irregular mass is produced, which clinically simulates carcinoma. The process has been termed fibrous mastopathy or fibrous disease of the breast, and may well represent an uneven involutionary change.

ADENOSIS

Unqualified, the term adenosis is usually used to describe an enlargement of lobules which otherwise exhibit no cytological or structural abnormalities. Different planes of section will produce an apparent variation in lobular size, and genuine variations may be caused by involution occurring after pregnancy and lactation or with advancing years. Bonser *et al.* (1961) stated that normal lobules might contain from fewer than 10 to more than 100 acini. Despite these wide normal limits, some lobules attain a sufficiently large size to be regarded as pathological. Such a lobule is illustrated in Fig. 6.7.

The term blunt duct adenosis is usually used to describe a form of organoid lobular hypertrophy composed of two-layered, dilated tubules embedded in specialized cellular stroma (Fig. 6.8), which may show pseudoangiomatous hyperplasia (*see* p. 273). The epithelium may be flattened or cuboidal, or exhibit columnar cell metaplasia with large

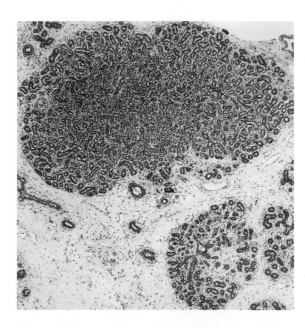

6.7 (Left) Adenosis. The lobule in the upper part of the picture is structurally and cytologically normal but is markedly enlarged, containing hundreds of acini. A normal lobule is included in the bottom right of the picture for comparison (H&E).

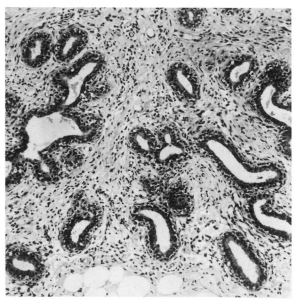

6.8 (Right) Blunt duct adenosis. The lobule consists of enlarged acini embedded in a cellular stroma (H&E).

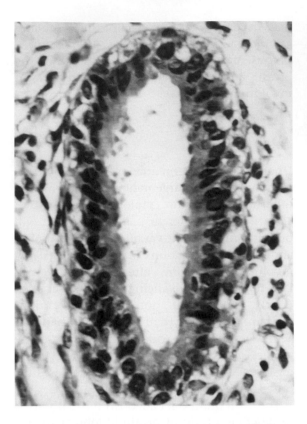

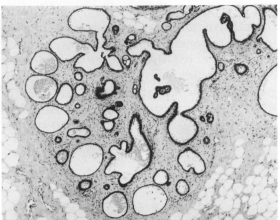

6.9 (Left) Higher-power view of Fig. 6.8. The epithelial cells lining this acinus are columnar and hypertrophic, exhibiting apical blebs suggestive of apocrine secretion (H&E).

6.10 (Right) Microcyst formation in blunt duct adenosis: the lobular architecture is retained, and there also appears to be dilatation of the terminal duct (top right) (H&E).

hyperchromatic ovoid nuclei (Fig. 6.9). The cytoplasm is rather basophilic and exhibits apical snouts, suggestive of apocrine secretion. These cells are, however, unlike the apocrine cells seen in cysts and occasionally exhibit atypical features. The lumina may contain calcified secretion, detectable by mammography as fine, non-branching calcifications.

Fraser *et al.* (1998) reported 42 cases with columnar cell alteration with prominent apical snouts and secretion (CAPSS), identified in 100 consecutive breast biopsies performed for microcalcification. At one end of the spectrum, the cells merely exhibited pronounced columnar cell metaplasia. At the other, tufts, bridges and micropapillae were seen composed of atypical cells. In extreme cases the features could arguably have constituted atypical ductal hyperplasia (ADH) or ductal carcinoma *in situ* (DCIS). Unequivocal DCIS was not, however, seen with greater frequency in biopsies containing CAPSS, although when DCIS co-existed with CAPSS, it was significantly more likely to be of the low-grade micropapillary–cribriform type. At the time of writing there is no evidence that this change is associated with an increased risk of developing breast cancer, but further studies are needed.

The acini in blunt duct adenosis may undergo some dilatation to form microcysts (Fig. 6.10). When this change is prominent, the picture merges with that seen in the more usual type of cyst formation described above. When minor it may resemble microcystic involution.

Sclerosing adenosis, apocrine adenosis, tubular adenosis and the various forms of microglandular adenosis are described under the heading of benign infiltrative epithelial lesions (*see* p. 88).

MYOEPITHELIOSIS

Myoepitheliosis is a multifocal process, usually located in the terminal duct lobular units. It is generally microscopic, but in aggregate the individual lesions may form a palpable mass (Tavassoli, 1991). It is characterized by a proliferation of myoepithelial cells that often assume a cuboidal or spindle-shaped appearance and may exhibit clear cytoplasm (Fig. 6.11). They may give rise to nodular or diffuse masses around the involved glandular structures, or intraluminal proliferations producing variable distension and sometimes occlusion of the lumina. In the latter case persistent luminal cells may be incorporated into the lesion. Small intraluminal papillae may be formed, which consist of central masses of myoepithelial cells covered by epithelium. The

6.11 (Left) Myoepitheliosis. There is a proliferation of cuboidal myoepithelial cells with clear cytoplasm, pushing the epithelial cells into the lumina, some of which are completely occluded (H&E).

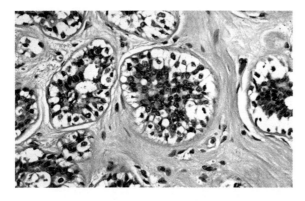

6.12 (Right) Several foci of squamous metaplasia within the walls of a cluster of cysts. The process has originated in the myoepithelial layer, pushing the metaplastic epithelium towards the lumen in a fashion reminiscent of pagetoid spread (H&E).

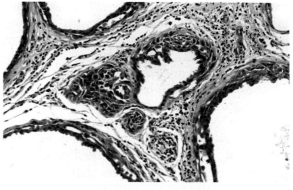

proliferating cells show no atypia or significant mitotic activity. They exhibit positive immunostaining for smooth muscle actin and cytokeratin 14, confirming their myoepithelial nature. None of the three cases reported by Tavassoli developed a recurrence during a follow-up period of 4–7.5 years.

SQUAMOUS METAPLASIA

This is an uncommon, small, focal, microscopic change that, in the author's experience, almost invariably involves the myoepithelial layer, pushing the epithelial cells towards the lumen. Its aetiology and pathogenesis are unknown, and it appears to have no prognostic significance. In the non-neoplastic breast it is usually seen in otherwise normal ducts or terminal duct–lobular units, although it is occasionally observed in the walls of cysts (Fig. 6.12). The main clinical significance of the change is that it is sometimes misdiagnosed as atypical hyperplasia. Squamous metaplasia may also occur in benign and malignant tumours, such as papillomas, phyllodes tumours and invasive carcinomas.

LACTATIONAL FOCI

These are focal secretory lobular lesions that resemble the lactating or pregnant breast at

6.13 (Left) Lactational focus. The lobule is enlarged, and the acini are dilated with secretion (H&E). (Illustration reproduced with permission from the *Journal of Pathology*.)

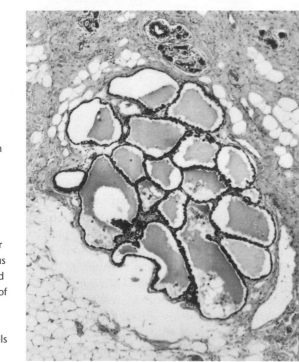

6.14 (Right) High-power view of a lactational focus showing hypertrophy and cytoplasmic vacuolation of the epithelial cells. Note that the cytoplasm is rather sparse in some cells (H&E).

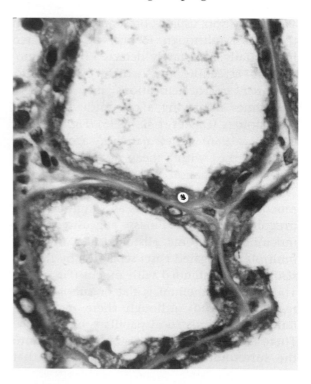

various stages of development. The lobules are enlarged and the acini dilated with secretion and lined by hypertrophic cells with large nuclei (Fig. 6.13). The cytoplasm is copious and vacuolated or sparse, giving the interior of the acini a hob-nailed appearance (Fig. 6.14). These two appearances presumably represent different phases of the secretory process as seen in normal lactation. The resemblance to the lactating breast is not only morphological as the lesions stain immuno-histochemically for the milk proteins α-lactal-bumin and casein (Earl, 1985).

Bailey *et al.* (1982) found these lesions in about 6% of breast biopsies, and a similar incidence has been reported in autopsy studies of patients with no history of breast disease (Frantz *et al.*, 1951; Sandison, 1962). They may be seen in young or elderly subjects, being in the former unrelated to the stage of the menstrual cycle. A failure of involution is not obviously the cause of the change as not all women give a history of pregnancy. Lactational foci do, however, appear to occur more frequently in patients receiving hormonal preparations (Bailey *et al.*,1982).

MUCOCOELE-LIKE LESION

This condition usually presents as a mass in the breast, although it may be discovered incidentally. It is rarely detected by mammographic screening, on which pleomorphic, clustered microcalcifications may be seen, sometimes displaying a crescentic ('tea-cup') morphology (Davies *et al.*, 1995) (Fig. 6.15). In Rosen's (1986) series patients' ages ranged from 25 to 61 with a mean of 40. All but one were premenopausal.

On macroscopic examination the mucocoele tumour appears as a multicystic or irregular gelatinous mass suggestive of a mucinous carcinoma. Histologically, there are multiple aggregated cysts separated by fibrous stroma and distended with mucin (Fig. 6.16). The lining epithelium is flat or cuboidal and regularly spaced, although there may be a tendency towards focal papillary hyperplasia. There is generally an extrusion of mucin into the surrounding stroma, forming lakes that

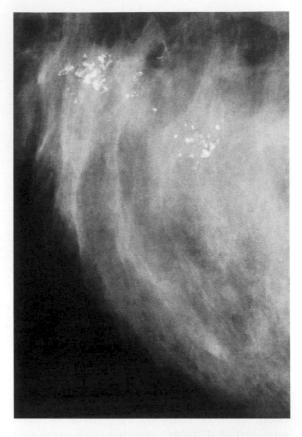

6.15 Clinical mammogram of a mucocoele-like tumour. Note the pleomorphic calcifications in the upper part of the picture.

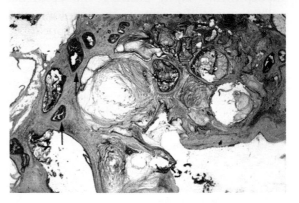

6.16 Mucocoele-like tumour showing numerous mucin-filled ducts, many of which have lost their epithelial lining. There is an extensive extrusion of mucin into the surrounding stroma. Some of the ducts (arrowed) show intraluminal proliferation, which at higher power amounted to atypical and non-atypical hyperplasia (H&E).

may contain fragments of epithelium derived from the cyst walls and simulating an invasive mucinous carcinoma. Features that help to exclude this possibility are the relative paucity of epithelial cells within the mucinous lakes and their lack of cytological features of malignancy. The absence of *in situ* carcinoma in the adjacent cysts is also a useful pointer. Mucocoele-like lesions should, however, be extensively sampled and examined carefully as similar mucinous changes have been found in association with intraduct papillomas, ADH and even DCIS (Komaki *et al.*, 1991; Ro *et al.*, 1991; Fisher and Millis, 1992). Haematoxyphilic microcalcifications may be seen within the distended terminal duct lobular units, in extruded mucin and in adjacent fibrous stroma.

Chinyama and Davies (1996) reviewed 962 breast cancers and 335 benign lesions, reporting mucin-filled ducts in 36 (3%) and mucin-filled ducts with mucin extrusion

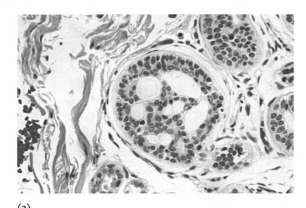

(a)

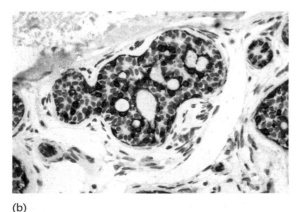

(b)

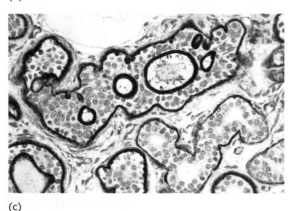

(c)

6.17 (a) Part of a lobule exhibiting collagenous spherulosis. The acinus in the centre of the illustration is dilated and contains several spherules surrounded by a barely perceptible thin eosinophilic basement membrane (H&E).
(b, c) The same lesion immunostained for cytokeratin 14 (b) and type IV collagen (c) to show the myoepithelium and basement membrane around the acini and the spherules.

(mucocoele-like lesions) in 27 (2%). Twelve of the latter were prototypic screen-detected cases, and eight showed atypical hyperplasia. A further twelve cases were incidental findings in association with screen-detected cancers, usually ductal (nst) but occasionally of mucinous type.

In their uncomplicated benign form, mucocoele-like lesions are usually cured by complete local excision. One of the patients reported by Hamele-Bena *et al.* (1996), however, experienced local recurrence. Chinyama and Davies (1996) recommended a close follow-up of patients with mucocoele-like lesions as they considered that mucin-filled ducts, mucocoele-like lesions, mucinous ADH, DCIS and invasive carcinoma might represent different stages of the same disease process. The lesions should clearly be completely excised and adequately sampled to exclude the possibility of atypia or malignancy.

The pathogenesis of the condition is not understood, but it is clear that the ability of breast epithelium to undergo metaplasia to cells capable of exporting a large volume of mucin is not invariably associated with invasive malignancy.

COLLAGENOUS SPHERULOSIS

This lesion was first reported by Clement *et al.* (1987), who described 15 cases in women between 39 and 55 years of age (mean 41). All the lesions were of microscopic size, being discovered incidentally in biopsy or mastectomy specimens. Eight cases were multiple. They consisted of clusters of generally discrete, acellular, eosinophilic, fibrillar spherules within the secondary lumina of lobular acini and ductules exhibiting non-atypical hyperplasia. The spherules measured 20–100 μm in diameter, were rich in collagen and also contained variable amounts of acidic mucin, basement membrane material and elastin. Some exhibited pale-staining or even hollow centres and darkly staining peripheries (Fig. 6.17a). Alcian blue–PAS staining revealed that some spherules were alcianophilic, some PAS positive and some positive for both. In

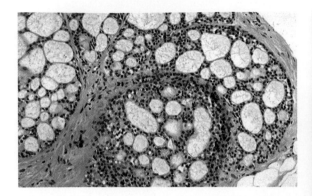

the last case the periphery of the spherules was typically PAS positive and the centre positive for alcian blue. Focal calcification was occasionally seen. The constituent fibrils were usually arranged in a concentric or laminated fashion. The number of spherules ranged from a few to about 50 in any given focus.

The cells immediately surrounding the spherules were positive for actin on immunostaining, indicating myoepithelial differentiation and raising the possibility that spherules are derived from myoepithelium-derived basement membrane material (Fig. 6.17b). This was later confirmed by Wells *et al.* (1990), who demonstrated laminin and collagens IV and III using immunohistology (Fig. 6.17c). The lesions were frequently associated with other benign proliferative processes such as papillomas, sclerosing adenosis and radial scars.

Clement *et al.* (1987) remarked on the similarity between collagenous spherulosis and adenoid cystic carcinoma in view of the presence of hyaline spherules in both lesions (Fig. 6.18). Furthermore, the cytological appearances, with myoepithelial differentiation, strengthen the resemblance. One of their 15 cases was mistaken for an adenoid cystic carcinoma. Collagenous spherulosis is, however, a microscopic lesion, does not exhibit stromal invasion and does not show the clearly dichotomous biphasic pattern with glandular spaces and stromal pseudocysts, the spherules having a highly variable staining reaction. Several of Clement's cases had been mistaken for the signet-ring variant of DCIS, but the mucin-positive material of the spherules is extracellular. The presence of the

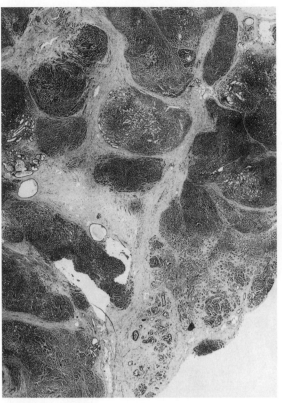

spherules and the lack of cytological features of malignancy exclude low nuclear grade cribriform DCIS.

Sgroi and Koerner (1995) described five cases in which collagenous spherulosis was involved by lobular carcinoma *in situ* giving an erroneous impression of low nuclear grade cribriform DCIS.

BENIGN PSEUDO-INFILTRATIVE EPITHELIAL LESIONS

Included under this heading are those lesions which, although benign, have the capacity to infiltrate locally and may thus be mistaken for invasive carcinoma. The lesions are not known to metastasize but they may have premalignant potential. The main feature that is common to all of them and distinguishes them from carcinoma is that they are cytologically benign.

Sclerosing adenosis

Sclerosing adenosis is a lobular proliferation in which the acini acquire distorted, spiky,

6.18 (Left) Florid collagenous spherulosis involving several grossly dilated acini and resembling adenoid cystic carcinoma. Malignancy is excluded by the benign cytological features, the lack of glandular lumina and the presence of a layer of myoepithelium around the acini (H&E).

6.19 (Right) Low-power view of florid sclerosing adenosis; the lobular architecture is retained despite the intensity of the proliferation (H&E).

6.20 (Left) Cellular phase of sclerosing adenosis involving three or four lobules apparently arising from the same interlobular duct (H&E). (Illustration reproduced with permission from Oxford University Press.)

6.21 (Right) Sclerotic phase of sclerosing adenosis: the epithelial elements are small with a large amount of intervening collagen (H&E).

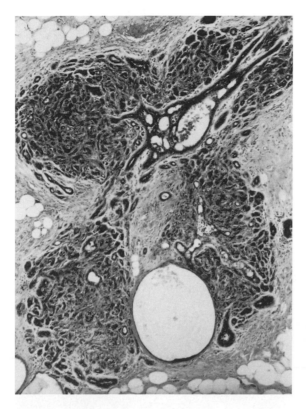

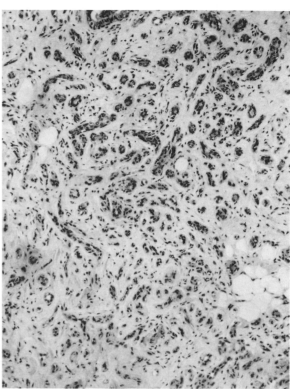

6.22 Immunostaining of a lobule showing sclerosing adenosis with an antibody (LLOO2) to cytokeratin 14, which reveals a strongly positive rim of myoepithelium around the epithelial cells.

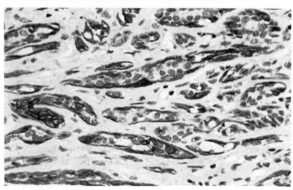

infiltrative margins. This infiltrative appearance may lead to a mistaken diagnosis of invasive carcinoma, particularly with the more florid examples, but the normal lobular architecture is retained and low-power examination is thus of great value in making the correct diagnosis (Fig. 6.19). Foote and Stewart (1945) recognized early cellular (Fig. 6.20) and late sclerotic (Fig. 6.21) phases of the process.

The proliferation involves both epithelial and myoepithelial cells, with a retention of the normal double-cell layer (Fig. 6.22), but stretching and distortion of the acini may lead to obliteration of the lumina. There are no cytological atypia, the cells having uniform normochromic nuclei. Mitoses are occasionally seen in the proliferative phase but are morphologically normal. The myoepithelium often predominates, and this can be more readily appreciated on immunohistochemical staining for smooth muscle actin or cytokeratin 14 (Fig. 6.22). Basement membrane material can almost invariably be demonstrated around the infiltrative cell masses using conventional PAS stains or immunohistochemical techniques for specific basement membrane components such as type IV collagen or laminin (Fig. 6.23).

In situ carcinoma may occasionally occur in lobules exhibiting sclerosing adenosis, the association occurring no more frequently than would be expected by chance. The resulting appearance, however, often leads to an erroneous diagnosis of invasive carcinoma (Fig. 6.24). As with uncomplicated sclerosing adenosis, the clue to the correct diagnosis is the retention of lobular architecture, myoepithelium and basement membrane (Rasbridge and Millis, 1995).

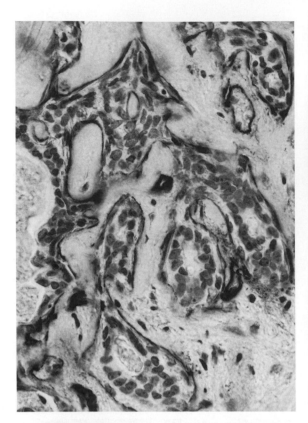

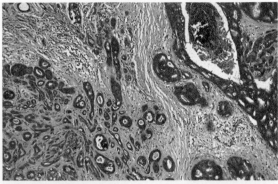

(a)

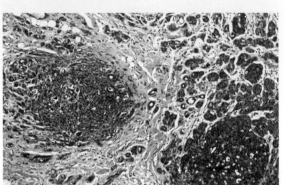

(b)

6.23 (Left) Methacarn-fixed section of sclerosing adenosis immunostained for the basement membrane component type IV collagen.

6.24 (Right) (a) A ductal carcinoma *in situ* exhibiting comedo and cribriform growth patterns is seen on the right of the picture. On the left is a lobule showing sclerosing adenosis. Extension of the *in situ* carcinoma into the sclerosing adenosis in the centre and upper left of the photograph gives a spurious impression of invasion. (b) Another field from the same case, in which the resemblance to invasive carcinoma is even more striking (H&E).

Ultrastructural studies confirm the normal cytological appearances and retention of the basement membrane, which may be normal or duplicated. Although elongated, the myoepithelial cells retain their hemidesmosomes, filaments and dense bodies (Ahmed, 1975).

In addition to the infiltration of the breast stroma, there may also be neural and vascular invasion (Fig. 6.25). Taylor and Norris (1967) found 20 examples of neural invasion in 1000 cases of sclerosing adenosis, and an incidence of 3.9% was reported by Davies (1973b). Invasion may be perineural or of the nerve bundle itself. Eusebi and Azzopardi (1976) found vascular invasion in a minority of cases. Only a single vein was usually involved, but in one case two veins and an artery were infiltrated. The infiltrating epithelium consisted of two cell-layered tubules surrounded by PAS-positive basement membrane material. The vessels showed advential or intimal fibrosis or irregular medial thickening.

The incidence of vascular or neural infiltration will clearly vary with the care with which

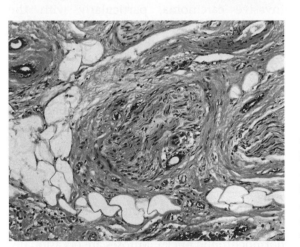

6.25 Perineural invasion in sclerosing adenosis. Several small tubules lined by a double layer of non-atypical cells infiltrate the nerves and surrounding tissue (H&E).

it is sought. There is no evidence, however, to suggest that the presence of either has any influence on the behaviour of the lesion.

The overall incidence of sclerosing adenosis was 12.5% of all benign breast biopsies in the study of Foote and Stewart (1945) and 25% in that of Davies (1973b). Sandison (1962) found sclerosing adenosis in 7%, and Bartow *et al.*

(1987) in up to 20%, of autopsies performed on subjects with no history of breast disease. In the latter study the change was more frequently encountered in women of European descent than in American Indians. In both these studies sclerosing adenosis was very rarely seen in women under the age of 35.

There is evidence that patients with significant sclerosing adenosis may have an increased risk of developing breast carcinoma. Jensen et al. (1989) found an increased relative risk of 2.1, which decreased to 1.7 when patients who also had atypical hyperplasia were excluded and rose to 6.7 when those with both sclerosing adenosis and atypical hyperplasia were analysed. A family history of breast cancer did not increase the risk for those with sclerosing adenosis alone. Tavassoli and Norris (1990) also found that sclerosing adenosis was associated with an increased risk of developing breast cancer but only in the presence of atypical hyperplasia. From the practical point of view, there is insufficient evidence for taking any clinical action when sclerosing adenosis is discovered.

Apocrine adenosis

The term apocrine adenosis is usually used to describe the superimposition of apocrine metaplasia, as seen in cysts (see above), on lobules exhibiting simple enlargement or sclerosing adenosis. It has also been used to describe the occurrence of apocrine metaplasia without cyst formation in radial scars or ductal adenomas and, as thus defined, is found in about 3% of unselected benign breast biopsies (Simpson et al., 1990).

Whole lobules are usually involved, but partial involvement may be seen in larger lesions. The combined effects of large cell size and distorted architecture can produce a disturbing appearance that may be mistaken for invasive carcinoma (Fig 6.26). The tubules are, however, surrounded by basement membrane and myoepithelium. Like apocrine cells lining cysts, those of apocrine adenosis have uniform nuclei and regular (although prominent) nucleoli. Furthermore, the architecture of the underlying lesion is still discernible, in contrast to invasive carcinoma. Like the cells of apocrine cysts, those of apocrine adenosis are positive for androgen receptors and negative for oestrogen and progesterone receptors (Selim and Wells, 1999).

In some cases, however, the apocrine cells are genuinely atypical and the process is then termed atypical apocrine adenosis, bearing an even stronger resemblance to invasive carcinoma (Carter and Rosen, 1991). Wells et al. (1995) found that 57% of cases showed positivity for c-erbB-2 and 29% for p53 on immunohistochemical staining, molecular characteristics that are usually associated with high-grade in situ or invasive carcinoma.

Seidman et al. (1996) regarded apocrine adenosis as atypical when the nucleoli were enlarged and there was a greater than 3-fold variation in nuclear area. Multiple nucleoli, variation in nucleolar size and mitotic activity were also present in some cases. Using this definition, which excluded the apocrine variant of DCIS, they followed up 37 women with the condition for an average of 8.7 years and found that the relative risk of developing carcinoma was 5.5 for all patients, although the confidence limits were very wide. This level of risk is, however, similar to that associated with atypical hyperplasia (see p. 105). The risk was particularly great in women over 60 and was probably low in younger women. Seidman et al. concluded that some cases might actually represent in situ apocrine carcinomas that are difficult to diagnose because of the lack of the usual architectural features. No carcinomas developed in the series of Carter and Rosen (1991), although the follow-up time was much shorter.

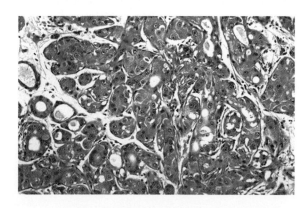

6.26 Apocrine adenosis. In this particular example, a focus of sclerosing adenosis exhibits extensive apocrine metaplasia. The apocrine cells produce a worrisome appearance, but close inspection reveals their uniformity and lack of pleomorphism (H&E).

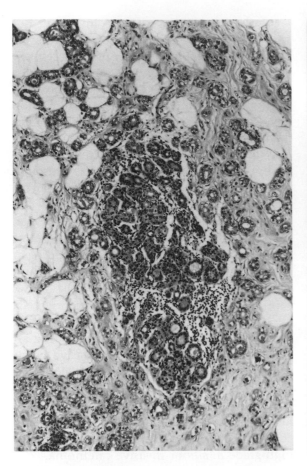

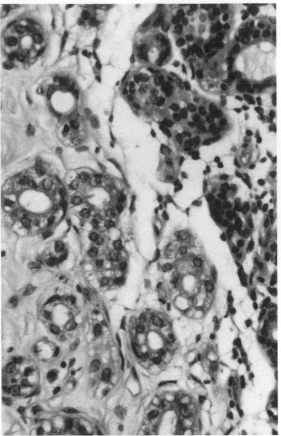

6.27 (Left) Microglandular adenosis. The collagenous and adipose stroma of the breast is infiltrated by numerous small, regular, rounded acinar structures. A residual normal lobule is seen in the centre (H&E).

6.28 (Right) Microglandular adenosis. The infiltrating acini are lined by a single layer of cells with vacuolated cytoplasm. Part of a normal lobule is included at the top right of the picture for comparison (H&E).

Microglandular adenosis

This is a rare lesion first illustrated by McDivitt *et al.* (1968) and later described in detail by Clement and Azzopardi (1983). In half the cases described the lesion was detected microscopically, whereas in the remainder there was a palpable mass, suggestive of malignancy. A distinctive mammographic pattern has not been described. The age range of patients in whom the condition has been diagnosed has ranged from 28 to 82, the mean being in the middle 50s (Millis and Eusebi, 1995).

The lesions vary from 3 to 40 mm in size and may occur as multiple, relatively discrete foci or as more extensive confluent zones in which normal lobular remnants may be seen. The proliferation takes the form of small, rounded acinar structures that infiltrate the breast stroma and adipose tissue (Fig. 6.27); to the author's knowledge, perineural or vascular invasion has not been described. The acini are lined by a single layer of cuboidal or flattened cells with bland nuclei, inconspicuous nuclei and scanty vacuolated or eosinophilic cytoplasm, usually containing demonstrable quantities of glycogen (Fig. 6.28). The cells have a characteristic immunophenotype, being positive for S100 and cytokeratin and negative for epithelial membrane antigen, GCDFP-15, progesterone receptor and c-erbB-2 (Millis and Eusebi, 1995). The lumina are usually open and rounded, often containing hyaline or granular PAS-positive, diastase-resistant secretion; calcospherites may also be seen on rare occasions. The luminal membranes are truncated and lack the apical snouts or blebs seen in tubular carcinomas. Myoepithelial cells are lacking, but immunostaining with antibodies to collagen IV and laminin reveals the presence of a basement membrane.

The cytological features are benign; the nuclei are uniform and normochromic, and mitoses are rare, with no atypical forms. *In situ* carcinoma, of either the lobular or the ductal type, has not been identified in any of the lesions so far studied, and there has been no evidence of malignant behaviour, although the longest follow-up period so far is only about 3.5 years. Clement and Azzopardi (1983) considered that the histogenesis was most likely to relate to the lobules, although there was some evidence that the lesion might sometimes be derived from small ducts. Co-existent classic sclerosing adenosis was found in only one of six cases, suggesting that microglandular adenosis is not a variant of this condition.

The distinction of microglandular adenosis from other forms of adenosis, including sclerosing adenosis and tubular adenosis, lies in the absence of an organoid or truly lobular pattern, the lack of myoepithelial cells and the absence of glandular distortion or dilatation. Distinction from tubular carcinoma rests on the benign cytological features, the multifocality or lobular clustering, the smaller more uniform glands, the lack of apical snouts and blebs, the absence of bridges across the lumina and the immunopositivity for S100, cytokeratin and basement membrane components. The stroma of tubular carcinoma is more cellular than that of microglandular adenosis, and elastosis may be seen. *In situ* carcinoma may be seen in tubular carcinoma but is absent in microglandular adenosis.

James *et al.* (1993) described 60 patients with microglandular adenosis in 14 of whom carcinoma was also present. This is likely to be an overestimation of the frequency of this association as the cases included personal consultations. The age of the patients with cancer ranged from 26 to 68 (mean 47). All had a mass, and six had a family history of breast cancer. Nodal metastases were detected in 3 of 11 patients who had an axillary dissection. All 10 patients treated with mastectomy were recurrence-free after a median follow-up period of 57 months. Two of three treated by local excision were free of recurrence after 12 and 105 months; the third developed bone metastases. Carcinoma arose in the microglandular

adenosis in 13 patients, *in situ* carcinoma being identified within expanded microglandular adenosis glands. In the remaining patient, the carcinoma developed in the opposite breast.

The carcinomas tended to have a distinctive morphological pattern, to be positive for S100 and cathepsin D, and to be associated with a relatively favourable outlook despite having histological features usually associated with an adverse prognosis. However, too few cases of microglandular adenosis have been described to make an accurate assessment of the risk of developing carcinoma in patients in whom the uncomplicated form is diagnosed. Rosenblum *et al.* (1986) recommended complete excision and follow-up for patients with microglandular adenosis and that lesions with atypical but not unequivocally malignant features should be treated with the same caution as other atypical hyperplasias.

Tubular adenosis

This term has been used to describe a condition characterized by the haphazard proliferation of elongated, narrow, non-crowded, sometimes branching tubules with collapsed, slit-like, well-defined or even dilated lumina. They are lined by bland-looking epithelial cells (without apical snouts) and myoepithelial cells. The growth pattern is non-lobular or only vaguely lobular, and there is an occasional infiltration of fat. The stroma may be sclerotic or oedematous (Oberman, 1984; Lee *et al.*, 1996). The lesion thus has an appearance intermediate between that of sclerosing adenosis and microglandular adenosis, being distinguished from the former by the non-lobular growth pattern and from the latter by the presence of a myoepithelial layer and the irregularity of the tubules.

Too few cases have been reported to determine whether the lesion is premalignant, the main importance of recognizing it being so that it can distinguished from invasive carcinoma. Lee *et al.* (1996) described three cases that were involved by DCIS, making the distinction from invasive carcinoma even more difficult. Tubular adenosis may be extensive enough to produce a palpable mass, but most reported examples have been detected incidentally.

Radial scar/complex sclerosing lesion

This group of lesions has received many different names in the past, but the above terminology is now generally accepted. Many of the lesions described as sclerosing papillary proliferations by Fenoglio and Lattes (1974) fall into this category. Others have used the terms benign sclerosing ductal proliferation (Tremblay *et al.*, 1977), non-encapsulated sclerosing lesion (Fisher *et al.*, 1979), infiltrating epitheliosis (Azzopardi, 1979) and indurative mastopathy (Rickert *et al.*, 1981).

Classically, the lesions have a stellate appearance, tubular structures radiating out from a central core of sclerosis and elastosis (Fig. 6.29). Elastosis may also be seen around the ducts radiating out from this area. The tubular structures may be two layered but

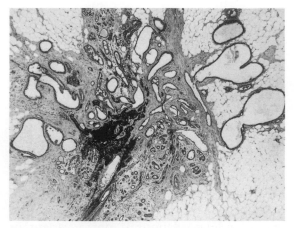

6.29 Radial scar stained by the Weigert method for elastin. There is a central core of elastosis from which tubular structures radiate out. There is only minor and focal hyperplasia of usual type in the upper left of the lesion.

commonly exhibit intraluminal hyperplasia (Fig. 6.30). In the centre they are often entrapped within the fibroelastotic material, where they exhibit a more random, non-organoid and infiltrative appearance (Figs 6.31 and 6.32). Vascular and neural invasion may rarely be seen, as in sclerosing adenosis. The features have been likened to those of a daisy head. Radial scars and complex sclerosing

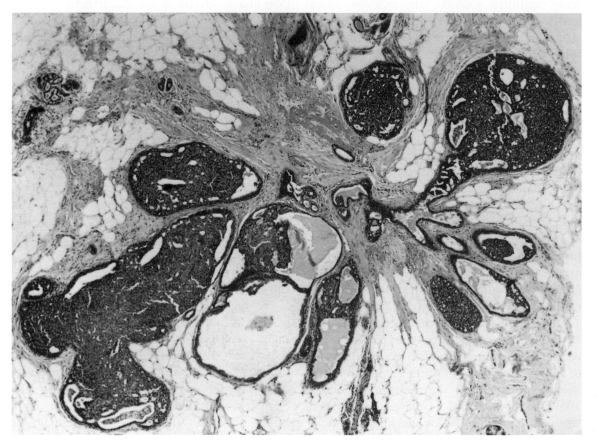

6.30 Radial scar with pronounced hyperplasia of usual type (H&E).

6.31 (Left) A small poorly cellular radial scar in which the central zone of fibroelastosis contains dispersed infiltrative-looking tubules (H&E).

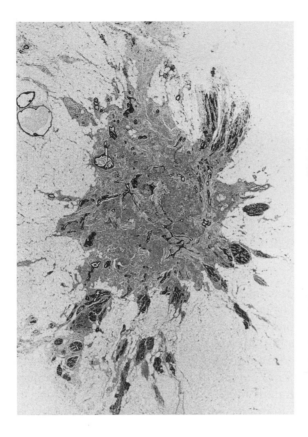

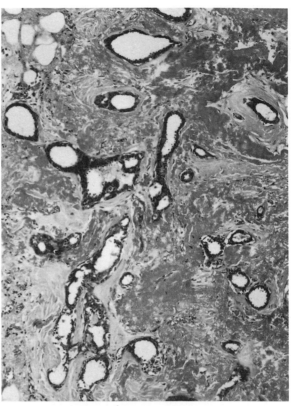

6.32 (Right) Higher-power view of Fig. 6.31. The tubules appear infiltrative, but they lack cytological features of malignancy and are surrounded by basement membrane and myoepithelium. Note the dense elastosis on the right of the picture (H&E).

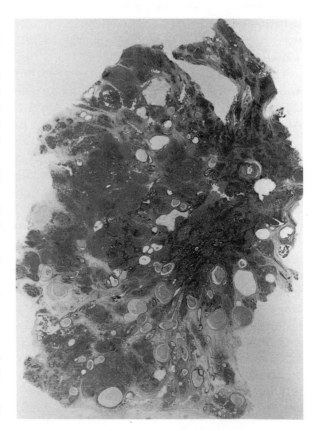

6.33 A complex sclerosing lesion. This example is very large and cellular. The fibroelastotic core is in the mid-right of the picture. Radiating from this area are numerous nodular masses of epithelium showing sclerosing adenosis and cystic change (H&E).

lesions are virtually indistinguishable from invasive carcinomas on macroscopic and radiological examination.

The term radial scar is applied to lesions less than 10 mm in maximal dimension. Complex sclerosing lesions are, however, not only larger than this, but also exhibit a more complex appearance, usually with nodular masses around the periphery showing papilloma formation, apocrine cysts and sclerosing adenosis (Fig. 6.33). Makanura *et al.* (1994) described a case exhibiting apocrine adenosis (see above), which gave rise to a false-positive diagnosis of malignancy on cytological examination. Some of the larger examples give the impression of being formed by the coalescence of several adjacent sclerosing lesions. There is some morphological overlap with ductal adenomas showing central scarring.

Most radial scars are small, measuring only a few millimetres across. Consequently, they are generally incidental findings in benign or malignant biopsies or resection specimens. Between 5 and 10 per cent achieve a size large enough to present as a clinical lump (Sloane and Mayers, 1993). Following the widespread introduction of breast cancer screening, an increasing number of cases are being detected by mammography, on which they appear as stellate lesions indistinguishable from invasive carcinoma (Fig. 6.34). Microcalcification may also be seen.

Several histological features distinguish radial scars and complex sclerosing lesions from carcinoma. First, the cells lining the tubules lack cytological atypia (*see* Fig. 6.32 above), and where intraductal proliferation is present, it generally exhibits the features of hyperplasia rather than carcinoma (*see* Fig 6.30 above). Second, basement membrane and a layer of myoepithelial cells surround the tubules. Third, carcinomas rarely exhibit the characteristic growth pattern of radial scars. Finally, the stroma of carcinomas is usually more cellular and fibroblastic than that of radial scars, where it is poorly cellular and extensively elastotic (*see* Fig. 6.32 above). In a large study of diagnostic consistency undertaken in the UK National Breast Screening Programme, 2.9% of diagnoses were of invasive carcinoma in cases where radial scar was the majority diagnosis (Sloane *et al.*, 1994).

The reported incidence of radial scars has varied significantly, largely according to the diligence with which they have been sought. Anderson and Gram (1984) found them in 1.7% of benign surgical biopsies, but only one or two blocks per case were examined. In a study of 83 consecutive, unselected female autopsies in which 57–166 blocks per specimen were examined, Nielsen *et al.* (1985) found an incidence of 28%. The lesions were multicentric in two thirds of cases and bilateral in nearly half. Jacobs *et al.* (1999) found radial scars in 7.1% of benign breast biopsy specimens from 1396 women enrolled in the Nurses' Health Study in the USA. Only 1 lesion per biopsy was found in 61% of cases, 2 in 21% and more than 2 in the remainder.

It has been suggested that radial scars may be preneoplastic or even represent early tubular carcinomas because of their morphological appearance. Linell *et al.* (1980)

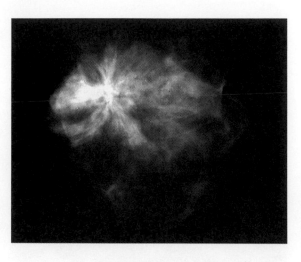

6.34 A specimen radiograph of a localization biopsy containing a radial scar (top left).

described naked tubular structures scattered in fat in some radial scars, which they interpreted as developing tubular carcinoma. In addition, ducts exhibiting an intraluminal cribriform proliferation suggestive of DCIS were described. Bahrmann (1962) also illustrated radial scars exhibiting transition to carcinoma. More recently, Sloane and Mayers (1993) found a high incidence of carcinoma and atypical hyperplasia in radial scars detected by mammographic screening (Figs 6.35 and 6.36). There was no relationship to the presence of carcinoma in the remaining breast when cases showing direct extension were excluded. The carcinomas identified included DCIS (of high and low nuclear grades), lobular carcinoma *in situ* and invasive carcinoma of tubular and ductal types. The malignant zones occupied a very variable proportion of the scars. The high incidence in screen-detected cases appeared to be explained by the greater size of the lesions and the older age of the patients in whom they were detected. Thus malignancy was rare in lesions under 6 mm in size and in patients under 50. This also applied to non-screen-detected cases. In a later study Douglas-Jones and Pace (1997) found 8 of 46 (17%) screen-detected radial scars to contain foci of DCIS.

Evidence derived from studies of benign and malignant breasts is less clear. In the study of Nielsen *et al.* (1985), radial scars were found in the breasts of 28% of unselected female autopsies, the frequency being significantly

6.35 (Left) A radial scar containing invasive (long arrow) and *in situ* (short arrow) carcinoma (H&E).

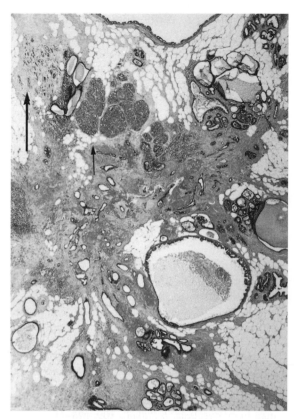

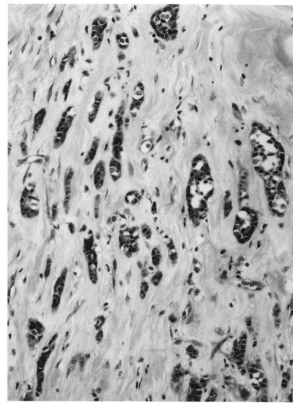

Fig 6.36 (Right) Higher-power view of the small (3 mm) focus of invasive carcinoma seen at the top-left of Fig. 6.35 (H&E).

increased in women with fibrocystic change but not with carcinoma. Similar findings were obtained in the contemporaneous study of Anderson and Battersby (1985), which found a relationship between radial scar and benign breast changes but not to parity, menopausal status, contraceptive pill usage or the presence of cancer. Wellings and Alpers (1984) extensively sampled breasts from unselected autopsies by the subgross slice method. They found a significantly higher incidence of radial scars in breasts containing, or contralateral to those containing, cancer than in those from noncancerous breasts from low-risk women. Furthermore, the mean number of scars was higher in the cancer-associated group.

Very few follow-up studies have been published. Fenoglio and Lattes (1974) followed up a number of patients with 'sclerosing papillary proliferations', many of which would now fall into the category of radial scar. An increased incidence of carcinoma was not found, but nearly half the 54 patients were lost to follow-up, and the period of observation was rather short, averaging 6.3

years. In a later study with a longer follow-up period averaging 19.5 years, Anderson and Gram (1984) found that only 1 of 32 patients with radial scar developed cancer, an incidence slightly lower than that expected in the general population.

Most recently, however, Jacobs *et al.* (1999) found that women with radial scars had a risk of developing breast cancer 1.8 times that of women without scars regardless of accompanying benign breast changes. When women who had proliferative disease without atypia were compared with those without proliferative disease, the relative risk of developing breast cancer was 1.5 for those without and 3.0 for those with radial scars. When women with atypical hyperplasia were compared with those without proliferative disease, the relative risk of cancer was 3.8 for those without and 5.8 for those with radial scars. In this very thorough and exhaustive study, the radial scar was thus found to be an independent risk factor for breast cancer. The risk of cancer development was unrelated to the size of the radial scar and the number detected in the biopsy. Of all the prospective studies carried out so far, this has the greatest statistical power.

There thus seem to be two types of cancer risk associated with radial scars. The first relates to the origin of cancer within the scar itself, particularly when it is large and occurring in an older patient. This situation seems analogous to that seen with in colorectal adenomas. The second relates to a slight general increase in breast cancer risk, a situation more like that associated with hyperplasia of usual type and other low-risk lesions.

In view of the above it is the author's opinion that all stellate lesions detected by mammography should be excised regardless of cytological or needle biopsy findings. In the study of Douglas-Jones and Pace (1997), the cytological findings were strongly suspicious of malignancy (C4 or 5) in only 1 of 8 mammographically detected radial scars containing foci of DCIS.

REFERENCES

Ahmed A. (1975) Apocrine metaplasia in cystic hyperplastic mastopathy: histochemical and ultrastructural observations. *J. Pathol.*, **115**, 211–20.

Andersen J.A., Gram J.B. (1984) Radial scar in the female breast. *Cancer*, **53**, 2557–60.

Anderson T.J., Battersby S. (1985) Radial scars of benign and malignant breasts: comparative features and significance. *J. Pathol.*, **147**, 23–32.

Azzopardi J.G. (1979) Problems in breast pathology. In Bennington J.L. (ed.) *Major Problems in Pathology*, vol. II. London, W.B. Saunders.

Bahrmann E. (1962) Die Mastopathie als Vorläufer des Mamma-Karzinoms. *Dtsch. Gesundh.-Wis.*, **17**, 1762–5.

Bailey A.J., Sloane J.P., Trickey B.S., Ormerod M.G. (1982) An immunocytochemical study of a-lactalbumin in human breast tissue. *J. Pathol.*, **137**, 13–23.

Bartow S.A., Pathak D.R., Black W.C., Key C.R., Teaf S.R. (1987) Prevalence of benign, atypical, and malignant lesions in populations at different risk for breast cancer. *Cancer*, **60**, 2751–60.

Berkowitz G.S., Kelsey J.L., Livolsi V.A. *et al.* (1984) Exogenous hormone use and fibrocystic breast disease by histopathologic component. *Int. J. Cancer*, **34**, 443–9.

Bonser G.M., Dossett J.A., Jull J.W. (1961) *Human and Experimental Breast Cancer*. London, Pitman Medical.

Cahn M.D., Tran T., Theur C.P., Butler J.A. (1997) Hormone replacement therapy and the risk of breast lesions that predispose to cancer. *Am. Surg.*, **63**, 858–60.

Carter D.J., Rosen P.P. (1991) Atypical apocrine metaplasia in sclerosing lesions of the breast: a study of 51 patients. *Mod. Pathol.*, **4**, 1–5.

Chinyama C.N., Davies J.D. (1996) Mammary mucinous lesions: congeners, prevalence and important pathological associations. *Histopathology*, **29**, 533–9.

Ciatto S., Biggeri A., Rosselli del Turco M., Bartoli D., Iossa A. (1990) Risk of breast cancer subsequent to proven gross cystic disease. *Eur. J. Cancer*, **26**, 555–7.

Clement P.B., Azzopardi J.G. (1983) Microglandular adenosis of the breast: a lesion simulating tubular carcinoma. *Histopathology*, **7**, 169–80.

Clement P.B., Young R.H., Azzopardi J.G. (1987) Collagenous spherulosis of the breast. *Am. J. Surg. Pathol.*, **11**, 411–17.

Davies J.D. (1973a) Hyperelastosis, obliteration and fibrous plaques in major ducts of the human breast. *J. Pathol.*, **110**, 13–26.

Davies J.D. (1973b) Neural invasion in benign mammary dysplasia. *J. Pathol.*, **109**, 225–31.

Davies J.D., Kutt E., Kulka J., Farndon J.R., Webb A.J. (1995) Mucoele-like lesions detected by the mammographic presence of suspicious clustered microcalcifications. *Breast*, **5**, 135–40.

Dixon J.M., McDonald C., Elton R.A., Miller W.R., (1999) Risk of breast cancer in women with palpable breast cysts: a prospective study. *Lancet*, **353**, 1742–5.

Douglas-Jones A.G., Pace D.P. (1997) Pathology of R4 spiculated lesions in the breast screening programme. *Histopathology*, **30**, 214–20.

Dupont W.D., Page D.L. (1985) Risk factors in women with proliferative breast disease. *N. Engl. J. Med.*, **312**, 146–51.

Earl H.M. (1985) Markers of human breast differentiation and breast carcinomas and characterization of monoclonal antibodies to human casein. PhD thesis, London University.

Eusebi V., Azzopardi J.G. (1976) Vascular infiltration in benign breast disease. *J. Pathol.*, **118**, 9–25.

Fenoglio C., Lattes R. (1974), Sclerosing papillary proliferations in the female breast: a benign lesion often mistaken for carcinoma. *Cancer*, **33**, 691–700.

Fisher C.J., Millis R.R. (1992) A mucocoele-like tumour of the breast associated with both atypical ductal hyperplasia and mucoid carcinoma. *Histopathology*, **21**, 69–71.

Fisher E.R., Palekar A.S., Kotwal, N., Lipana N. (1979) A nonencapsulated sclerosing lesion of the breast. *Am. J. Clin. Pathol.*, **71**, 240–6.

Foote F.W., Stewart F.W. (1945) Comparative studies of cancerous versus noncancerous breasts. *Ann. Surg.*, **121**, 6–53.

Frantz V.K., Pickren J.W., Melcher G.W., Auchincloss H. (1951) Incidence of chronic cystic disease in so-called 'normal breasts': a study based on 225 postmortem examinations. *Cancer*, **4**, 762–83.

Fraser J.L., Raza S., Chorny K., Connolly J.L., Schnitt S.J. (1998) Columnar alteration with prominent apical snouts and secretions. A spectrum of changes frequently present in breast biopsies performed for microcalcifications. *Am. J. Surg. Pathol.*, **22**, 1521–7.

Gatalica Z. (1997) Immunohistochemical analysis of apocrine breast lesions. Consistent over-expression of androgen receptor accompanied by the loss of estrogen and progesterone receptors in apocrine metaplasia and apocrine carcinoma *in situ*. *Pathol. Res. Pract.*, **193**, 753–8.

Hamele-Bena D., Cranor M.L., Rosen P.P. (1996) Mammary mucocele-like lesions. Benign and malignant. *Am. J. Surg. Pathol.*, **20**, 1081–5.

Ironside J.W., Guthrie W. (1985) The galactocoele: a light and electron microscopic study. *Histopathology*, **9**, 457–67.

Jacobs T.W., Byrne C., Colditz G., Connolly J.L., Schnitt S.J. (1999) Radial scars in benign biopsy specimens and the risk of breast cancer. *N. Engl. J. Med.*, **340**, 430–6.

James B.A., Cranor M.L., Rosen P.P. (1993) Carcinoma of the breast arising in microglandular adenosis. *Am. J. Clin. Pathol.*, **100**, 507–13.

Jensen R.A., Page D.L., Dupont W.D., Rogers L.W. (1989) Invasive breast cancer risk in women with sclerosing adenosis. *Cancer*, **64**, 1977–83.

Komaki K., Sakamoto G., Sugano H. *et al.* (1991) The morphologic feature of mucus leakage appearing in low papillary carcinoma of the breast. *Hum. Pathol.*, **22**, 231–6.

Lee K., Chan J.K.C., Gwi E. (1996) Tubular adenosis of the breast: a distinctive lesion mimicking invasive carcinoma. *Am. J. Surg. Pathol.*, **20**, 46–54.

Linell F. Ljungberg O., Andersson I. (1980) Breast carcinoma: aspects of early stages, progression and related problems. *Acta Pathol. Microbiol. Scand. (A).*, **272** (suppl.), 1–233.

McDivitt R.W., Stewart F.W., Berg J.W. (1968) Tumors of the breast. In *Atlas of Tumor Pathology, 2nd series, Fascicle II*. Washington, DC, Armed Forces Institute of Pathology.

Makunura C.N., Curling O.M., Yeomans P., Perry N., Wells C.A. (1994) Apocrine adenosis within a radial scar: a case of false positive breast diagnosis. *Cytopathology*, **5**, 123–8.

Millis R.R., Eusebi V. (1995) Microglandular adenosis of the breast. *Adv. Anat. Pathol.*, **2**, 10–18.

Nielsen M., Jensen J., Andersen J.A. (1985) An autopsy study of radial scar in the female breast. *Histopathology*, **9**, 287–95.

Oberman H.A. (1984) Benign breast lesions confused with carcinoma. In: McDivitt R.W., Oberman H.A., Ozzello L., Kaufman N. (eds) *The Breast*. United States–Canadian Academy of Pathology Monographs in Pathology vol. 25. Baltimore, Williams & Wilkins.

Pastides H., Kelsey J.L., LiVolsi V.A., Holford T.R., Fischer D.B., Goldenberg I.S. (1983) Oral contraceptive use and fibrocystic breast disease with special reference to histopathology. *J. Natl Cancer Inst.*, **71**, 5–9.

Pearlman W.H., Giueriguian J.D., Sawyer M.E. (1973) A specific progesterone-binding component of human breast cyst fluid. *J. Biol. Chem.*, **248**, 5736–41.

Rasbridge S.A., Millis R.R. (1995) Carcinoma *in situ* involving sclerosing adenosis: a mimic of invasive breast carcinoma. *Histopathology*, **27**, 269–73.

Rees B.I., Gravelle I.H., Hughes L.E. (1977) Nipple retraction in duct ectasia. *Br. J. Surg.*, **64**, 577–80.

Rickert R.R., Kalisher L., Hutter R.V.P. (1981) Indurative mastopathy: a benign sclerosing lesion of breast with elastosis which may simulate carcinoma. *Cancer*, **47**, 561–71.

Ro J.Y. Sneige N., Sahin A.A., Silva E.G., del Junco G.W., Ayala A.G. (1991) Mucocele-like tumor of the breast associated with atypical ductal hyperplasia or mucinous carcinoma. *Arch. Pathol. Lab. Med.*, **115**, 137–40.

Rosen P.P. (1986) Mucocele-like tumors of the breast. *Am. J. Surg. Pathol.*, **10**, 464–9.

Rosenblum M.K., Purrazzella R., Rosen P.P. (1986) Is microglandular adenosis a precancerous disease? A study of carcinoma arising therein. *Am. J. Surg. Pathol.*, **10**, 237–45.

Sandison A.T. (1962) *An Autopsy Study of the Adult Human Breast*. National Cancer Institute Monograph No. 8. Washington, DC, US Department of Health, Education and Welfare.

Seidman J.D., Ashton M., Lefkowitz M. (1996) Atypical apocrine adenosis of the breast: a clinicopathologic study of 37 patients with 8.7 year follow-up. *Cancer*, **77**, 2529–37.

Selim A.-G.A., Wells C.A. (1999) Immunohistochemical localisation of androgen receptor in apocrine metaplasia and apocrine adenosis of the breast: relation to oestrogen and progesterone receptors. *J. Clin. Pathol.*, **52**, 838–41.

Sgroi D., Koerner F.C. (1995) Involvement of collagenous spherulosis by lobular carcinoma *in situ*: potential confusion with cribriform ductal carcinoma in situ. *Am. J. Surg. Pathol.*, **19**, 1366–70.

Simpson J.F., Page D.L., Dupont W.D. (1990) Apocrine adenosis – a mimic of mammary carcinoma. *Surg. Pathol.*, **3**, 289–99.

Sloane J.P., Mayers M.M. (1993) Carcinoma and atypical hyperplasia in radial scars and complex sclerosing lesions: importance of lesion size and patient age. *Histopathology*, **23**, 225–31.

Sloane J.P., Ellman R., Anderson T.J. *et al.* (1994) Consistency of histopathological reporting of breast lesions detected by screening: findings of the UK National EQA Scheme. *Eur. J. Cancer*, **30A**, 1414–19.

Tavassoli F.A. (1991) Myoepithelial lesions of the breast. Myoepitheliosis, adenomyepithelioma and myoepithelial carcinoma. *Am. J. Surg. Pathol.*, **15**, 554–68.

Tavassoli F.A., Norris H.J. (1990) A comparison of the results of long-term follow-up for atypical intraductal hyperplasia and intraductal hyperplasia of the breast. *Cancer*, **65**, 518–29.

Taylor H.B., Norris H.J. (1967) Epithelial invasion of nerves in benign diseases of the breast. *Cancer*, **20**, 2245–9.

Tremblay G., Buell R.H., Seemayer T.A. (1977) Elastosis in benign sclerosing ductal proliferation of the female breast. *Am. J. Surg. Pathol.*, **1**, 155–9.

Walsh P.V., McDicken I.W., Bulbrook R.D., Moore J.W., Taylor W.H., George W.D. (1984) Serum oestradiol-17B and prolactin concentrations during the luteal phase in women with benign breast disease. *Eur. J. Cancer Clin. Oncol.*, **20**, 1345–51.

Wellings S.R., Alpers C.E. (1984) Subgross pathologic features and incidence of radial scars in the breast. *Hum. Pathol.*, **15**, 475–9.

Wells C.A., Wells C.W., Yeomans P., Vina M., Jordan S., d'Ardenne A.J. (1990) Spherical connective inclusions in epithelial hyperplasia of the breast ('collagenous spherulosis'). *J. Clin. Pathol.*, **43**, 905–8.

Wells C.A., McGregor I.L., Makunura C.N., Yeomans P., Davies J.D. (1995) Apocrine adenosis: a precursor of aggressive breast cancer? *J. Clin. Pathol.*, **48**, 737–42.

7 Benign intraductal proliferations

7.1 (Left) Hyperplasia of usual type in an interlobular duct. Although the duct is significantly enlarged and the lumen completely occluded, the cells are a mixture of epithelial cells with rounded vesicular nuclei, myoepithelial-like spindle cells with smaller, dark ovoid nuclei and occasional lymphocytes with small, dark round nuclei and clear haloes. The secondary lumina are irregular, varying from small and indistinct to large and clear cut. The nuclei are unevenly spaced and show streaming; they have indiscernible nucleoli and show no evidence of mitotic activity. Necrosis is absent (H&E). (Illustration reproduced with permission from Oxford University Press.)

7.2 (Right) Hyperplasia of usual type in two acini. The secondary lumina are more regular and truncated than in Fig. 7.1, but there is a mixture of cell types, and atypia and mitotic activity are lacking. The nuclei are unevenly spaced and stream across the bridges with their long axes parallel to the direction of the bridge (H&E).

HYPERPLASIA OF USUAL TYPE

Hyperplasia of usual type (HUT) is the term used to describe benign, non-atypical proliferations contained within the mammary glandular tree (Figs 7.1–7.3). It is also known by other names, such as non-atypical hyperplasia and proliferative disease without atypia. The lesions are sometimes large enough to suggest an origin within the interlobular ducts, but, as discussed below, most are probably derived from the terminal duct–lobular units.

One of the essential features of HUT is the lack of cytological atypia. The epithelial cells are uniform, with normochromic nuclei that are usually vesicular and have easily discernible but delicate nuclear membranes. Nucleoli are generally inconspicuous. Mitotic activity varies but is usually low, and mitotic figures are morphologically normal. The cells are cohesive, often appearing syncytial. The nuclei are not evenly spaced and often overlap. Haemorrhage and necrosis are rare but may occasionally be seen in very florid examples.

A population of smaller cells with darker ovoid nuclei is also usually present (Figs 7.1–7.3). They were, in view of their high

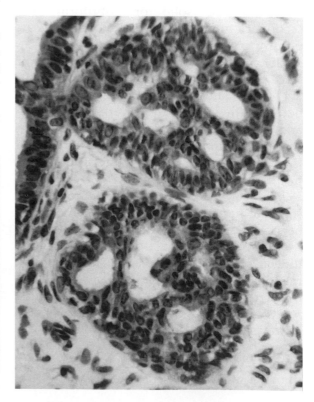

alkaline phosphatase activity (Ahmed, 1974) and ultrastructural appearance, long thought to be myoepithelial cells (Ahmed, 1980). More recent immunohistological studies, however, have shown that while they exhibit keratin (14+/19–) and S100 profiles (S100-β+/S100-α-), in keeping with myoepithelial cells, they lack smooth muscle actin and consequently appear to be basal keratin-type epithelial cells. These cells are thought to be post-stem cells or intermediate cells (Boecker *et al.*, 1992; Ichihara *et al.*, 1997). Very rarely, however, spindle cell metaplasia may be seen, the spindle cells having a true myoepithelial phenotype on immunostaining. Myoepithelial cells are invariably present in their normal location around the periphery of the involved structures. Intraepithelial lymphocytes and histiocytes are also present and may be identified using the appropriate immunohistological staining techniques (Lwin *et al.*, 1985). HUT is thus a polymorphic proliferation, the mixture of cell types being an important feature in distinguishing it from *in situ* carcinoma.

Ductal enlargement may be slight or massive, and the cells may totally or partially occlude the lumen. The proliferation may be solid or cribriform. The secondary lumina in the cribriform areas are usually irregular in outline and may show evidence of apocrine secretion, although the large eosinophilic apocrine cells seen in cysts are rare. The cellular bridges extending between the lumina are of variable thickness and usually exhibit a tapering appearance, the nuclei tending to 'stream' with their long axes parallel to the direction of the bridge.

Solid, finger-like processes may project into the duct lumen. The term papillomatosis has been used by some authors (particularly in the USA) to describe this appearance (and indeed HUT in general). This type of micropapillary hyperplasia may in some cases resemble that seen in the male breast in gynaecomastia (*see* Fig. 16.3). In this book, however, 'papillomatosis' is reserved for those proliferations exhibiting a true fibrovascular core. Some of the processes join the duct wall at both ends to form peripheral

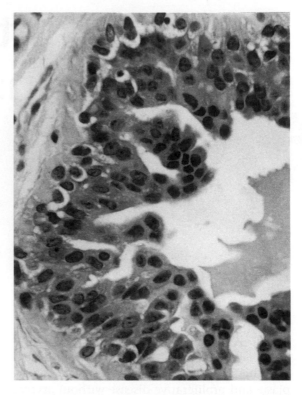

7.3 Hyperplasia of usual type. Some of the epithelial cell nuclei are large with discernible nucleoli, but they are normochromic and regular. All other features indicate a non-atypical proliferation. There is a mixture of cell types and the secondary lumina are irregular in size and shape. The nuclei are unevenly spaced and tend to stream across the peripheral bridges. Mitoses and necrosis are absent (H&E).

bridges (*see* Fig. 7.3 above); in such cases the cells tend to 'stream' across as described above. Periductal fibrosis, elastosis and inflammation are not usually seen, although foam cells may be present in the lumen. Microcalcification is uncommon, and consequently HUT is rarely detected by mammography.

Ultrastructural studies of the epithelial cells confirm their benign nature. They contain occasional lipid and secretory droplets, as well as aggregates of glycogen particles. Rough endoplasmic reticulum is sparse, and intracytoplasmic lumina are not observed. Desmosomes are present, and occasional myoepithelial cells exhibit myofilaments with focal densities. The basal lamina is intact and may appear normal or thickened. The histological differences between HUT, atypical ductal hyperplasia (ADH) and the low nuclear grade variants of ductal carcinoma *in situ* (DCIS) are summarised in Table 7.1.

There has been much recent interest in the level of consistency that can be achieved by

TABLE 7.1 Comparison of histological features of ductal hyperplasia and ductal carcinoma *in situ* (DCIS), major diagnostic features being shown in bold type

Histological features	Hyperplasia of usual type	Atypical ductal hyperplasia	Low nuclear grade DCIS
Size	Variable size but rarely extensive unless associated with other benign processes such as papilloma or radial scar	Usually small (less than 2–3 mm) unless associated with other benign processes such as papilloma or radial scar	Rarely less than 2–3 mm and may be very extensive
Cellular composition	**Mixed epithelial and spindle-shaped cells. Lymphocytes and macrophages may also be present. Myoepithelial hyperplasia may occur around the periphery**	May be uniform cell population but merges with areas of usual type hyperplasia within the same duct space. Spindle-shaped cells may be intermingled with the proliferating cells	**Single cell population.** Spindle-shaped cells not seen. Myoepithelial cells usually in normal location around duct periphery but may be attenuated
Architecture	Variable	Micropapillary, cribriform or solid patterns but may be rudimentary	**Well developed micropapillary, cribriform or solid patterns**
Lumina	**Irregular, often ill-defined**	May be distinct, well formed rounded spaces in cribriform type. Irregular, ill-defined lumina may also be present	**Well delineated, regular punched out lumina in cribriform type**
Cell orientation	**Often streaming with long axes of nuclei arranged parallel to direction of cellular bridges, which often have a 'tapering' appearance**	Cell nuclei may be at right angles to bridges in cribriform types, forming 'rigid' structures	**Cell bridges 'rigid' in cribriform type with nuclei orientated towards the luminal space. Micropapillary structures with indiscernible or poorly developed fibro-vascular cores. Cells tend to show orientation around lumina or over papillae**
Nuclear spacing	**Uneven**	May be even or uneven	**Even**
Epithelial cell appearance	**Small ovoid normochromic nuclei.** Variation in shape	**Uniform small or medium sized cells with hyper-chromatic nuclei present at least focally**	**Uniform cell population** with small or medium-sized, monotonous, hyperchromatic nuclei
Nucleoli	Indistinct	Single small	Single small
Mitoses	Infrequent with no abnormal forms	Infrequent, abnormal forms rare	Infrequent, abnormal forms rare
Necrosis	Rare	Rare	Uncommon. If present, confined to small particulate debris in cribriform and/or luminal spaces

N.B. All the features of a lesion should be taken into account when making a diagnosis. No criterion is reliable alone.
(Reproduced with permission from the NHS National Breast Screening Programme and the European Commission.)

pathologists in diagnosing intraductal hyperplasias, particularly the atypical variants. In a recent study it was shown that HUT can be diagnosed with a reasonable level of consistency, the κ value of 0.54 being intermediate between those associated with DCIS and those with ADH (Elston *et al.*, 2000).

In the autopsy study of Frantz *et al.* (1951), intraductal proliferation was found in 16% of the general population. All cases were associated with cysts, which were macroscopically visible in about half the cases. Only 19% of subjects with intraductal hyperplasia were premenopausal. In his study of 800 autopsies, Sandison (1962) found a rather similar (22%) incidence of hyperplasia and noted that the change was rare below the age of 40. In a study of 519 forensic autopsies performed on women with no history of breast disease, Bartow *et al.* (1987) found epithelial hyperplasia in up to 40% of cases, although this incidence fell to 15% for those considered to be moderate in severity and to less than 5% for those held to be severe. For all grades of severity, the incidence rose markedly in women over 35.

Kramer and Rush (1973) examined the breasts of 70 women over the age of 70 at autopsy and found intraductal hyperplasia in 69%, in 43% of which the change was considered to be severe. This higher incidence seems to be explained partly by the greater age of the subjects and partly by extensive sampling, as 40 75 mm × 25 mm microscopic sections were examined from each breast. Regardless of the precise incidence, some degree of HUT is clearly common in normal women.

There have been many studies investigating the possible preneoplastic significance of HUT. Dupont and Page (1985) followed up a large number of patients who had had benign breast biopsies and found that those with proliferative disease without atypical hyperplasia had a risk of developing cancer that was 1.9 times that of women with non-proliferative lesions. In later studies by Carter *et al.* (1988), London *et al.* (1992), McDivitt *et al.*

(1992), Bodian *et al.* (1993) and Marshall *et al.* (1997), the relative risk for proliferative disease without atypia was 1.9, 1.6, 1.8, 2.1 and 1.7, respectively. In two studies a family history of breast cancer was associated with a further increase in risk (Dupont and Page, 1985, ×2.5; Carter *et al.*, 1992, ×1.8), but this was not seen in the others. In the study of Tavassoli and Norris (1990), 6 (5%) of 117 patients with non-atypical ductal hyperplasia developed carcinoma after an average follow-up period of 14 years. The malignancies occurred in either breast. These levels of risk are generally not considered to be high enough to justify increased surveillance or any form of treatment. For a further discussion of the precancerous significance of proliferative lesions, *see* Chapter 10.

Immunohistochemical and genetic studies of HUT have revealed molecular and cellular heterogeneity, but, at the time of writing, only two aspects have been reported to have diagnostic or prognostic value. The first is the demonstration of the basal keratin cells (see above), which may be useful in distinguishing HUT from atypical hyperplasia and DCIS, where they are absent. The second is the expression of transforming growth factor-β type II receptor, which Gobbi *et al.* (1999) found to be related to the risk of developing breast cancer. Thus women with HUT exhibiting 25–75% or fewer than 25% positive cells had an odds ratio of invasive breast cancer of 1.98 and 3.41, respectively, compared to those with HUT exhibiting more than 75% positive cells. This observation requires independent verification.

HUT usually exhibits immunopositivity for the oestrogen receptor, the proportion of cells being higher than that in the normal breast but showing the normal increase with age. Two patterns may be observed: one in which, like the normal breast, positive and negative cells are intimately mixed, and the other in which virtually all the cells are positive (Shoker *et al.*, 1999a). Cells abnormally co-expressing oestrogen receptors and Ki67 are found in a small proportion of cases (Shoker *et al.*, 1999b; Iqbal *et al.*, 2000). Some cases of HUT thus share a pattern of

7.4 Allelic imbalance in hyperplasia of usual type. (a) These foci of hyperplasia of usual type were microdissected from formalin-fixed, paraffin-embedded sections. (b) The DNA was extracted and amplified using the polymerase chain reaction (PCR) with fluorescent primers spanning polymorphic microsatellite repeat sequences on chromosome 17. The PCR products were then run on a gel and scanned for fluorescence intensity. The resulting traces are illustrated. The figures in the boxes give the molecular size (in base pairs) of the products, the maximum height of the trace and the area under it. The bottom trace is of normal breast DNA, in which the two polymorphic alleles are normally represented. (The spikes represent PCR products of differing molecular weight resulting from the imperfect replication of the repeated DNA sequences by the DNA polymerase.) The top tracing from the upper lesion shows both alleles normally represented. The middle trace is from the lower lesion and reveals the loss of one allele (arrow).

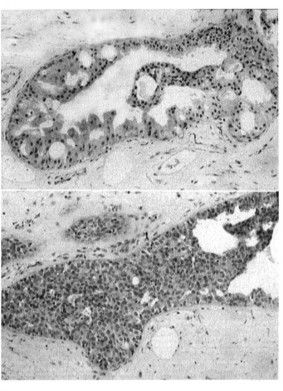

(a)

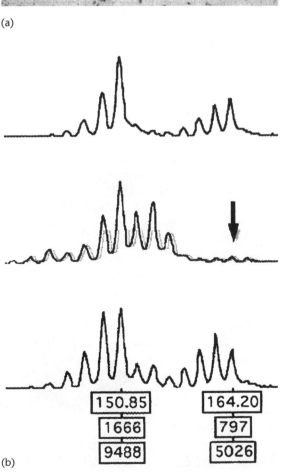

(b)

150.85		164.20
1666		797
9488		5026

oestrogen receptor expression with atypical hyperplasia and DCIS but the clinical significance of this is not yet known. An increase in Ki67+ and cyclin D1+ cells is common, but a changes in p21, p53 and c-erbB-2 immunostaining is rare and of uncertain significance (Mommers *et al.*, 1998). Poremba *et al.* (1998) did not detect telomerase activity in HUT, in contrast to carcinomas.

Molecular genetic studies of HUT have shown that about one third of cases exhibit allelic imbalance (AI) if a large number of loci are investigated, although it is rare and inconsistent at any one locus (Lakhani *et al.*, 1996; O'Connell *et al.*, 1998) (Fig. 7.4). This suggests that at least a proportion of cases are clonal (neoplastic) rather than hyperplastic as the name implies. AI can only be demonstrated by this method if the great majority of cells in the proliferation exhibit the change. It is highly unlikely that all cells would have acquired the abnormality independently and therefore probable that all the cells were derived from a single precursor in which a certain profile of AI had occurred. Lesions from cancerous breasts often share AI with the cancer, supporting their precursor status. The prognostic significance of AI in general or at any locus in particular is not yet known. Fluorescence *in situ* hybridization studies have shown a borderline or true aneusomy of chromosomes 16, 17, 18 and X in a proportion of cases (Micale *et al.*, 1994), providing further evidence that at least some are likely to be precancerous.

ATYPICAL DUCTAL HYPERPLASIA

Atypical ductal hyperplasia is the term used by many workers to describe *in situ* proliferations that have some but not all the morphological features of DCIS. There is a spectrum of changes linking HUT with DCIS, and distinguishing the two is often more quantitative than qualitative. As hyperplasia may fall short of DCIS for different reasons, ADH has been regarded by many as a heterogeneous group of disorders rather than a single entity. It is hardly surprising, therefore, that diagnosing the condition has been associated with a low level of interobserver consistency, with κ statistics often being as low as 0.25 (Swanson Beck *et al.*, 1985; Sloane *et al.*, 1994; Wells *et al.*, 1998). Problems are encountered in distinguishing ADH from both HUT and DCIS, the latter mainly the low nuclear grade forms (Sloane *et al.*, 1994). The pronounced cytological atypia associated with the high nuclear grade forms makes diagnosing DCIS relatively straightforward regardless of growth pattern or other associated features (*see* Chapter 8).

In an attempt to improve diagnostic consistency, Page and Rogers (1992) laid down clear criteria for diagnosing ADH, thus making it a positive diagnosis rather one of exclusion. Using these criteria Page and various associates demonstrated that women whose breasts harbour ADH have an increased risk of developing carcinoma (e.g. Dupont and Page, 1985). There were three categories of criterion: cytological features, histological patterns and

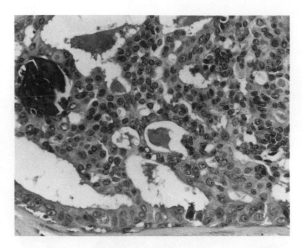

the semi-quantitative extent of the change. The cells are evenly spaced and uniform with oval or rounded hyperchromatic nuclei. They are indistinguishable from those of the low nuclear grade forms of DCIS (*see* Chapter 8) but comprise only part of the cell population in any given basement-bound space.

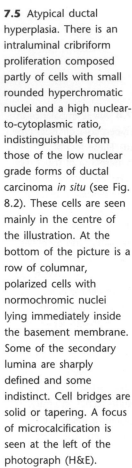

7.5 Atypical ductal hyperplasia. There is an intraluminal cribriform proliferation composed partly of cells with small rounded hyperchromatic nuclei and a high nuclear-to-cytoplasmic ratio, indistinguishable from those of the low nuclear grade forms of ductal carcinoma *in situ* (see Fig. 8.2). These cells are seen mainly in the centre of the illustration. At the bottom of the picture is a row of columnar, polarized cells with normochromic nuclei lying immediately inside the basement membrane. Some of the secondary lumina are sharply defined and some indistinct. Cell bridges are solid or tapering. A focus of microcalcification is seen at the left of the photograph (H&E).

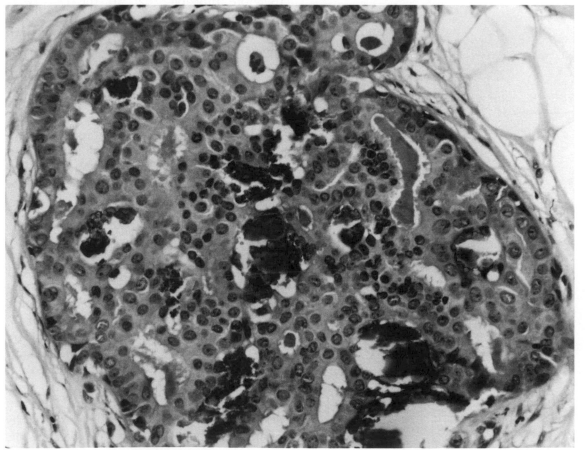

7.6 Atypical ductal hyperplasia. Cells similar to those of the low nuclear grade forms of ductal carcinoma *in situ* are seen, particularly in the centre. Polarized cells with normochromic nuclei are seen around the periphery of the duct at the left and right of the picture. Secondary lumina are truncated or indistinct. In this example most of the cellular bars are rigid. There are several clusters of microcalcification (H&E).

To distinguish ADH from HUT, the atypical cells should comprise an entire non-tapering bar crossing a space or a group of cells at least six across. The non-atypical cells often consist of a row of columnar, polarized cells lying immediately above the basement membrane (Figs 7.5 and 7.6). Secondary lumina may be ragged and sharply defined, even within the same primary lumen. The lesions of ADH are generally small and rarely measure more than 2–3 mm in maximal dimension. Where there is significant doubt about distinguishing ADH

from DCIS, then the more benign diagnosis is appropriate. The main features distinguishing ADH from HUT and DCIS are listed in Table 7.1.

Even following these explicit criteria, diagnostic consistency remains unacceptably low, at least among a reasonable number of pathologists (Sloane *et al.*, 1999). By comparing the level of consistency obtained on histological sections with that on medium- or high-power images of small parts of the sections, Elston *et al.* (2000) found that intralesional heterogeneity was not a major cause of the inconsistency, which was due to the inability of observers to agree on the interpretation of selected histological appearances.

Another problem with the Page and Rogers' criteria is that they may be too exclusive as there appear to be some proliferations (excluding those resembling the proliferations in Fig. 7.9 below) that are partially composed of more pleomorphic atypical cells, unlike those of low nuclear grade DCIS (Fig. 7.7). Other proliferations may not fall within the Page and Rogers definition even though they are composed of small uniform cells (Fig. 7.8). Little is known about the clinical significance of such changes, particularly about any associated cancer risk. One way of reporting these lesions while retaining the Page and Rogers' criteria for ADH is to classify them as 'hyperplasia with atypical features'.

At the time of writing there is no obvious solution to the problem of diagnostic inconsistency associated with ADH. It seems unlikely that morphological criteria of sufficient robustness can be devised, and further advances may depend on identifying certain molecular features that are associated with risk – a not improbable scenario given that much is currently being learned about the molecular pathology of precancerous breast lesions.

From a practical point of view the following advice is offered. If a diagnosis of ADH is contemplated, extensive sampling should be undertaken to search for evidence of unequivocal DCIS, with which it frequently co-exists. In the case of needle core biopsies, this may necessitate open biopsy. A diagnosis of ADH

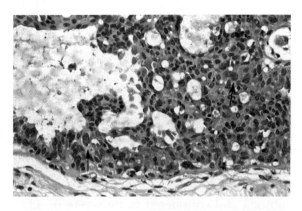

7.7 Intraluminal proliferation of unevenly distributed polymorphic cells associated with poorly delineated secondary lumina. The architectural features are those of hyperplasia of usual type, but some of the epithelial cells have large pleomorphic nuclei (arrows). This lesion was not accompanied by carcinoma. It does not fall easily into any of the present categories of intraductal proliferation (H&E).

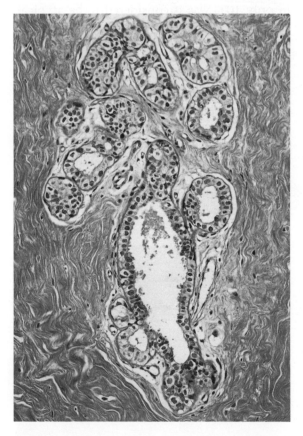

7.8 A terminal duct and lobule lined by abnormal monotonous cells with rounded hyperchromatic nuclei and a high nuclear-to-cytoplasmic ratio. The cells comprise the whole proliferation and exhibit a clinging growth pattern with little intraluminal proliferation. The change was very extensive, involving an area of many centimetres. Although the lesion does not obviously fit the Page and Rogers criteria, the majority diagnosis of a group of European experts was atypical ductal hyperplasia and was made by 65% of group members.

should be restricted to those cases in which DCIS is being seriously considered but cannot be identified with confidence. Only rarely should it be made where the diagnostic features extend for more than 2–3 mm or involve multiple duct spaces. A criterion for distinguishing ADH from DCIS used by the Armed Forces Institute of Pathology is that lesions less than 2 mm in diameter are not regarded as DCIS unless they exhibit high-grade cytology or necrosis (Tavassoli, 1998). Pathologists should participate in multidisciplinary meetings, where appropriate management decisions, taking into account all the clinical, radiological and pathological data, can be made. Multidisciplinary team working can greatly minimize the adverse effects of pathological diagnostic uncertainty.

DCIS may occasionally spread along the duct system, mingling with non-neoplastic epithelial cells (Fig. 7.9). Zones of pre-existing hyperplasia may sometimes be involved in this fashion, and the subpopulation of malignant cells may be difficult to identify. In cases of doubt further sampling should be undertaken. These cases should not be diagnosed as ADH.

ADH may exhibit microcalcification and consequently be detected by screening mammography. The calcifications are usually finely granular rather than branching and may be difficult to visualize in specimen radiographs (see Figs. 7.5 and 7.6 above, and Fig. 7.10).

Dupont and Page (1985) followed up a large number of patients with benign breast biopsies and found that those with atypical hyperplasia (either ductal or lobular) had a risk of developing cancer 5.3 times that seen in women without proliferative lesions. The risk applied to any site in either breast. In later studies by Carter *et al.* (1988), London *et al.* (1992), McDivitt *et al.* (1992), Bodian *et al.* (1993) and Marshall *et al.* (1997), the relative risk for atypical hyperplasia was 3.0, 3.7, 2.6, 3.0 and 2.4, respectively. Diagnostic inconsistency is a major reason for the variable risk reported in these studies. A family history of breast cancer further increased the risk by a factor of 2.5 in the study of Dupont and Page

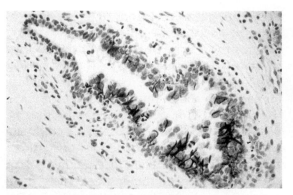

and 1.8 in that of Carter *et al.* but had no effect in the other investigations. Tavassoli and Norris (1990) followed 82 patients with ADH for an average of 12.4 years; invasive carcinoma subsequently developed in 8 (9.8%), 6 in the ipsilateral and 2 in the contralateral breast (see Table 10.1).

Atypical hyperplasia is a much less common autopsy finding than HUT in women without a history of breast disease. Although, in the detailed study of Kramer and Rush (1973), intraductal hyperplasia was found in 69% of subjects and considered to be severe in 43%, in only 10% was it considered to be atypical. About half the breasts containing ADH also contained DCIS or infiltrating carcinoma.

The difficulty of distinguishing ADH from the low nuclear grade variants of DCIS has prompted molecular studies aimed at elucidating the relationship between the two disorders. Evidence for continuing to separate ADH and low nuclear grade DCIS has been provided by Weinstat-Saslow *et al.* (1995) and Gillett *et al.* (1998), who used *in situ* hybridization and immunohistochemistry respectively to detect cyclin D1 mRNA and protein in

7.9 Partial involvement of an interlobular duct by high nuclear grade ductal carcinoma *in situ*. The immunopositivity of the malignant cells for c-erbB-2 in this immuno-peroxidase stain makes their recognition easy, but in ordinary H&E-stained sections a picture like this may be incorrectly interpreted as atypical ductal hyperplasia because of the mixture of cell types. The presence of frank cytological malignancy in a subpopulation of mixed cell types often means that *in situ* carcinoma is nearby.

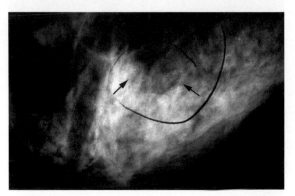

7.10 Clinical mammogram containing clusters of granular microcalcification, mostly within the area encircled by the chinagraph mark made by the radiologist (arrows). A zone of similar calcification is also seen in the upper-right of the picture. A histological examination of both these zones showed intraductal proliferation focally fulfilling the Page and Rogers criteria.

biopsy specimens. They found a similar level in ADH and benign lesions, and a much higher level in low- and high-grade DCIS and invasive carcinoma. Other studies, however, have found a graded increase in cyclin D1 overexpression from normal to invasive carcinoma via HUT, ADH and DCIS, a significant difference not always being seen between consecutive stages (Alle *et al.*, 1998; Mommers *et al.*, 1998; Zhu *et al.*, 1998; Monaghan *et al.*, 1999). Shoker *et al.* (1999b) have shown that cases of ADH fulfilling the Page and Rogers criteria show patterns of oestrogen receptor expression and dysregulation similar to those seen in low-grade DCIS.

AI has been found in nearly half the cases studied, an incidence comparable to that seen in low-grade DCIS and greater than that in HUT. The incidence at any one locus is, however, low (Lakhani *et al.*, 1995; O'Connell *et al.*, 1998) (see above and Fig. 7.4 above). ADH from cancerous breasts frequently shares AI of at least one locus with the cancer. The finding of AI has the same implications as in HUT. Not only is AI an early change in the development of human breast cancer, but its occurrence in ADH also indicates that it is likely to be a monoclonal (neoplastic) proliferation rather a polyclonal (hyperplastic) one as its name suggests.

There is thus a case for grouping the various forms of *in situ* proliferation together as a spectrum of mammary *in situ* neoplasia (MIN) or ductal *in situ* neoplasia (DIN), as has been suggested by Rosai (1991) and Tavassoli (1998) respectively. Tavassoli proposed dividing DIN into three main groups, DIN1 including HUT, ADH and low-grade DCIS (DIN 1a, 1b and 1c respectively), DIN2 intermediate-grade DCIS, and DIN3 high-grade DCIS.

In the author's opinion a classification based on *in situ* neoplasia would be preferable to the current one based on hyperplasia and *in situ* carcinoma, providing international agreement could be reached. First, it would be more in keeping with current evidence on the biological nature of the proliferations. Second, it would be consistent with that used in other organs (e.g. cervix, prostate and larynx). Third, it would have the main clinical advantage of indicating to clinicians a continuous spectrum of proliferative change and eliminating the hyperplasia/cancer dichotomy. Merely changing the terminology would not, however, improve diagnostic consistency or prognostication, although it would provide a more flexible framework within which to refine diagnostic indications by morphological or molecular criteria. The most important factor in determining whether individual patients are managed appropriately is communication between pathologists, radiologists and clinicians to ensure that all aspects of a case are taken into consideration before any decision is made.

SOLITARY INTRADUCT PAPILLOMA

Clinically manifest intraduct papillomas are not very common: Sandison (1958) identified them in only 3.7% of over 1000 surgical specimens of breast. In the study of Cahn *et al.* (1997), they were found to be more common in women on hormone replacement therapy. Although usually occurring in middle age, they may also be seen in adolescents and the elderly. They are the most common cause of discharge from the nipple, and about 80% of patients present with this symptom, the discharge being blood-stained in half the cases. A mass can often be palpated, but nipple retraction is uncommon. Bilateral tumours are rare.

Macroscopically, a papilloma may appear as an elongated structure, usually a few millimetres in diameter, extending along a major duct or as a more spheroidal lesion. The latter type results in greater distension of the duct, which may assume a cyst-like appearance (Fig. 7.11). The terms cystadenoma and intracystic papilloma have been used by some authors to describe this form. Even with this type of lesion, the size is rarely greater than 30 mm. Some intraduct papillomas involve smaller ducts and may be of microscopic size; many blocks may be required to identify them.

The histological differences between intraduct papilloma and encysted papillary carcinoma are summarized in Table 7.2. Intraduct papillomas exhibit an arborescent

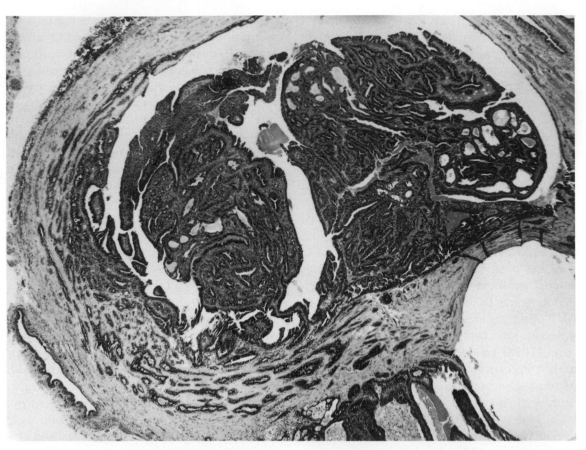

7.11 Intraduct papilloma. The tumour is contained within a dilated interlobular duct and consists of arborescent fibrovascular structures covered by epithelial cells. There is peripheral fibrosis with epithelial entrapment at the bottom right of the picture, giving a false impression of invasion (H&E).

growth pattern with branching fibrovascular cores covered by epithelial and myoepithelial cells (Fig. 7.12). The epithelial cells usually form a single layer, but there may be zones of HUT (Fig. 7.13). The cores are usually well developed (Figs 7.11 and 7.12) but may sometimes be delicate and poorly formed. However, they are rarely, if ever, absent, and the epithelial cells do not show a true 'back-to-back' appearance.

The cytological features are benign (Fig. 7.12). The cells are uniform and their nuclei normochromic, with delicate nuclear membranes and usually inconspicuous nucleoli. Mitoses are infrequent, and abnormal forms are not seen. Apical snouts are often present on the luminal surface, and apocrine metaplasia, as seen in breast cysts, is common (Fig. 7.14). Two cell types are usually identified: an outer epithelial and an inner myoepithelial layer (Fig. 7.12). Necrosis and haemorrhage are, however, not infrequent and thus do not have the same diagnostic

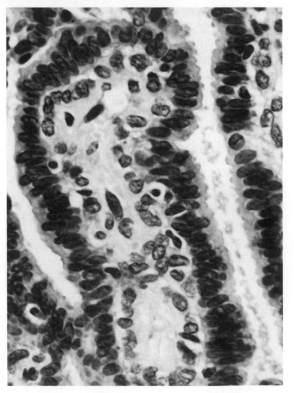

7.12 Intraduct papilloma. Well-developed fibrovascular cores are covered by an inner layer of myoepithelial cells with rounded vesicular nuclei and an outer layer of columnar epithelial cells with more darkly staining nuclei (H&E).

TABLE 7.2 Distinction of papilloma from encysted papillary carcinoma

Histological features	Papilloma	Encysted papillary carcinoma
1) Fibrovascular cores	Usually broad and extend throughout the lesion	Very variable, usually fine and may be absent in at least part of the lesion
2) Cells covering papillae		
a) basal	Myoepithelial layer always present	Myoepithelial cells usually absent but when present usually form a discontinuous layer
b) luminal	Single layer of regular luminal epithelium OR features of usual type hyperplasia	Cells often taller and more monotonous with oval nuclei, the long axes of which lie perpendicular to stromal core of papillae. Nuclei may be hyperchromatic. Epithelial multi-layering frequent, often producing cribriform and micropapillary patterns of DCIS overlying the papillae or lining the cyst wall.
3) Mitoses	Infrequent with no abnormal forms	More frequent; abnormal forms may be seen
4) Apocrine metaplasia	Common	Rare
5) Surrounding tissue	Benign changes may be present including hyperplasia of usual type	Surrounding ducts may show DCIS
6) Necrosis and haemorrhage	May occur in either. Not a useful discriminating feature.	
7) Periductal and intra-tumoural fibrosis	May occur in either. Not a useful discriminating feature.	

N.B. All the features of a lesion should be taken into account when making a diagnosis. No criterion is reliable alone.
Abbreviation: DCIS = Ductal carcinoma *in situ*
(Reproduced with permission from the NHS Breast Screening Programme and the European Commission.)

significance as in solid intraduct proliferations. Papillomas may rarely exhibit chondroid or osseous metaplasia (Smith and Taylor, 1969).

Ultrastructural studies (Fisher, 1976; Ahmed, 1980) have confirmed the benign appearance of the cells. The cell membranes have normal luminal microvilli, desmosomes and junctional complexes; cytoplasmic organelles are sparse. The outer myoepithelial cells are often elongated and exhibit prominent cytoplasmic filaments. The basement membrane is intact but may be thickened. Cells exhibiting apocrine metaplasia show ultrastructural features similar to those seen in cysts.

Sclerosing papillomas are those which exhibit zones of fibrosis, sometimes appearing to result

7.13 (Left) Intraduct papilloma stained with an antibody to smooth muscle actin using the immunoperoxidase technique. The brown reaction product identifies the myoepithelial layer on which there are multiple layers of cytologically non-atypical epithelial cells.

7.14 (Right) Intraduct papilloma. There is a zone of apocrine metaplasia on the right of the picture (H&E).

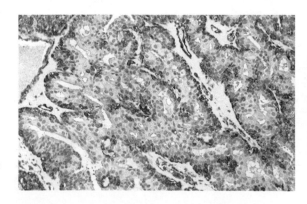

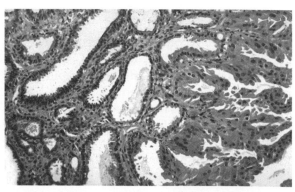

from necrosis or haemorrhage. Fibrotic zones may occur at the periphery and partially replace the tumour in an uneven fashion. Entrapped irregular masses of epithelium are often left behind, which may exhibit an infiltrative appearance and be mistaken for infiltrating carcinoma (*see* Fig. 7.11 above, and Fig. 7.15). The epithelial cells, however, have benign cytological features (Fig. 7.16). Furthermore, although the duct wall is often obscured, its outline can often be traced outside the apparently infiltrative tissue from the neighbouring intact wall (Fig. 7.15).

Many authors, particularly in the USA, have used the term papillomatosis synonymously with HUT or sometimes more specifically to describe benign intraductal proliferations exhibiting solid intraluminal finger-like projections. These structures, however, lack a true fibrovascular core and are classed in this book as HUT. The term papillomatosis does, however, appear to be justified to describe benign intraductal proliferations that are identical in structure and cytological appearance to papillomas except that they are multiple and microscopic in size (Fig. 7.17). As thus defined papillomatosis is very uncommon, rarely causes symptoms and is usually associated with other forms of intraductal hyperplasia and benign epithelial alterations. It is important to distinguish papillomatosis from multiple intraduct papilloma (see below).

In his study of 800 autopsies performed on patients with no history of breast disease, Sandison (1962) found intraduct papillomas in the breasts of 13 cases, an incidence of 1.6%; 10 were solitary and 3 multiple. None was found in women aged under 35. Using very extensive sampling techniques on a group of patients all over 70 years of age, Kramer and Rush (1973) found intraduct papilloma in 21%, the tumours being bilateral in 6%. Nearly all the cases were associated with other forms of intraductal proliferation. Although intraduct papilloma is not very common in clinical practice, small lesions appear to be not infrequent at a subclinical level, especially in older women.

There has been some dispute about the premalignant potential of intraduct papillomas. In some publications (see, for example,

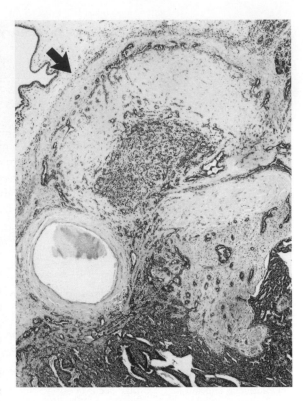

7.15 Fibrosis in a large intraduct papilloma, giving the impression of invasion. The fibrotic, but intact, duct wall (arrowed) can be traced around the periphery of the lesion (H&E).

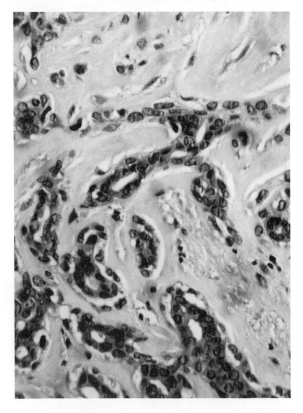

7.16 Detail of the fibrotic zone shown in Fig. 7.15; note the double cell layer and the lack of cytological atypia (H&E).

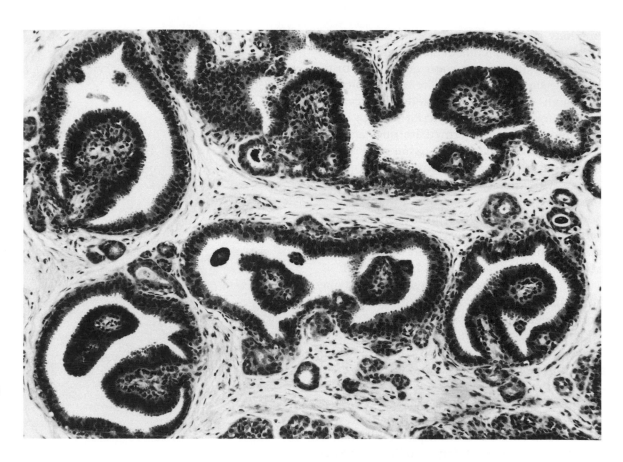

7.17 Papillomatosis. There are multiple microscopic papillary ingrowths with fibrovascular cores. There was no macroscopically visible tumour in this specimen (H&E).

Kilgore *et al.*, 1953; Moore *et al.*, 1961), in which an increased incidence of subsequent carcinoma has been found, the initial diagnosis has been questioned, and many of the tumours would nowadays be regarded as intraduct papillary carcinomas *ab initio*. Other studies, such as those of Lewison and Lyons (1953), Hendrick (1957) and Kraus and Neubecker (1962), have failed to find an increased risk of carcinoma.

More recently, Page *et al.* (1996), studied biopsies containing papillomas from 368 women and found that the relative risk of developing invasive carcinoma was in general similar to that for proliferative disease without atypia. The presence of HUT within the papilloma did not increase the chance of developing carcinoma. The relative risk was, however, significantly increased for women whose papillomas contained foci of atypical hyperplasia, being more than 4 times that of women whose papillomas were unassociated with this change, either in the papilloma itself or in the neighbouring breast.

MULTIPLE INTRADUCT PAPILLOMA

This is a rare entity that Haagensen (1971) found to be significantly less common than solitary intraduct papilloma. The condition differs from the solitary variety in that the lesions are multiple and much less frequently subareolar in location. Discharge from the nipple is thus less common, and most patients present with a palpable mass, which may sometimes involve an entire sector of the breast. The condition is bilateral in about 25% of cases and tends to occur in a somewhat younger age group than solitary papilloma; a few cases have been reported in adolescents. Multiple intraduct papilloma is distinguished from papillomatosis, as defined above, by the extent and macroscopic size of the proliferation.

Histologically, the lesions are identical to ordinary papillomas (Fig. 7.18). Apocrine metaplasia and pseudo-infiltration of the capsule may be seen. Between one-quarter and one-third of patients, however, have associated carcinoma, which is usually intraductal but may rarely be infiltrative. The size of the carcinoma varies considerably but is usually small and often microscopic. Extensive histological sampling is therefore indicated. Although any type of intraduct carcinoma may be found, it is usually cribriform or papillary and of low or intermediate nuclear grade (Fig. 7.19). The malignant tissue may appear to be separate from the papillomas or may merge with them. There may also be borderline foci linking the benign and malignant zones, which exhibit multilayering, cellular monomorphism, nuclear hyperchromasia, a partly cribriform appearance or a focal loss of stroma (Ohuchi *et al.*, 1984; Papotti *et al.*, 1984). One or more of these features may sometimes be seen in cases without any definite evidence of malignancy.

Ohuchi *et al.* (1984) graphically reconstructed 15 cases of multiple papilloma using 200–300 5 μm semi-serial sections. The findings were compared with 10 solitary intraduct papillomas examined in the same way. The terminal duct–lobular units were involved in all cases of multiple papilloma but in only one of the solitary papillomas, which were otherwise confined to the interlobular ducts. This explains the difference in anatomical location and clinical presentation of the two forms of the disease. It is also consistent with the widely held view that terminal duct–lobular units have a greater potential for malignant change than do interlobular ducts.

The actual number of papillomas varies considerably from case to case: Papotti *et al.* (1984) found between 5 and 153 per patient. These authors gathered their cases from a large series of quadrantectomy and mastectomy specimens removed for carcinoma. They found 18 examples in 2500 malignant breasts, giving an incidence of 0.7%. In about half the mastectomy specimens, the papillomas were confined to the quadrant containing the carcinoma, but in the other half they were distributed evenly throughout the breast.

There is a risk of recurrence after local excision, even in patients in whom there is no definite evidence of malignancy. Murad *et al.* (1981) found that 5 of 11 cases of multiple intraduct papilloma recurred after local

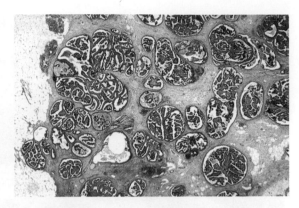

7.18 Multiple intraduct papilloma. There is extensive benign intraduct papillary proliferation involving the whole field (H&E).

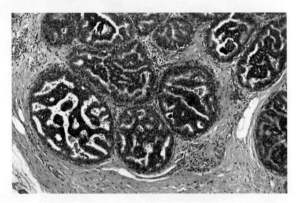

7.19 Multiple intraduct papilloma; this photograph is taken from a separate area of the same section illustrated in Fig. 7.18 and shows a zone of cribriform, low nuclear grade ductal carcinoma *in situ* (H&E).

excision. The recurrent lesions resembled the original ones except for an exaggeration of epithelial stratification. Of Haagensen's 13 patients followed for more than 10 years, nine recurred locally, between 5 and 16 years later.

The risk of subsequent carcinoma in patients in whom all the papillomas appear to be benign is difficult to assess but is almost certainly increased. In Haagensen's series of 39 cases of multiple intraduct papilloma, 15 were associated with carcinoma. In 9 of these the malignancy was co-existent, but in the other 6 it apparently evolved after previous local excision. The time from the presentation with papilloma to the diagnosis of carcinoma varied from 4 to 9.5 years.

JUVENILE 'PAPILLOMATOSIS' (SWISS CHEESE DISEASE)

This is an uncommon entity characterised by intraductal proliferation, cysts, duct ectasia and sclerosing adenosis (Fig. 7.20) (Rosen *et al.*, 1980, 1985). The age at presentation has

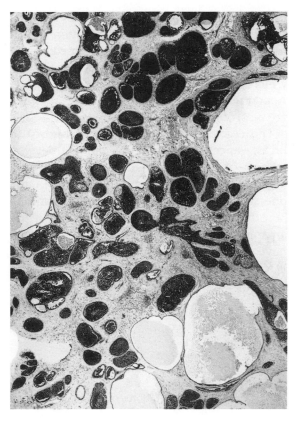

7.20 Section of a breast lump from a 19-year-old girl showing juvenile papillomatosis. Note the extensive cyst formation and hyperplasia. Some of the ducts with hyperplasia show a small amount of central necrosis. There was no sclerosing adenosis in this example (H&E).

ranged from 12 to 48 years, with a median of 21; 70% of the patients are aged under 26.

Although none of the individual histological changes is specific for juvenile papillomatosis, the combination of features and the age at presentation make it a distinctive disorder. The lesion is usually a localized, multinodular, firm, mobile mass that may vary between 10 and 80 mm in diameter and is often mistaken clinically for fibroadenoma. It is generally situated in the upper outer or inner quadrant and rarely in the subareolar region. The cut surface is firm and nodular, a large number of cysts and dilated ducts giving the lesion its characteristic Swiss cheese appearance. The condition is bilateral in about 4% of cases.

Although described as papillomatosis, the intraductal proliferation is not truly papillary and would be regarded as HUT using the terminology employed in this book. In some cases the proliferating cells show atypia and undergo necrosis, making the distinction from DCIS difficult. In such instances, the whole clinicopathological picture should be taken into account. Mitoses are not usually numerous, and apocrine metaplasia is often seen within the zones of hyperplasia. Foam cells may be identified within the lumina of the ducts. The cysts and ectatic ducts vary in size, often measuring up to 10 mm in diameter. The cysts may exhibit apocrine metaplasia and papillary apocrine hyperplasia. Sclerosing adenosis is a common accompaniment.

The condition has no relationship with parity, menstrual disorders, age at menarche or hormone use by the patient or by her mother during pregnancy.

Of the 180 patients reported by the Juvenile Papillomatosis Registry (Rosen *et al*., 1985), 28% had a family history of breast cancer, but this could be an underestimate in view of their young age. Persistent or recurrent lesions were found in 25 (14%) who had a subsequent biopsy, although it was concluded that wide local excision was usually adequate to control the condition. Seven patients (4%) had breast carcinoma (some of the juvenile secretory type) at presentation, two in the contralateral breast.

In a later study, Rosen and Kimmel (1990) reviewed a series of 41 patients with a median follow-up period of 14 years in order to determine the risk of developing cancer after a diagnosis of juvenile papillomatosis. DCIS developed in four (10%) between 5 and 15 years later and was associated with microinvasion in one. All these patients were, however, unusual in that they had recurrent and bilateral juvenile papillomatosis and a family history of breast cancer. The carcinoma developed in the juvenile papillomatosis in three cases and in the contralateral breast in one. Present evidence thus indicates that patients with juvenile papillomatosis are not at great risk of developing breast cancer, particularly if they have unilateral disease and lack a family history.

PAPILLARY LESIONS IN CHILDREN AND YOUNG ADULTS

Papillomas and papillomatosis are usually encountered in adults but may rarely occur in children. Rosen (1985) described papillary lesions occurring in 38 children and young women between 10 and 26 years of age. Six were younger than 14, and 31 younger than 20. Three patterns were identified: papilloma, sclerosing papillomatosis and papillomatosis. Histologically, the lesions did not differ from those occurring in older women. All the papillomas were single, localized lesions limited to one duct or a limited number of contiguous ducts, and no multiple types were seen. Sclerosing papillomas were those in which the ductal outline was distorted and disrupted by fibrosis within and external to the ducts (*see* Fig. 7.15 above). The papillomatosis would be classified as HUT using the terminology employed in this book, although some cases

exhibited small papillary processes with a fibrovascular core. The distinction from juvenile papillomatosis is mainly based on the lack of the characteristic cystic component, which produces the 'Swiss cheese' appearance. Apocrine metaplasia and sclerosing adenosis are also not usually encountered.

Thirteen per cent had a family history of breast cancer, but carcinoma did not develop in any of the 38 patients after a follow-up period varying from 14 to 307 months. Only one subsequent carcinoma was found among 36 other cases in the literature, this occurring after an interval of 22 years. These lesions thus have no greater adverse prognostic significance in children than they do in adults. Treatment should be restricted to local excision.

REFERENCES

Ahmed A. (1974) The myoepithelium in cystic hyperplastic mastopathy. *J. Pathol.*, **113**, 209–15.

Ahmed A. (1980) Ultrastructural aspects of human breast lesions. *Pathol. Ann.*, **15**, 411–43.

Alle K.M., Henshall S.M., Field A.S., Sutherland R.L. (1998) Cyclin D1 protein is overexpressed in hyperplasia and intraductal carcinoma of the breast. *Clin. Cancer Res.*, **4**, 847–54.

Bartow S.A., Pathak D.R., Black W.C., Key C.R., Teaf S.R. (1987) Prevalence of benign, atypical, and malignant lesions in populations at different risk for breast cancer. *Cancer*, **60**, 2751–60.

Bodian C.A., Perzin K.H., Lattes R., Hoffman P., Abernathy T.G. (1993) Prognostic significance of benign proliferative breast disease. *Cancer*, **71**, 3896–907.

Boecker W., Bier B., Freytag G. *et al.* (1992) An immunohistochemical study of the breast using antibodies to basal and luminal keratins, alpha-smooth muscle actin, vimentin, collagen IV and laminin. I: Normal breast and benign proliferative lesions. *Virchows Archiv. A, Pathol. Anat.*, **421**, 315–22.

Cahn M.D., Tran T., Theur C.P., Butler J.A. (1997) Hormone replacement therapy and the risk of breast lesions that predispose to cancer. *Am. Surg.*, **63**, 858–60.

Carter C.L., Corle D.K., Micozzi M.S., Schatzkin A., Taylor P.R. (1988) A prospective study of the development of breast cancer in 16,692 women with benign breast disease. *Am. J. Epidemiol.*, **128**, 467–77.

Dupont W.D., Page D.L. (1985) Risk factors in women with proliferative breast disease. *N. Engl. J. Med.*, **312**, 146–51.

Elston C.W., Sloane J.P., Amendoeira I. *et al.* (2000) Causes of inconsistency in diagnosing and classifying intraductal proliferations of the breast. *Eur. J. Cancer*, **36**, 1769–72.

Fisher E.R. (1976) Ultrastructure of the human breast and its disorders. *Am. J. Clin. Pathol.*, **66**, 291–374.

Frantz V.K., Pickren J.W., Melcher G.W., Auchincloss H. (1951) Incidence of chronic cystic disease in so-called 'normal breasts': a study based on 225 postmortem examinations. *Cancer*, **4**, 762–83.

Gillett C.E., Lee A.H.S., Millis R.R., Barnes D.M. (1998) Cyclin D1 and associated proteins in mammary ductal carcinoma *in situ* and atypical ductal hyperplasia. *J. Pathol.*, **184**, 396–400.

Gobbi H., Dupont W.D., Simpson J.F. *et al.* (1999) Transforming growth factor-beta and breast cancer risk in women with mammary epithelial hyperplasia. *J. Natl Cancer Inst.*, **91**, 2096–101.

Haagensen C.D. (1971) *Diseases of the Breast*, 2nd edn. London, W.B. Saunders.

Hendrick J.W. (1957) Intraductal papilloma of the breast. *Surg. Gynecol. Obstet.*, **105**, 215–23.

Ichihara S., Koshikawa T., Nakamura S., Yatabe Y., Kato K. (1997) Epithelial hyperplasia of usual type expresses both S100-α and S100-β in a heterogeneous pattern but ductal carcinoma *in situ* can express only S100-α in a monotonous pattern. *Histopathology*, **30**, 533–41.

Iqbal M., Davies M.P.A., Shoker B.S., Jarvis C., Sibson D.R., Sloane J.P. (2000) Subgroups of non-atypical hyperplasia of breast defined by proliferation of estrogen receptor positive cells (submitted for publication).

Kilgore A.R., Fleming R., Ramos M.M. (1953) The incidence of cancer with nipple discharge and the risk of cancer in the presence of papillary disease of the breast. *Surg. Gynecol. Obstet.*, **96**, 649–60.

Kramer W.M., Rush B.F. (1973) Mammary duct proliferation in the elderly: a histopathologic study. *Cancer*, **31**, 130–7.

Kraus F.T., Neubecker R.D. (1962) The differential diagnosis of papillary tumors of the breast. *Cancer*, **15**, 444–55.

Lakhani S.R., Collins N., Stratton M.R., Sloane J.P. (1995) Atypical ductal hyperplasia of the breast: a clonal proliferation with loss of heterozygosity on chromosomes 16q and 17p. *J. Clin. Pathol.*, **48**, 611–15.

Lakhani S.R., Slack D.N., Hamoudi R.A., Collins N., Stratton M.R., Sloane J.P. (1996) Detection of allelic imbalance indicates that a proportion of mammary hyperplasia of usual type are clonal, neoplastic proliferations. *Lab. Invest.*, **74**, 129–35.

Lewison E.F., Lyons J.G. (1953) Relationship between benign breast disease and cancer. *Arch. Surg.*, **66**, 94–114.

London S.J., Connolly J.L., Schnitt S.J., Colditz G.A. (1992) A prospective study of benign breast disease and the risk of breast cancer. *JAMA*, **267**, 941–4.

Lwin K.Y., Zuccarini O., Sloane J.P., Beverley P.C.L. (1985) An immunohistological study of leucocyte localisation in benign and malignant breast tissue. *Int. J. Cancer*, **36**, 433–8.

Marshall L.M., Hunter D.J., Connolly J.L. *et al.* (1997) Risk of breast cancer associated with atypical hyperplasia of lobular and ductal types. *Cancer Epidemiology, Biomarkers and Prevention*, **6**, 297–301.

McDivitt R.W,. Stevens J.A., Lee N.C., Wingo P.A., Rubin G.L., Gersell D. (1992) Histologic types of benign breast disease and the risk for breast cancer. The Cancer and Steroid Hormone Study Group. *Cancer*, **69**, 1408–14.

Micale M.A., Visscher D.W., Gulino S.E., Wolman S.R. (1994) Chromosomal aneuploidy in proliferative breast disease. *Hum. Pathol.*, **25**, 29–35.

Mommers E.C.M., van Diest P.J., Leonhart A.M., Meijer C.J.L.M., Baak J.P.A. (1998) Expression of proliferation and apoptosis-related proteins in usual ductal hyperplasia of the breast. *Hum. Pathol.*, **29**, 1539–45.

Monaghan H., Scott D., Schrimankar J. *et al.* (1999) Cyclin D1 expression in usual hyperplasia, atypical ductal hyperplasia and low nuclear grade ductal carcinoma in situ of the breast: an immunohistochemical study. *J. Pathol.*, **187**(suppl.), 25A.

Moore S.W., Pearce J., Ring E. (1961) Intraductal papilloma of the breast. *Surg. Gynecol. Obstet.*, **112**, 153–8.

Murad T.M., Contesso G., Mouriesse H. (1981) Papillary tumors of large lactiferous ducts. *Cancer*, **48**, 122–33.

O'Connell P.O., Pekkel V., Fuqua A.W. *et al.* (1998) Analysis of loss of heterozygosity in 399 premalignant breast lesions at 15 genetic loci. *J. Natl Cancer Inst.*, **90**, 697–703.

Ohuchi N., Abe R., Kasai M. (1984) Possible cancerous change of intraductal papillomas of the breast: a 3-D reconstruction study of 25 cases. *Cancer*, **54**, 605–11.

Page D.L., Rogers L.W. (1992) Combined and cytologic criteria for the diagnosis of mammary atypical ductal hyperplasia. *Hum. Pathol.*, **23**, 1095–7.

Page D.L., Salhany K.E., Jensen R.A., Dupont W.D. (1996) Subsequent breast carcinoma after biopsy with atypia in a breast papilloma. *Cancer*, **78**, 258–66.

Papotti M., Gugliotta P., Ghiringhello B., Bussolati G. (1984) Association of breast carcinoma and multiple intraductal papillomas: an histological and immunohistochemical investigation. *Histopathology*, **8**, 963–75.

Poremba C., Boecker W., Willenbring H. *et al.* (1998) Telomerase activity in proliferative breast lesions. *Int. J. Oncol.*, **12**, 641–8.

Rosai J. (1991) Borderline epithelial lesions of the breast. *Am. J. Surg. Pathol.*, **15**, 209–21.

Rosen P.P. (1985) Papillary duct hyperplasia of the breast in children and young adults. *Cancer*, **56**, 1611–17.

Rosen P.P., Kimmel M. (1990) Juvenile papillomatosis of the breast; a follow up study of 41 patients having biopsies before 1979. *Am. J. Clin. Pathol.*, **93**, 599–603.

Rosen P.P., Cantrell B., Mullen D.L., DePalo A. (1980) Juvenile papillomatosis (Swiss cheese disease) of the breast. *Am. J. Surg. Pathol.*, **4**, 3–12.

Rosen P.P., Holmes G., Lesser M.L., Kinne D.W., Beattie E.J. (1985) Juvenile papillomatosis and breast carcinoma. *Cancer*, **55**, 1345–52.

Sandison A.T. (1958) A study of surgically removed specimens of breast, with special reference to sclerosing adenosis. *J. Clin. Pathol.*, **11**, 101–9.

Sandison A.T. (1962) *An Autopsy Study of the Adult Human Breast*. National Cancer Institute Monograph No. 8. Washington, DC, US Dept. of Health, Education and Welfare.

Shoker B.S., Jarvis C., Sibson R., Walker C., Sloane J.P. (1999a) Oestrogen receptor expression in the normal and pre-cancerous breast. *J. Pathol.*, **188**, 237–244.

Shoker B.S., Jarvis C., Clarke R.B. *et al.* (1999b) Estrogen receptor positive proliferating cells in the normal and precancerous breast. *Am J Pathol.*, **155**, 1811–15.

Sloane J.P. and members of the National Coordinating Group for Breast Screening Pathology (1994) Consistency of histopathological reporting of breast lesions detected by screening: findings of the UK National EQA Scheme. *Eur. J. Cancer*, **30A**, 1414–19.

Sloane J.P., Amendoeira I., Apostolikas N. *et al.* (1999) Consistency achieved by 23 European pathologists from 12 countries in diagnosing breast disease and reporting prognostic features of carcinomas. *Virchows Archiv.*, **434**, 3–10.

Smith B.H., Taylor H.B. (1969) The occurrence of bone and cartilage in mammary tumors. *Am. J. Clin. Pathol.*, **51**, 610–18.

Swanson Beck J. and members of the Medical Research Council Breast Tumour Pathology Panel (1985) Observer variability in reporting of breast lesions. *J. Clin. Pathol.*, **38**, 1358–65.

Tavassoli F.A. (1998) Ductal carcinoma *in situ*: introduction of the concept of ductal *in situ* neoplasia. *Mod. Pathol.*, **11**, 140–54.

Tavassoli F.A., Norris H.J. (1990) A comparison of the results of long-term follow-up for atypical intraductal hyperplasia and intraductal hyperplasia of the breast. *Cancer*, **65**, 518–29.

Weinstat-Saslow D., Merino M.J., Manrow, R.E. *et al.* (1995) Overexpression of cyclin D mRNA distinguishes invasive and in situ breast carcinoma from non-malignant lesions. *Nat. Med.*, **1**, 1257–60.

Wells W.A., Carney P.A., Eliassen M.S., Tosteson A.N., Greenberg E.R. (1998) Statewide study of diagnostic agreement in breast pathology. *J. Natl Cancer Inst.*, **90**, 142–5

Zhu X.L., Hartwick W., Rohan T., Kandel R. (1998) Cyclin D1 gene amplification and protein expression in benign breast disease and breast carcinoma. *Mod. Pathol.*, **11**, 1082–8.

8 Ductal carcinoma *in situ*

INTRODUCTION

Ductal carcinoma *in situ* (DCIS) is not a single morphological entity but a heterogeneous group of proliferations that vary in cytology and architecture. The frequency with which it is encountered in biopsy and excision specimens has dramatically increased since the introduction of mammographic screening, accounting for about 18% of screen-detected cancers in the UK National Breast Screening Programme (Moss *et al.*, 1995) compared with about 5% of those in symptomatic women. A significantly higher proportion of DCIS is encountered in some North American series and UK breast screening units, largely because of a greater detection of low nuclear grade forms. Symptomatic patients may present with a palpable mass, especially if the tumour is extensive and associated with periductal inflammation and fibrosis. If the major ducts are involved, there may be nipple discharge or Paget's disease.

CLASSIFICATION

Cytological features

At one extreme the cells may be of *high nuclear grade* (Fig. 8.1), exhibiting irregularly spaced, very pleomorphic nuclei with coarse, clumped chromatin, prominent nucleoli and frequent mitoses. The amount of cytoplasm is variable; it is usually palely eosinophilic but may exhibit apocrine, clear cell or, very rarely, signet-ring change (see below). The nuclear-to-cytoplasmic ratio is generally between 1:1 and 1:3. The growth pattern in these cases is usually solid or comedo but may be cribriform, micropapillary or even clinging (see

8.1 Ductal carcinoma *in situ* of high nuclear grade. The nuclei are grossly pleomorphic and exhibit uneven chromatin distribution, prominent nucleoli and thick nuclear membranes. There is individual cell necrosis but no comedo pattern. The surrounding stroma is densely infiltrated by chronic inflammatory cells (bottom) (H&E). (Illustration reproduced with permission from *Human Pathology*).

119

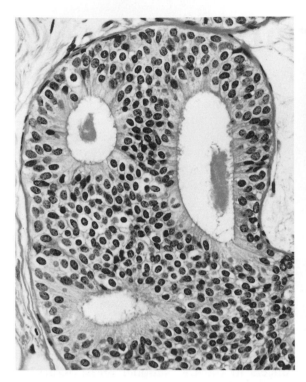

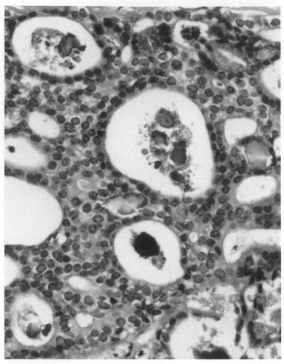

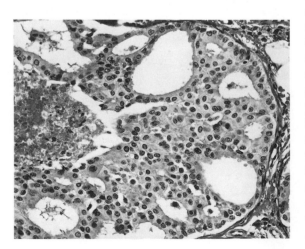

below). Some degree of necrosis is usually present, however, even in the non-comedo cases. Calcification, when present, is dystrophic and amorphous.

At the other extreme the cells may be of *low nuclear grade* (Fig. 8.2), exhibiting monomorphic, regularly spaced and usually hyperchromatic nuclei, with a fine chromatin pattern, inconspicuous nucleoli and few mitoses. The nuclear-to-cytoplasmic ratio is high, almost invariably exceeding unity. The growth pattern is cribriform, micropapillary or clinging, although a solid variant also occurs. Necrosis is uncommon and tends to affect individual cells or small groups. Comedo necrosis is very rare. Calcification, when present, is usually focal and psammomatous (Fig. 8.3).

Not all cells fit the above the descriptions and are said to be of *intermediate nuclear grade*. They show some pleomorphism, but this is not as marked as in those of high nuclear grade (Figs 8.4 and 8.5).

Architectural features

DCIS is described as *solid* when the lumen is replaced by solid masses of neoplastic cells (*see*

Fig. 8.1 above). *Comedo* DCIS exhibits a prominent central zone of necrosis (Fig. 8.6), usually in association with a solid growth pattern but sometimes with a micropapillary or cribriform background (Fig. 8.4). The *cribriform* type is characterized by the presence of secondary luminal spaces, which produce a sieve-like appearance (Figs. 8.2–8.4).

Micropapillary DCIS exhibits finger-like papillary structures that project from the walls of dilated duct-like spaces into the lumina. The papillae may exhibit a fibrovascular core

8.2 (Left) Low nuclear grade ductal carcinoma *in situ*. The cells have small, regular, hyperchromatic nuclei, inconspicuous nucleoli and a high nuclear-to-cytoplasmic ratio. The growth pattern is cribriform, and the cells show marked polarization around the secondary lumina (H&E). (Illustration reproduced with permission from *Human Pathology*.)

8.3 (Right) Low nuclear grade ductal carcinoma *in situ* with a well-developed cribriform growth pattern. The nuclei are slightly larger and less hyperchromatic than in Fig. 8.2, but they are uniform and the nuclear-to-cytoplasmic ratio is high. Many of the larger secondary lumina contain focal deposits of hydroxyapatite. There is cell polarization around the secondary lumina, but it is not as pronounced as in Fig. 8.2. (H&E).

8.4 Intermediate nuclear grade ductal carcinoma *in situ*. Some of the nuclei resemble those in Figs 8.2 and 8.3, but others are larger and more vesicular with discernible small nucleoli. Note that the growth pattern is predominantly cribriform, but there is comedo necrosis on the left of the picture. Cell polarization is present around the secondary lumina (H&E). (Illustration reproduced with permission from *Human Pathology*.)

8.5 Intermediate nuclear grade ductal carcinoma *in situ*. The cells have larger, more vesicular and more pleomorphic nuclei than those in Figs 8.2 and 8.3, and the nuclear-to-cytoplasmic ratio is lower. However, the cells lack the gross pleomorphism seen in the high nuclear grade variants. The lumen is filled with foamy macrophages. This appearance should not be mistaken for comedo necrosis (H&E). (Illustration reproduced with permission from *Human Pathology*.)

8.6 Ductal carcinoma *in situ* of comedo type. The cells have large, pleomorphic nuclei with easily discernible nucleoli. There is an extensive central, comedo-type necrosis (bottom). A small focus of necrosis is also seen among the epithelial cells (arrow). The presence of nuclear debris in the lumen helps to distinguish comedo necrosis from eosinophilic secretion, which is found in some examples of ductal carcinoma *in situ* (H&E).

8.7 Micropapillary ductal carcinoma *in situ* of low nuclear grade. The papilla on the right has a well-developed fibrovascular core covered by polarized, multilayered epithelium, but there is no evidence of a myoepithelial layer. The papillae on the left lack a fibrovascular core (H&E).

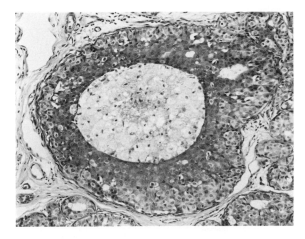

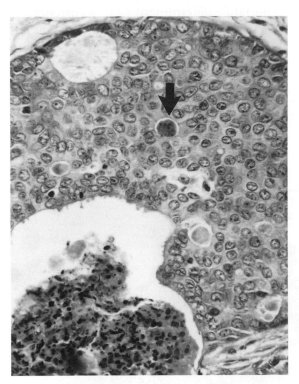

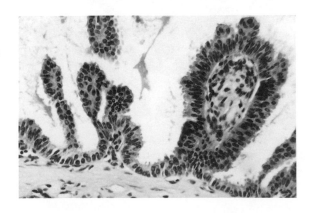

(Fig. 8.7), but generally these are lacking. Papillary processes devoid of epithelium may fuse in the lumen to form peripheral or Roman bridges (Fig. 8.8). The cells do not stream across the bridges as in hyperplasia and are more regularly arranged, often in a double layer. When the nuclei are ovoid they may be arranged at right angles to the direction of the bridge. Most cases of micropapillary DCIS are of low or intermediate nuclear grade but high-grade cases are also encountered (Fig. 8.9).

Encysted papillary DCIS (Fig. 8.10) is a localized tumour in a dilated duct, usually close to the nipple. The papillae in this type often exhibit a fibrovascular core (see below). Azzopardi (1979) drew attention to a type of DCIS that he termed *clinging carcinoma*, which is composed of one or just a few layers of cells lining dilated ducts; the lumen is usually empty, although a few peripheral bridges or micropapillae may be observed (Fig. 8.11). This pattern may merge with other types, making the diagnosis straightforward, but when the low nuclear grade variant occurs alone, it may easily be misinterpreted as benign unless the malignant cytological features are recognized.

Periductal inflammation (*see* Fig. 8.1 above), fibrosis and elastosis may be seen around DCIS, particularly around the high nuclear grade variants. Elastosis is seen less frequently than in infiltrating carcinomas, and its presence should therefore prompt the search for foci of infiltration. The basal lamina surrounding the ducts is usually intact but may be irregularly thickened or highly attenuated. In some places there are gaps in the basal lamina that cannot be identified by conventional light microscopy but may be seen using immunohistological stains for basement membrane components or electron microscopy. At the site of the gaps the tumour cells may show no specific features or may protrude through the defect (Ozzello, 1971) (Fig. 8.12). This should not be interpreted as microinvasion (see below).

Classification systems

The increased detection of DCIS as a result of mammographic screening has been

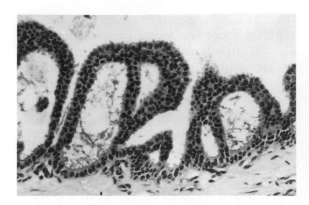

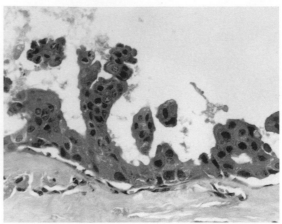

accompanied by an increase in the use of breast-conserving surgery, which, although having an undoubted cosmetic benefit, runs the risk of not eradicating the disease. If left untreated DCIS will develop into invasive carcinoma in a significant proportion of cases, generally within about 10 years of diagnosis (see below). Local recurrence as *in situ* or invasive disease after breast-conserving surgery has been reported in 4–23% of cases depending on the choice of adjuvant treatment (Schnitt *et al.*, 1988). The most important determinant of recurrence is clearly the adequacy of surgical excision, but the pathological assessment of the excision margins is problematic, for the reasons discussed later in this chapter. Histological classifications have thus been devised with the objective of predicting clinical outcome and consequently shaping patient management. In addition to being able to predict the prognosis, an acceptable classification

8.9 (Right) Micropapillary ductal carcinoma *in situ* of high nuclear grade. Note the gross pleomorphism of the nuclei (H&E).

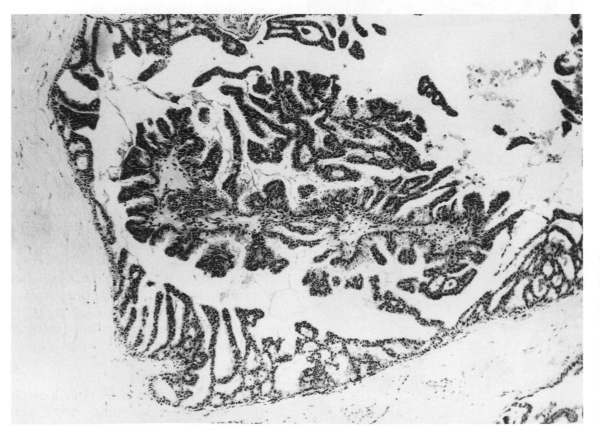

8.10 Encysted papillary ductal carcinoma *in situ*. The wall of the duct can be seen at the left and at the bottom of the picture. The dilated lumen is filled with a papillary proliferation with some fibrovascular cores, mainly in the centre of the lesion (H&E).

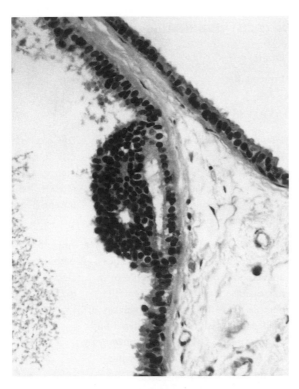

8.11 Clinging variety of ductal carcinoma *in situ* of low nuclear grade. One or two layers of monotonous cells with hyperchromatic nuclei line two adjacent dilated ducts. A solitary multilayered peripheral cellular bridge is seen in the centre of the field (H&E). (Illustration reproduced with permission from Oxford University Press.)

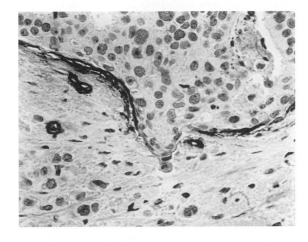

8.12 Paraffin-embedded section of ductal carcinoma *in situ* fixed in methacarn and stained for type IV collagen. There is a breach in the basement membrane through which a small tongue of epithelium protrudes.

al., 1989; Poller *et al.*, 1994; Fisher *et al.*, 1995). Micropapillary types have been found to be more extensive (Patchefsky *et al.* 1989; Bellamy *et al.*, 1993; Lennington *et al.*, 1994).

Architecture is not, however, independent of cytology. About 90% of comedo carcinomas, for example, are of high nuclear grade. Several workers have observed that nuclear grade correlates better with tumour size, microinvasion and local recurrence after surgical excision than with growth pattern (Patchefsky *et al.*, 1989; Lagios 1990), although the relationship between micropapillary architecture and extent of spread may be independent of nuclear grade (Bellamy *et al.*, 1993).

The major problem with architecture-based classification is that more than one growth pattern is found in at least 50% of tumours (Lennington *et al.*, 1994; Fisher *et al.*, 1995). In such cases, most authors classify according to the dominant pattern, generally at least 60–70% of the tumour. Patchefsky *et al.* (1989), however, found that as many as 29% of tumours were difficult to classify as there was no clear dominance of any one pattern; this was more likely to be encountered in larger lesions. Harrison *et al.* (1996) found that 84% of DCIS had a single nuclear grade, whereas only 39% showed a single architectural pattern. Quinn and Ostrowski (1997) also found intralesional nuclear grade to vary significantly less than growth pattern. Furthermore, in DCIS associated with invasive disease, nuclear grade correlates better with the grade of the invasive component than with growth pattern (Goldstein and Murphy, 1996). Given these considerations it is not surprising that classification based on architecture alone is associated with a low level of observer consistency (see below).

In view of these considerations, many new classifications have been proposed over the past 10 years, the histological criteria of the main ones being summarized in Table 8.1 with reference to the illustrations where possible.

Lagios classification
Lagios was one of the first workers to demonstrate that cytological features were more

must also be quick and easy to apply, be in line with current concepts of the nature of the disease and be consistently applicable by many pathologists.

The accepted method of classifying DCIS for many years was based entirely on architecture, and several studies have demonstrated a relationship between this feature and behaviour. Comedo carcinomas have been found to be larger, more frequently associated with microinvasion and more likely to recur after local excision than other types (Patchefsky *et*

TABLE 8.1. Summary of ductal carcinoma *in situ* (DCIS) classifications

Classification (feature[s] assessed)	Grade		
	High	Intermediate	Low
Lagios (nuclear grade, mitoses, necrosis)	*High grade*. Large nuclei (2 red blood cells in diameter) with vesicular chromatin, 1 or more nucleoli and a high mitotic index (2+ mitoses/10 hpf). Extensive linear coagulative necrosis of comedo type is present (**Fig. 8.6**)	*Intermediate grade*. Intermediate nuclei (1–2 red blood cells in diameter) with coarse chromatin, infrequent nucleoli and an intermediate mitotic index (1–2 mitoses/10 hpf). Punctate necrosis may be present (**Fig. 8.5**)	*Low grade*. Small nuclei (1–1.5 red blood cells in diameter) with diffuse chromatin, inapparent nucleoli and a low mitotic index (<1 mitosis/10 hpf) Necrosis absent (**Figs 8.2, 8.3, 8.7, 8.8**)
Tavassoli (cytological atypia, necrosis)	*High grade*. DCIS showing cytological atypia and necrosis. Includes all comedo carcinomas and signet-ring cell variants of intraductal carcinoma and many intraductal apocrine carcinomas. (**Fig. 8.6**)	*Moderate grade*. This category contains three groups. 1) DCIS lacking cellular atypia and forming solid, cribriform or micropapillary patterns with central necrosis. 2) Cribriform, micropapillary or solid patterns with cytologic atypia but no necrosis. 3) DCIS variants showing an admixture of two uniform cell types +/- necrosis. (**Figs 8.4, 8.5**)	*Low grade*. Cribriform and micropapillary patterns. Uniform population of cells lacking necrosis or atypia. (**Figs 8.2, 8.3, 8.7, 8.8, 8.11**)
European Pathologists Working Group (differentiation =nuclear grade & cell polarisation)	*Poorly differentiated*. Nuclei very pleomorphic with irregular outlines and spacing. Chromatin coarse and clumped with prominent nucleoli. Mitoses often seen. Cell polarization absent or minimal. Central necrosis and individual cell necrosis usually present, often associated with amorphous calcification. (**Figs 8.1, 8.6**)	*Intermediately differentiated*. Nuclei mildly or moderately pleomorphic with some variation in size, outline and spacing. Chromatin fine to coarse and nucleoli evident. Occasional mitoses. Cell polarization seen. Central necrosis variable. Individual cell necrosis may be present. Calcifications amorphous or laminated (**Figs 8.4, 8.5**)	*Well differentiated*. Evenly spaced monomorphic nuclei of uniform size and regular outline. Chromatin uniform and fine, nucleoli insignificant and mitoses rare. Polarization of cells marked. Necrosis absent or minimal. Calcifications usually laminated and rarely amorphous (**Figs 8.2, 8.3, 8.7, 8.8, 8.11**)
European Breast Screening Groups (nuclear grade)	*High nuclear grade*. Pleomorphic cells with irregularly spaced and usually large nuclei exhibiting marked variation in size, irregular nuclear contour, coarse chromatin and prominent nucleoli. Mitoses frequent and abnormal forms may be seen. Growth patterns variable but often solid or comedo. Cell polarization rare (**Figs 8.1, 8.6, 8.9**)	*Intermediate nuclear grade*. Mild to moderate nuclear pleomorphism, less than that in high-grade DCIS but without the monotony of the low-grade type. Nucleo-cytoplasmic ratio often high. One or two nucleoli may be identified. Growth pattern usually solid, cribriform or micropapillary. Some degree of cell polarization. (**Figs 8.4, 8.5**)	*Low nuclear grade*. Monomorphic, evenly spaced cells with roughly spherical centrally placed nuclei and inconspicuous nucleoli. Mitoses few. Individual cell necrosis rare. Architecture often micropapillary and cribriform with polarized cells (**Figs 8.2, 8.3, 8.7, 8.8, 8.11**)
Nottingham (necrosis and morphology)	*Pure comedo*. Central lumina containing necrotic debris surrounded by large pleomorphic viable cells in solid masses (**Fig. 8.6**)	*DCIS with necrosis (non-pure comedo)*. Necrotic neoplastic cells within duct lumina but lacking a pure comedo pattern and often showing a cribriform or micropapillary architecture (**Fig. 8.4**)	*DCIS without necrosis*. No necrosis or necrosis limited to a few necrotic or desquamated cells within intraductal lumina. Includes majority of classic cribriform, papillary and micropapillary subtypes (**Figs 8.2, 8.3, 8.5, 8.7, 8.8, 8.11**)

continued

TABLE 8.1. *continued*

Classification (feature[s] assessed)	Grade		
	High	Intermediate	Low
Van Nuys (nuclear grade, necrosis)	*High grade.* Nuclei greater than two red blood cells in diameter, with vesicular chromatin and one or more nucleoli. Comedo necrosis (DCIS with central lumina containing necrotic debris surrounded by large pleomorphic cells or necrotic neoplastic cells within ducts with other architectural patterns e.g. cribriform or micropapillary) usually present but not essential (**Figs 8.1, 8.6, 8.9**)	*Non-high grade with necrosis.* Low-grade nuclei (1–1.5 red blood cells in diameter with diffuse chromatin and inapparent nucleoli) or intermediate-grade nuclei (1–2 red blood cells in diameter with coarse chromatin and infrequent nucleoli) and comedo-type necrosis. No minimum requirement for comedo necrosis but individual necrotic cells not scored (**Fig. 8.4**)	*Non-high grade without necrosis.* Low- or intermediate-grade nuclei and no comedo necrosis (**Figs 8.2, 8.3, 8.5, 8.7, 8.8, 8.11**)
Ottesen *et al* (size, circumscription, stromal fibrosis)	*Tumour forming.* DCIS macroscopically larger than 5 mm with closely related *in situ* formations and the surrounding stroma showing confluent fibrosis	*Diffuse.* DCIS macroscopically and microscopically ill delimited, larger than 5 mm and exhibiting segmental-like extensions. Stromal fibrosis varies from little to moderate	*Microfocal.* DCN measuring 5 mm or less in diameter. Localized to one or a few lobules or ducts

(Reproduced with permission from *Histopathology*.)

predictive of recurrence than was architecture. The system uses a combination of nuclear grade, mitotic activity and necrosis. It was first published with four categories (Lagios *et al.*, 1989) and later revised with three: (1) high grade, (2) intermediate grade, and (3) low grade (Lagios, 1995).

The Armed Forces Institute of Pathology Classification

There are three categories: (1) high grade, (2) moderate grade, and (3) low grade. They are based on cytological atypia and necrosis, the worst group having both, the best neither and the middle category various combinations of these two features (Tavassoli, 1998).

European Pathologists Working Group (EPWG) classification (Holland *et al.*, 1994)

There are three categories: (1) poorly differentiated, (2) intermediately differentiated, and (3) well differentiated, based on nuclear grade

and cell polarization. The second feature refers to the orientation of cells around secondary lumina or over papillae with their apical borders directed towards the lumen.

Classification of the UK National Health Service Breast Screening Programme (NHSBSP) and European Commission (EC) Working Groups (National Coordinating Group for Breast Screening Pathology, 1995; European Commission, 1996).

This is the simplest classification and is derived from that of the EPWG. The lesions are divided into: (1) high nuclear grade, (2) intermediate nuclear grade, and (3) low nuclear grade using exactly the same criteria, but cell polarization is not taken into account. It was felt that this criterion does not always correlate with nuclear grade and might therefore be difficult to apply consistently. At the time of writing, this system is in use in both the UK national and EC-supported breast-screening programmes.

Nottingham classification (Poller *et al.*, 1994)

There are three categories based primarily on necrosis: (1) pure comedo, (2) DCIS with necrosis (non-pure comedo), and (3) DCIS without necrosis. The comedo category, however, also exhibits high nuclear grade cells.

Van Nuys classification (Silverstein *et al.*, 1996)

There are three groups according to nuclear grade and necrosis: (1) high grade (with or without comedo-type necrosis), (2) non-high grade with comedo-type necrosis, and (3) non-high grade without comedo-type necrosis.

Danish Breast Cancer Co-operative Group Classification (Ottesen *et al.*, 1992)

There are three groups according to growth pattern and size: (1) microfocal, (2) diffuse, and (3) tumour-forming. The main problem with this classification is that combinations of growth pattern, particularly of groups (2) and (3), are common. Furthermore, nuclear grade varies significantly within groups.

Ability of classifications to predict clinical outcome

The most important manifestation of treatment failure is arguably the development of metastatic carcinoma, but the most frequently studied is local recurrence as it is generally the only clinical event that occurs with sufficient frequency to obtain statistically significant data. In up to half the cases, however, local recurrence includes an invasive component (Solin *et al.*, 1993; Lagios, 1995; Badve *et al.*, 1998). Using the classification of Lagios (1995) on a series of patients treated with breast-conserving surgery without irradiation and followed up for a mean of 10 years, high-grade DCIS was associated with a local recurrence rate of 32% compared to 10% for intermediate grade and 0% for low grade.

Badve *et al.* (1998) compared the ability of four classifications of DCIS to predict recurrence up to 20 years after local excision. They found an association between local recurrence

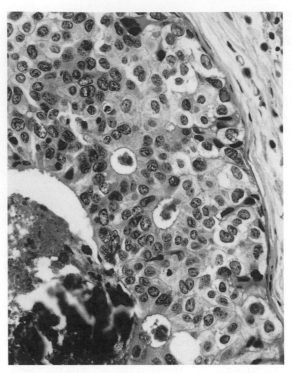

8.13 High nuclear grade ductal carcinoma *in situ* with calcified comedo necrosis at the bottom left of the illustration. This example also shows a marked polarization of cells around the secondary lumina (H&E). (Illustration reproduced with permission from *Human Pathology*.)

and differentiation as defined by the EPWG, but it just failed to reach statistical significance at the 5% level. A stronger and statistically significant correlation was, however, found using the classification of the NHSBSP and EC Working Groups in which nuclear grade is used alone and cell polarization is disregarded. This was caused by a small number of recurring cases with high-grade nuclei being downgraded as a consequence of exhibiting polarized cells (Fig. 8.13). Whether the tumour recurred as *in situ* or invasive carcinoma was unrelated to nuclear grade. A statistically significant difference in recurrence rate after local excision was not found among the three groups of the Nottingham classification. A highly significant correlation with local recurrence rate was, however, found with the three groups of the Van Nuys classification, confirming the earlier findings of Silverstein *et al.* (1995), in which 8-year actuarial disease-free survival was statistically significantly different, at 61%, 84% and 93% respectively. Despite the heterogeneity of nuclear grade in the three groups defined by growth pattern by Ottesen *et al.* (1992), there was a statistically significant correlation with recurrence over a median follow-up period of 53 months. Thus recurrences were seen in 9% of the microfocal, 28% of the diffuse and 38% of the tumour-forming cases.

The time course over which DCIS recurs locally varies with grade. Lagios *et al.* (1989) and Schwartz *et al.* (1992) found the mean time to recurrence to be 24 and 26 months respectively for high-grade DCIS, and 87 and 85 months for low grade. Irradiation appears to delay the recurrence of high-grade DCIS, the mean time to recurrence in the series of Silverstein *et al.* (1990) and Solin *et al.* (1993) being 40 and 42 months, respectively.

Local recurrences occur as either *in situ* or invasive carcinoma, usually in roughly equal number (Silverstein *et al.*, 1998), although no classification to date has been found to be able to determine the probability of developing invasive disease.

In conclusion, most studies have shown nuclear grade to be the best predictor of local recurrence, together with necrosis in some classifications. Specifically identifying comedo necrosis, however, does not appear to be useful. Architecture, including cell polarization, also appears to have little value. The findings of Ottensen *et al.* (1992) are more difficult to interpret in this context, but their scheme relies less on histological features than on lesion size and circumscription. The former has been found to have independent prognostic significance in other studies (see below).

Consistency with which classifications are applied

There is little information at the time of writing on the consistency with which histopathologists can classify DCIS using any of the above schemes. Of the small number of studies that have been undertaken, most have involved few pathologists. Although such studies may be useful in determining the level of agreement that can be achieved within a laboratory, they are inadequate for assessing interlaboratory variation and for determining the reliability of data generated by breast-screening programmes.

In a large study involving 186–251 pathologists over a 3-year period, Sloane *et al.* (1994) found an unacceptably low level of consistency using the architectural classification with an overall κ statistic (*see* Chapter 2) of 0.23. More recently, the 23 pathologists of the EC Working Group on Breast Screening Pathology categorized 33 cases of DCIS and obtained overall κ statistics of 0.37, 0.35 and 0.42 using the EPWG, NHSBSP/EC and Van Nuys classifications respectively (1998). These findings were essentially similar to those of Bethwaite *et al.* (1998), who also found a higher level of consistency using nuclear grade and the Van Nuys system than architecture. In all three-way systems, the lowest values are obtained for the middle categories (Sloane *et al.*, 1998). Consequently, when the NHSBSP/EC system was condensed to two groups (high nuclear grade versus other), a higher κ value of 0.46 was obtained (Sloane *et al.*, 1998). A more recent study (Sloane *et al.*, 1999) has shown that intralesional heterogeneity is a significant cause of inconsistency when classifying by nuclear grade as well as by growth pattern, indicating that an improvement in consistency could be achieved by a stricter assessment of the proportions present.

The relatively high κ value obtained for the Van Nuys classification is probably explained the fact that it involves two dichotomous decisions (high grade versus other, and necrosis versus no necrosis) rather than defining the three groups on a continuous spectrum. A low κ statistic of 0.34 was obtained using the Nottingham classification even when it was condensed to two categories (comedo versus other). The surprising inability to identify comedo DCIS consistently resulted from the difficulty in distinguishing comedo necrosis from eosinophilic secretion in the duct lumen and from non-comedo necrosis.

The most robust histological features thus appear to be high- and low-grade nuclei and necrosis as long as the latter does not involve the recognition of a comedo growth pattern. These features also appear to be most effective in predicting clinical outcome.

Without endorsing any particular system of classification of DCIS, a Consensus Conference Committee meeting in Philadelphia,

USA, concluded that DCIS should be stratified primarily by nuclear grade (Consensus Conference Committee, 1997).

SPECIAL SUBTYPES OF DCIS

Encysted papillary carcinoma

This is a distinctive form of DCIS (*see* Fig. 8.10 above) that represents the malignant counterpart of the intraduct papilloma and usually presents with similar clinical features. The distinction from papilloma may be very difficult and should not be attempted on frozen sections (Haagensen, 1971). Even unequivocally benign-appearing tumours may exhibit malignant zones on further sampling.

The essential points of distinction from papilloma are summarized in Table 7.2. The proliferation usually consists of epithelial cells only; myoepithelial cells are generally lacking and, if present, form only a discontinuous layer. The complete failure to detect a myoepithelial layer, even using appropriate immunohistochemical techniques, almost invariably rules out a papilloma. Fibrovascular cores are often absent and when present are finer than those in intraduct papillomas. The papillomatous processes are covered by a variable number of cells, and the consistent two-layered structure of the papilloma is not seen; even where there is a double cell layer, this is not usually caused by myoepithelial differentiation (*see* Figs 7.11–7.13, and Figs 8.7 and 8.10 above). Immunostaining for smooth muscle actin used to detect myoepithelial cells should be interpreted cautiously as the pericytes of small blood vessels may be very close to the epithelium. Consequently, it is best also to use an antibody to cytokeratin 14 (Fig. 8.14).

In common with other forms of DCIS, encysted papillary carcinomas exhibit the cytological features of malignancy. Nuclear grade is variable: about half the cases exhibit nuclei of intermediate grade, the remainder being approximately equally divided between high and low nuclear grades (Lefkowitz *et al.*, 1994). In some lesions the papillae are covered by tall, pseudostratified, columnar cells with long slender hyperchromatic nuclei (*see* Fig.

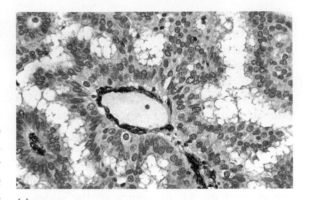

(a)

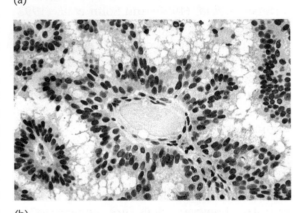

(b)

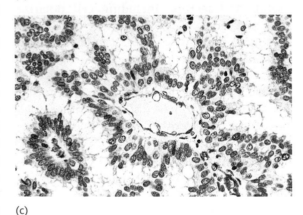

(c)

8.14 (a) Papillary ductal carcinoma *in situ* immunostained for smooth muscle actin. There is a strongly positive layer of cells closely applied to the epithelium, giving the impression of a myoepithelial layer. (b) Same field stained for the myoepithelial marker cytokeratin 14 (LLOO2). (c) Same field immunostained for CD34, revealing a layer of endothelial cells at the site of the actin positivity, which in this case was caused by the pericytes of the dilated vessel in the centre of the fibrovascular core.

8.7 for similar cells). Epithelial multilayering is common, often producing cribriform and micropapillary patterns, as described above. Where glandular spaces occur they have more truncated margins than in papillomas, and apocrine metaplasia is absent. Mitoses vary from few to numerous, abnormal forms occasionally being seen. Necrosis and haemorrhage may be present, but these have little diagnostic significance as they may also be seen in papillomas. The surrounding ducts and terminal duct–lobular units may exhibit more usual forms of DCIS, particularly the micropapillary and cribriform variants.

In short, the major points of distinction from papilloma are the paucity or lack of stroma, the presence of only one cell type, the cytological features of malignancy, the lack of apocrine metaplasia and the presence of obvious DCIS in the neighbouring breast.

Encysted papillary carcinomas, as well as all other types of DCIS, should be adequately sampled in order to search for microscopic foci of invasion. Invasion is, of course, a valuable feature in clinching a diagnosis of malignancy in an equivocal tumour.

In the study by Lefkowitz *et al.* (1994) of 77 cases, 10-year survival was 100% and disease-free survival 91%. Curiously, recurrence did not appear to be related to tumour size or stromal invasion, although the latter could have been caused by undersampling. None of the low nuclear grade tumours recurred. Carter *et al.* (1983) noted that recurrence and the development of invasive disease were related to the presence of DCIS extending from the encysted lesion into the adjacent small and medium-sized ducts.

Apocrine DCIS

Some degree of apocrine differentiation is not uncommon in *in situ* and infiltrating breast carcinomas, but pure apocrine DCIS is rare (Fig. 8.15). The cells exhibit abundant granular eosinophilic cytoplasm, large pleomorphic nuclei and prominent nucleoli. Apical blebbing is, however, not usually seen. Mitoses and necrosis may be present.

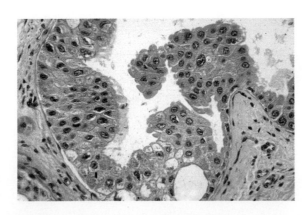

8.15 Apocrine ductal carcinoma *in situ*. The cells have copious granular eosinophilic cytoplasm and large vesicular nuclei. In contrast to the metaplastic cells that line the cysts, however, they exhibit gross nuclear pleomorphism (H&E).

The main diagnostic problem with this variant is distinguishing it from fibrocystic change exhibiting apocrine metaplasia and papillary hyperplasia as benign apocrine cells exhibit large nuclei and prominent nuclei. Benign apocrine cells are, however, uniform and malignant ones pleomorphic, showing a significant variation in the size and shape of nuclei and nucleoli, and and uneven chromatin pattern. Mitoses, particularly abnormal forms, and necrosis are also very useful pointers to malignancy.

Abati *et al.* (1990), studied 55 patients with apocrine DCIS. Local recurrence occurred in 3 of 20 patients treated by biopsy alone but not in 2 patients who received irradiation after the biopsy. All patients treated by mastectomy remained disease free. The authors concluded that the prognosis associated with apocrine DCIS is not significantly different from that associated with the usual forms of the disease. There are, however, significant problems of assessing nuclear grade in this form of intraductal carcinoma given the appearance of non-malignant apocrine cells (see above). The assessments of the extent of disease and the clearance of excision margins are thus especially important (see below).

Like the cells of apocrine cysts, those of apocrine DCIS are usually positive for androgen receptor and negative for oestrogen receptor on immunohistochemical staining (Gatalica, 1997).

Clear cell DCIS

Focal clear cell change is not uncommon in the various types of DCIS, particularly the high nuclear grade forms, but it is rare for the whole lesion to exhibit this appearance (Fig. 8.16). Clear cell DCIS may occur alone or in association with clear cell variants of invasive carcinoma, such as lipid- and glycogen-rich carcinomas. The prognosis associated with clear cell DCIS appears to be the same as that of other forms of DCIS of similar nuclear grade and size.

Neuroendocrine DCIS

This variant is the *in situ* equivalent of the invasive neuroendocrine carcinoma described on p. 191 and was first described by Cross *et al.* (1985). It appears to be less heterogeneous than the invasive form. In the author's experience it causes significant diagnostic difficulties and is not infrequently mistaken for a benign lesion. Clinical presentation is often as a breast lump or nipple discharge (Ashworth and Haqqani, 1986), usually in older women. The average age in the series of Tsang and Chan (1996) was about 70.

The lesion is composed mainly of solid, compact masses of cells permeated by a framework of vascular connective tissue around which the neoplastic cells tend to palisade to form pseudo-rosettes (Fig. 8.17). Elsewhere there may be cellular ribbons, trabeculae and tubular structures (Fig. 8.18). Microglandular spaces and rosettes may be seen. Polypoid masses of tumour cells sometimes project into dilated spaces and may be covered by a layer of attenuated 'normal' epithelium, producing a pagetoid appearance. Pagetoid spread into adjacent ducts may be seen. Necrosis is not a feature, and periductal inflammation and fibrosis are not usually encountered. The cells exhibit uniform, rounded or ovoid nuclei with punctate chromatin and inconspicuous nucleoli (Fig. 8.18). The cytoplasm is eosinophilic and faintly granular or clear; rarely is there a significant quantity of mucin. Some degree of spindle cell differentiation is fairly common. Mitoses are infrequent, with no abnormal forms. Non-endocrine DCIS may be seen in the adjacent ducts.

Grimelius staining is positive in the majority of cases and is generally present in between 30 and 100% of cells (Fig. 8.19). Immunostaining is usually positive for chromogranin A (8.20), synaptophysin and neurone-specific enolase, the reaction being strongest in the areas exhibiting argyrophilia. Variable positivity has been reported for β-human chorionic gonadotrophin, ACTH, corticotrophin-like intermediate lobe peptide and neurotensin. There is usually immunopositivity for oestrogen and progesterone receptors and negativity for p53 and c-erbB-2 (Tsang and Chan, 1996). Ultrastructural examination reveals the presence of typical dense-core granules (Cross *et al.*, 1985).

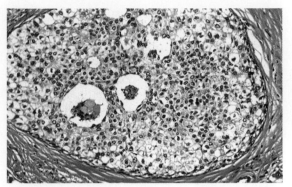

8.16 Clear cell ductal carcinoma *in situ*. There is a largely solid proliferation of high nuclear grade cells with copious clear cytoplasm. There are two small foci of necrosis in the centre of the duct (H&E).

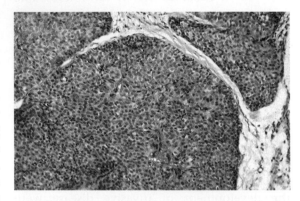

8.17 Neuroendocrine ductal carcinoma *in situ*. The ducts are greatly distended with a solid proliferation of uniform cells permeated by several fibrovascular cores around which the neoplastic cells tend to palisade (H&E).

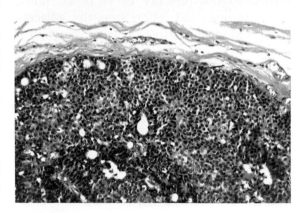

8.18 Neuroendocrine ductal carcinoma *in situ*. In this field there is significant tubule formation (H&E).

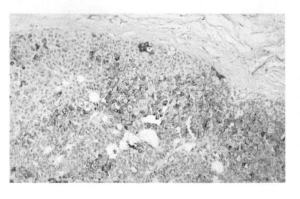

8.19 Neuroendocrine ductal carcinoma *in situ* stained by the Grimelius method. Many of the cells at the periphery of the duct exhibit cytoplasmic argyrophilia.

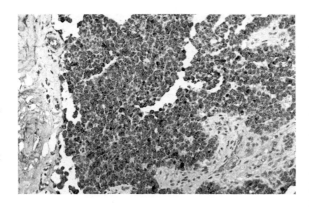

At the time of writing insufficient cases have been reported to make a reliable assessment of prognosis in terms of local recurrence or progression to invasive disease. One of the five patients reported by Tsang and Chan followed for 3–10 years developed *in situ* recurrence. As with other forms of DCIS complete excision should be achieved, and this requires a careful assessment of the excision margins.

Where there is accompanying invasive carcinoma, it tends to be of the neuroendocrine or mucinous type (Tsang and Chan, 1996).

Cystic hypersecretory DCIS

This is a very rare form originally described by Rosen and Scott (1984). Macroscopically, it forms masses generally measuring between 10 and 100 mm composed of multiple cystic structures containing gelatinous material. The gross appearance is occasionally likened to that of juvenile papillomatosis. Histologically, the ducts are markedly distended by densely eosinophilic material, giving a resemblance to

thyroid follicles (Fig. 8.21). The lining epithelium may in some places appear cytologically benign, being composed of flattened, cuboidal or columnar cells, the latter frequently exhibiting vacuolated, eosinophilic cytoplasm. In one case the ducts were lined by columnar mucinous epithelium similar to that seen in the endocervix. Elsewhere there are cytologically malignant cells, usually of low nuclear grade and exhibiting a micropapillary growth pattern (Fig. 8.22). There may occasionally be a leakage of cyst contents into the surrounding stroma, associated with an intense inflammatory reaction.

A diagnosis of malignancy should not be made unless there is unequivocal evidence of DCIS. If only the cytologically benign type of epithelium is found, the term cystic hypersecretory hyperplasia should be used. This is, of course, a diagnosis of exclusion that can only be made after complete excision of the lesion and extensive sampling. Guerry *et al.* (1988) identified four cases of cystic hypersecretory hyperplasia in which the epithelium was at least focally atypical with epithelial crowding, nuclear enlargement and hyperchromasia but no formation of micropapillary carcinoma. These lesions were designated as cystic hypersecretory hyperplasia with atypia. No case was associated with invasive carcinoma.

Of the 29 patients with cystic hypersecretory carcinoma reported by Guerry *et al.* (1988), four also had invasive carcinoma which in three was of high grade and largely devoid of the hypersecretory characteristics. These patients had regional lymph node involvement at presentation, and one had systemic

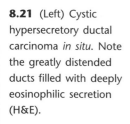

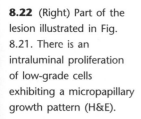

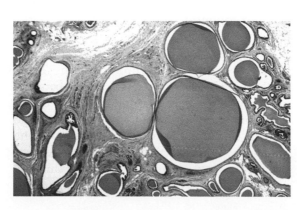

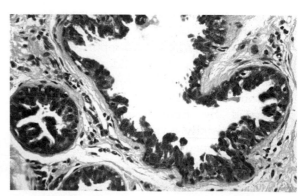

metastases. Where there was intermingling of the *in situ* and invasive components, the cytological features of the two phases exhibited similar features. Patients without invasive disease had an excellent prognosis, none experiencing recurrence. This accords with the generally low nuclear grade of the lesions, but nearly all were treated by mastectomy. Prognostication should be somewhat guarded where patients have undergone local excision.

Secretory (juvenile) DCIS

This is different from the above and represents the *in situ* form of invasive secretory carcinoma. It is an extremely rare variant of DCIS, accounting for only a tiny proportion of secretory carcinomas, of which there are fewer than 100 cases in the literature. Like the invasive form, it is composed of cells of rather bland appearance exhibiting little variation in nuclear size, shape or staining intensity (Fig. 8.23). The cytoplasm is abundant and pale, vacuolated or clear. It usually contains periodic acid–Schiff-positive secretory material and, like the invasive carcinoma, shows positive immunostaining for α-lactalbumin (Fig. 8.24). Mitoses and necrosis are rare.

Mucinous DCIS

Several types of DCIS exhibiting mucinous change have been described, but all are uncommon. Some cases are composed of cells similar to those seen in infiltrating mucinous carcinomas and are associated with a large amount of extracellular, intraductal mucin (Fig. 8.25). Rarely, mucocoele-like tumours may result from mucinous DCIS (*see* p. 86). Intracellular and extracellular mucin may also be seen in tumours exhibiting neuroendocrine differentiation.

Maluf and Koerner (1995) reported a type of DCIS that they called 'solid papillary carcinoma of the breast'. This tumour exhibited a predominantly solid growth pattern but was permeated by fibrovascular cores around which the mildly atypical, small-to-medium-sized cells tended to palisade. Mitotic figures were commonly found, but necrosis was rare. Most tumours contained variably sized extra-

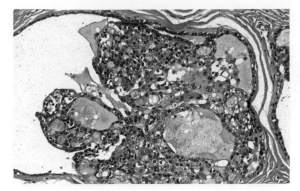

8.23 Secretory (juvenile) ductal carcinoma *in situ*. Note the bland appearance of the nuclei, the copious vacuolated cytoplasm and the large amount of extracellular secretion (H&E).

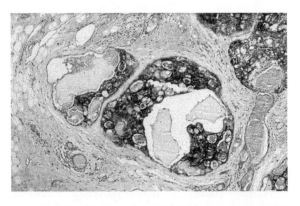

8.24 Same case as in Fig. 8.23 stained for α-lactalbumin by the immunoperoxidase method.

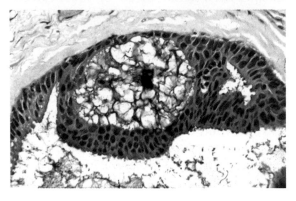

8.25 Mucinous ductal carcinoma *in situ*. The cells have a cytological appearance similar to that of invasive mucinous carcinoma, and there is a large amount of extracellular mucin (H&E).

cellular mucin pools, and intracellular mucin was also common, sometimes being associated with the formation of signet-ring cells. Eleven of 17 cases stained positive for Grimelius, and 8 of 14 positive for chromogranin. These tumours highlight the relationship between mucin production and neuroendocrine differentiation in breast neoplasms, which is also seen in invasive tumours, particularly of the mucinous type. Furthermore, they demonstrate that not all lesions that exhibit a neuroendocrine type of growth pattern show

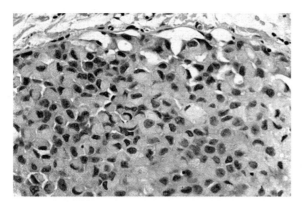

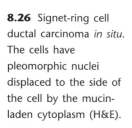

8.26 Signet-ring cell ductal carcinoma *in situ*. The cells have pleomorphic nuclei displaced to the side of the cell by the mucin-laden cytoplasm (H&E).

neuroendocrine differentiation at the cellular level, at least by currently available methods.

Pure signet-ring DCIS has been described but is extremely rare and is characterized by proliferating signet-ring cells, generally arranged in a papillary or solid growth pattern (Fig. 8.26).

As with other special types prognostic data on mucinous variants of DCIS are lacking. They should therefore be evaluated by nuclear grade, size and the adequacy of excision, as for other variants of DCIS.

OTHER PATHOLOGICAL FEATURES OF DCIS THAT ARE RELATED TO RECURRENCE AFTER LOCAL EXCISION

Adequacy of excision

This is clearly the most important determinant of recurrence given that DCIS is almost invariably a unicentric process. Complete local excision is curative, but defining the precise limits of the disease may be difficult or impossible even using combined radiological and histological techniques because of extensive microscopic spread along the duct system. Consequently, the pathological assessment of excision margins, although important, has limitations. Residual tumour may not be present when the margins appear to be involved as the lesion may merely have reached a margin and not actually extended beyond it, or it may have been destroyed by the surgical procedure. A false impression of complete excision may be obtained when the relevant part of the tumour is not included in the sections examined. This is particularly

likely to occur with poorly circumscribed lesions that appear to be multicentric in two-dimensional sections. Re-excision specimens sometimes appear not to contain residual tumour owing to sampling error, giving an erroneous impression that the lesion was originally completely excised.

Using a stereoscopic technique, Faverly *et al.* (1994) found that 8% of DCIS have a multi-focal distribution with gaps greater than 10 mm between foci. This phenomenon was seen exclusively in the low nuclear grade DCIS, the high-grade variant showing continuous growth. They concluded, however, that, with careful examination, the phenomenon is unlikely to lead to a false assessment margin status and should not discourage the use of conserving treatment for eradicable DCIS.

Fisher *et al.* (1995) reviewed histological material from the United States National Surgical Adjuvant Breast Project and divided cases into those in which the margins were thought to be involved and those in which they were not. Margin involvement was regarded as transection of the tumour; lesions that were described as 'close' or 'too close' were regarded as being completely excised. During a mean follow-up period of 48 months, recurrences were observed after lumpectomy alone in 11% of patients with free margins and in 25% of those where they were involved. For patients who had received adjuvant radiotherapy, the corresponding figures were 4% and 10%. Similar findings were obtained by Lagios *et al.* (1989), a recurrence rate of 10% being encountered in non-irradiated patients in whom excision was considered to be complete by histological examination, radiographic–pathological correlation and post-operative mammography.

Solin *et al.* (1993) reviewed cases from many centres and found that where DCIS extended to within 2 mm of the margin, recurrence occurred in 12% compared to 4% of those whose tumour was greater than this distance away. The difference was not, however, statistically significant. In the study of Silverstein *et al.* (1990), 26 patients with DCIS underwent re-excision of their disease. In 10 the initial biopsy had clear but close margins and none exhibited residual tumour in the re-excision specimens. The remaining 16 patients had involved margins, and in five of these residual tumour was found.

It has thus generally been found that the pathological assessment of margin involvement correlates with the presence of residual DCIS in the breast and clinical recurrence, although the correlation is far from perfect. The accuracy of prediction depends upon a number of factors, including the care with the specimen is examined, the number of blocks taken, the length of time the patient is followed up and how adequacy of excision is defined.

Lesion size

Lagios *et al.* (1989) found a relationship between lesion size and recurrence after local excision of DCIS, but this was not confirmed by Fisher *et al.* (1995), probably because the number of tumours greater than 10 mm was relatively small in this study. Silverstein *et al.* (1996) found that size was an important determinant of recurrence after local excision (see below). The degree of circumscription of the tumour is also likely to be important, as circumscribed tumours are easier to excise; circumscription may, however, be difficult to evaluate.

Consistency studies have shown a wide range in size measurement in most cases of DCIS, but histograms generally show that the measurements are often tightly grouped and that the wide ranges are caused by a small number of outlying results. There is, however, a significant number of cases in which there is a genuine lack of agreement on size. In a large study carried out in the UK National Breast Screening Programme, 80% of the size estimates fell within 3 mm of the median in only 8 of 17 cases (Sloane *et al.*, 1994). In the remaining nine cases the measurements were more variable. A more recent study has shown that DCIS is measured less consistently than invasive carcinoma (Sloane *et al.*, 1998).

Several reasons for variation in size measurement were identified:

1. The lesion varied significantly in the different sections circulated to the participating pathologists.

2. The DCIS merged with atypical ductal hyperplasia, leading to uncertainty about whether to include the latter in the measurement and about where one process stopped and the other began.

3. Widely dispersed foci of tumour occurred rather than compact masses.

4. There were different dimensions in different planes.

5. A tendency existed to round measurements up or down, usually to the nearest 5 mm.

A prognostic index for DCIS

It is likely that the most accurate prognostication will be achieved using several features combined into some form of index akin to the Nottingham Prognostic Index used successfully for invasive carcinoma (*see* p. 223). Silverstein *et al.* (1996) recently devised an index based on tumour size, excision margin width and the Van Nuys classification (see above), each receiving a score of 1–3. For size a score of 1 was given for tumours 15 mm or less in diameter, 2 for those 16–40 mm and 3 for those over 40 mm. For excision margins a score of 1 was given where the tumour-free margin exceeded 10 mm, 2 where it was 1–9 mm and 3 where it was less than 1 mm. Using the Van Nuys classification, a score of 1 was given for non-high nuclear grade lesions without comedo-type necrosis, 2 for non-high nuclear grade with comedo-type necrosis and 3 for high nuclear grade lesions with or without comedo-type necrosis. Cases were then divided into three groups with an aggregate score of 3–4, 5–7 and 8–9 respectively.

Recurrence-free survival was predicted more accurately by the index than by any of the three constituent pathological variables alone. Furthermore, it was found that patients with a prognostic index score of 3–4 did not show a local disease-free survival benefit from breast irradiation, whereas those with a score of 5–7 benefited significantly from adjuvant radiotherapy. Although patients with scores of 8 and 9 also benefited from irradiation, the recurrence rate after local excision was extremely high, even where radiotherapy was given, suggesting that mastectomy is most appropriate for these patients. At the time of writing these findings are in need of independent validation.

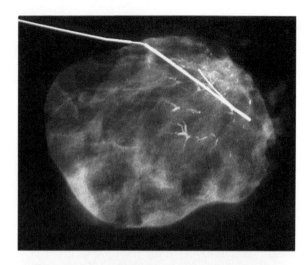

8.27 Specimen radiograph exhibiting a zone of coarse branching calcification. Histological examination revealed a high nuclear grade ductal carcinoma *in situ* with a predominantly comedo growth pattern.

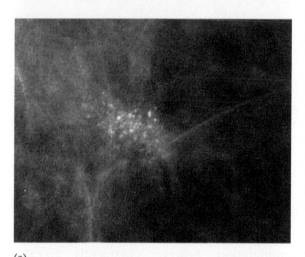

(a)

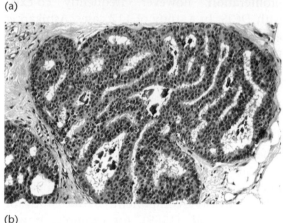

(b)

8.28 (a) Clinical mammogram showing a small zone of fine granular calcification. (b) Histological section of the calcified area showing low nuclear grade cribriform ductal carcinoma *in situ* with foci of intraluminal calcification.

RADIOLOGICAL FEATURES OF DCIS

DCIS is usually detected as microcalcification by clinical mammography. This, associated with the high nuclear grade variants, particu-

lar those of comedo growth pattern, is either coarsely granular or linear, the latter often with a branching pattern (Fig. 8.27). These correspond to the amorphous-type calcifications on histology (*see* Fig. 8.13 above). The low-grade variants usually exhibit finely granular calcification (Fig. 8.28), which corresponds to clusters of laminated, crystalline calcifications on histology (*see* Fig. 8.3 above). Encysted papillary carcinomas usually present as well-circumscribed radiological densities, sometimes with satellite nodules and occasionally with calcification (Soo *et al.*, 1995). Reiff *et al.* (1994) described seven cases of DCIS appearing as a stellate mass on radiography without calcification. In four cases the appearance was caused by a complex sclerosing lesion with associated DCIS, whereas in the other three it was due to the DCIS alone.

Based on the extent of calcification, mammography usually underestimates the extent of DCIS, the extent of the discrepancy being related to histological type. Holland *et al.* (1990) found a discrepancy of more than 20 mm in 16% of comedo DCIS and 47% of micropapillary/cribriform types. Specimen radiography should not therefore be used alone to assess either the size or adequacy of excision of DCIS.

MICROANATOMICAL ORIGIN OF DCIS

The term ductal carcinoma *in situ* implies that it arises from the breast ducts rather than the lobules. This is often assumed to be the case in view of the size of the structures involved and is sometimes undoubtedly true, particularly with encysted papillary lesions and some solid tumours associated with nipple discharge or Paget's disease. When DCIS is still relatively small and isolated, however, it usually has a lobular architecture, albeit markedly distended (Fig. 8.29).

Wellings *et al.* (1975) used a subgross technique to examine a large number of whole human breasts. Thin, stained slices of breast tissue were examined with a dissecting microscope, and the lesions identified were subjected to histological examination. They found that hyperplasia and DCIS generally exhibited a lobular architecture and that a continuous spectrum of change could be observed from normal lobules through varying grades of hyperplasia and atypical ductal hyperplasia to *in situ* carcinoma. In the progression to DCIS there was increasing distension and unfolding of the lobule, which came to resemble the interlobular ducts. Spread along the duct system undoubtedly occurs, making the point of origin more difficult to assess in more advanced lesions.

Despite the currently used terminology, the distinction between ductal and lobular carcinoma *in situ* is thus based on architectural and cytological features rather than the site of origin. The distinction is important in view of the significant difference in biological behaviour between the two entities (*see* Chapter 9).

MULTICENTRICITY IN DCIS

Multicentricity has been defined as foci of tumour more than 50 mm from the main tumour mass or as tumour in more than one quadrant. As thus defined it occurs in about one third of patients and is found more frequently in larger tumours, being uncommon in lesions less than 25 mm in size (Brown *et al.*, 1976; Lagios *et al.*, 1982). It is, however, extremely difficult or impossible in most cases to distinguish extensive intraductal spread from multicentricity in two-dimensional histological sections. This is particularly true if there is communication between glandular trees, as reported by Ohtake *et al.* (1995), who identified ductal anastomoses, mainly in the vicinity of the nipple. If DCIS were truly multicentric, bilaterality should be seen in a significant number of cases, and *in situ* or invasive recurrences should be common in the contralateral breast or in remote sites in the ipsilateral breast. Unlike lobular carcinoma *in situ*, however, DCIS is rarely bilateral. Two out of the 28 cases in the series of Millis and Thynne (1975) were bilateral, but there were none out of 58 in the combined series of Rosen *et al.* (1980) and Page *et al.* (1982). Recurrence after local excision of DCIS almost invariably occurs near the site of previous surgery (see below), and

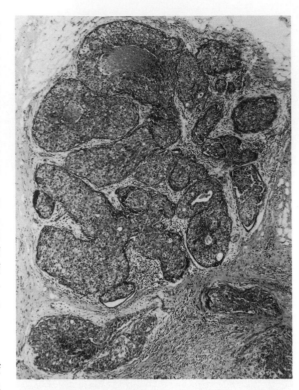

8.29 Small ductal carcinoma *in situ* of the comedo type. Note the lobular architecture (H&E).

initial and recurrent lesions show a high degree of concordance of genetic abnormalities, as determined by comparative genomic hybridization (Waldman *et al.*, 2000). It thus appears that DCIS is rarely multicentric.

Other forms of intraduct and intralobular proliferation, however, frequently co-exist with DCIS. In a study of 112 cases, Ashikari *et al.* (1971) found hyperplasia or atypical hyperplasia in 75% and lobular carcinoma *in situ* in 21%.

MICROINVASION

The term microinvasion has been used in different ways by different authors. Some have used it without definition, whereas others have stipulated precisely the maximum extent of the invasive component. In the study of Schwartz *et al.* (1989), for example, it was defined as comprising no more than 10% of the whole tumour mass. For the purposes of European breast screening programmes (UK National Co-ordinating Group for Breast Screening Pathology, 1995; European Commission, 1996), a microinvasive carci-

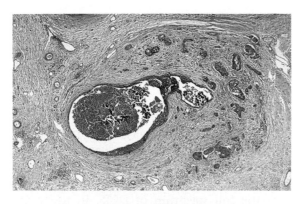

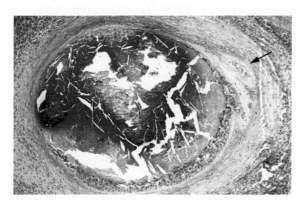

8.30 Comedo ductal carcinoma *in situ* partly surrounded by microinvasive carcinoma. In no place does the invasive component extend more than 1 mm from the basement membrane of the duct.

8.31 Comedo ductal carcinoma *in situ* surrounded by dense fibrosis and chronic inflammation. At one point the fibrosis has encroached on the duct wall, entrapping malignant epithelium and giving an impression of invasion (arrow) (H&E).

noma is defined as follows. It is a tumour in which the dominant change is DCIS but in which there are one or more clearly separate foci of infiltration of non-specialized interlobular or interductal stroma, none measuring more than 1 mm (approximately two high-power fields) in maximal diameter (Fig. 8.30).

This is a very restrictive definition, so tumours fulfilling the criteria are consequently rare, although the incidence is clearly dependent on the extent of sampling. Where there is sufficient doubt about the presence of invasion, the case should be regarded as DCIS. Where the evidence is equivocal, tumours should be regarded as possibly microinvasive. Possible microinvasion includes islands of apparently separate malignant epithelium embedded in periductal fibrosis or inflammation, where the true boundary of the specialized stroma is not clear. It excludes breaches in the basement membrane identified solely by electron microscopy, histochemistry or immunohistology (*see* Fig. 8.12 above) and lesions where there is demonstrable continuity between the putatively invasive focus and the parent DCIS (Fig. 8.31). Microinvasion is more frequently encountered in DCIS of high nuclear grade.

The prognosis of microinvasive carcinoma has not been extensively investigated as most centres are unable to assemble sufficient cases to obtain statistically significant data. Silverstein *et al.* (1993), however, compared the clinical outcome of 47 patients with microinvasive carcinoma defined as above with 285 patients with DCIS alone. They found that microinvasive carcinomas tended to be larger, had a slightly higher average nuclear grade and were more often of the comedo type. As a consequence of these features, they were more likely to be treated by mastectomy. No differences were observed between patients with non-invasive and microinvasive carcinomas in terms of recurrence and 7-year disease-free or overall survival.

Cases in which the invasive foci are significantly in excess of 1 mm should be classified as invasive carcinomas, but two tumour measurements should be given: the size of the invasive component and that of the whole lesion to include the DCIS. Together with a description of the number, size and distribution of the invasive foci, these measurements should give the clinician enough information on which to base an appropriate management strategy. Lagios *et al.* (1989) found that foci of occult invasion were more likely to be found in association with larger lesions, being confined to breasts in which the extent of DCIS exceeded 45 mm and occurring in 50% of breasts where the lesion was 55 mm or greater. Occult invasion was not seen where the lesion measured less than 25 mm. For a discussion of invasive carcinomas with an extensive intraduct component, the reader is referred to p. 173.

METASTASIS AND DCIS

Most studies report examples of metastatic spread, the precise incidence of which is difficult to assess although it appears to be about 1–2% (Ashikari *et al.*, 1971; Westbrook and Gallager, 1975; Lagios *et al.*, 1982). Invasion or microinvasion is not always found in these cases even after extensive sampling, but it is presumed to be present either in association with the DCIS itself or as a separate subclinical lesion. Perhaps the minute protrusions through the basement membrane seen on electron microscopy or immunohistochemistry give rise to metastases in very rare cases.

INCIDENCE OF DCIS

Pure DCIS is not a very common symptomatic lesion, accounting for about 5% of breast carcinomas that present clinically. It accounts, however, for about 15–20% of cancers detected by mammographic screening in the UK and most other European countries (see above). A higher proportion is encountered in some North American series and UK centres, apparently because of the detection of a larger number of low nuclear grade cases (Recht *et al.*, 1998). Sandison (1962) found DCIS in only 1 out of 776 autopsies performed on subjects of all ages without any history of breast disease. Wellings *et al.* (1975) used much more extensive sampling techniques in autopsy cases, cutting the breast into 5–150 2 mm slices. Suspicious lesions were then selected by staining the slides with haematoxylin and examining them under the dissecting microscope. DCIS was found in 4% of breasts examined in this way.

Kramer and Rush (1973) also used very extensive sampling and found DCIS in 5.7% of autopsies performed on women over the age of 70. This represented an incidence 19 times greater than that of clinically overt infiltrating carcinoma in patients of this age group. Welch and Black (1997) reviewed seven autopsy series of women not known to have had breast cancer in life and found a median prevalence of DCIS of 8.9%, which was highest in the 40–70-year-old age group. The number of slides examined per breast ranged from 9 to 275, and, not surprisingly, a higher level of scrutiny tended to discover more cases. The median incidence of invasive cancer was 1.3%. These findings indicate that, even in the presence of mammographic screening, most cases of DCIS remain undetected.

NATURAL HISTORY OF DCIS

The natural history of DCIS has been difficult to establish as all cases presenting clinically or mammographically have been treated by local excision or mastectomy. In two ingenious but laborious studies, DCIS was identified as a diagnostic error in a very large number of benign breast biopsies. As diagnostic errors these tumours were, not surprisingly, largely of low nuclear grade and thus did not represent the full spectrum of DCIS. In the series of Betshill *et al.* (1978), later updated by Rosen *et al.* (1980), 30 cases of DCIS were identified among 8000 benign breast biopsies. Follow-up data were available on 15 patients. Ten developed clinical carcinoma of the ductal type, on average 10 years after biopsy. This gives an incidence of 67% if only the patients who were followed up are included, or 33% if those without follow-up data are assumed not to have developed subsequent carcinoma.

Page *et al.* (1982) reviewed 11 760 biopsies and found 28 cases of DCIS. Follow-up data were available on all patients, seven developing invasive carcinoma 3–10 years later. The invasive tumours always appeared in the ipsilateral breast in the same or an adjacent quadrant. Three patients were followed for less than 3 years, and, if these were excluded, the incidence of subsequent invasive carcinoma was 28%. Quoting a previous study in which it was found that 40% of DCIS were removed in their entirety by the biopsy technique alone, Page *et al.* (1982) concluded that their best estimate of any residual DCIS becoming invasive was about 50%. This figure accords with studies of DCIS treated by local excision, in which about 50% of recurrent cases are associated with an invasive component (see above).

PAGET'S DISEASE OF THE NIPPLE

Paget's disease presents clinically with roughening, reddening and erosion of the nipple. Histologically, large, pale-staining malignant cells are seen singly or in nests within the epidermis, especially in the lower half (Fig. 8.32). The cells are also occasionally seen in

8.32 (Left) Paget's disease of the nipple. The epidermis is extensively infiltrated by large, pale-staining malignant cells (H&E).

8.33 (Right) Paget's disease of the nipple. The malignant cells are not as readily distinguished from the epidermal cells as in Fig. 8.32, and there is some resemblance to Bowen's disease (H&E).

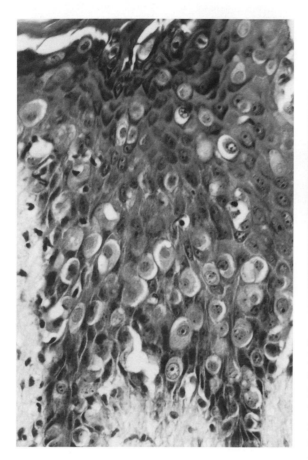

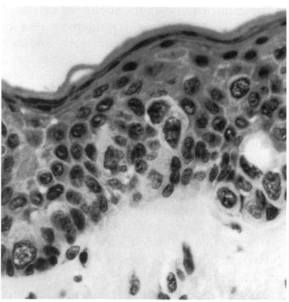

skin appendages and, in more advanced cases, may extend into the epidermis of the areola and adjacent breast skin.

The cells are usually easy to distinguish from normal epidermal cells by their clear cytoplasm and positive staining for mucin. Clear cytoplasm and mucin positivity are, however, not always present and the lesion may occasionally resemble Bowen's disease, exhibiting full-thickness epidermal dysplasia, a loss of nuclear polarity and marked cytological anaplasia (Rayne and Santa Cruz, 1992) (Fig. 8.33). Histological features that are useful in distinguishing anaplastic Paget's from Bowen's disease are the frequent presence of cleft-like acantholysis, the absence of dyskeratotic cells and the persistence of the basal layer in the former. Rare examples are associated with increased melanin pigmentation and may be mistaken for malignant melanoma, both clinically and histologically.

Immunohistological staining for low molecular weight keratins is very useful as the Paget cells are positive, in contrast to the negative keratinocytes that express keratins of higher molecular weight (Fig. 8.34). Immunostains for epithelial membrane antigen are also useful; the Paget cells exhibit intense membrane and cytoplasmic positivity compared to the weak or negative staining of the keratinocytes. Melanocytes are negative for epithelial membrane antigen and keratins. The great majority of cases show positive immunostaining for c-erbB-2 (Fig. 8.35), and about one third show immunopositivity for p53 (Kanitakis *et al.*, 1993).

Ultrastructurally, Paget cells exhibit fairly prominent cytoplasmic organelles and may contain occasional melanosomes. Desmosomes may be seen between adjacent Paget cells as well as between Paget cells and keratinocytes. Intracytoplasmic lumina are rare.

Paget's disease is almost invariably associated with an underlying DCIS involving the collecting ducts and lactiferous sinuses (Fig. 8.36). It is usually of high nuclear grade and may be associated with invasive carcinoma. There is occasionally also lobular *in situ* carcinoma. About 2% of breast carcinomas are associated with Paget's disease (Fisher *et al.*, 1975), most, not surprisingly, being subareolar in location. Paget's disease is associated with a greater frequency of apparently multicentric carcinoma (Fisher *et al.*, 1975).

There has been dispute about the origin of Paget cells. Some have considered them to arise locally within the epidermis, and the presence of occasional melanosomes and desmosomal contacts with keratinocytes would seem to support this view. The melanocyte colonization of infiltrating carcinomas has been observed, however, and neoplastic cells may acquire melanin pigment. Furthermore, there would seem to be no reason why Paget cells should not establish contact with adjacent keratinocytes. Ozzello (1971) concluded that the ultrastructural features of Paget cells were insufficiently distinctive to determine their origin. However, the almost invariable presence of an underlying breast carcinoma, the mucin positivity and the immunohistochemical staining profile tend to support the generally held view that they represent intraepidermal spread from underlying DCIS.

MOLECULAR STUDIES OF DCIS

Oestrogen and *progesterone* receptors are demonstrable by immunohistology in between a third and a half of all cases of DCIS, being significantly associated with low and intermediate nuclear grade and cribriform, solid and micropapillary growth patterns (Fig. 8.37). Steroid receptor expression is uncommonly seen in cases exhibiting high nuclear grade, comedo necrosis and c-erbB-2 or p53 expression (Giri *et al.*, 1989; Poller *et al.*, 1993; Bobrow *et al.*, 1995).

Studies of proliferation markers show, not surprisingly, that a low proliferation rate is associated with low nuclear grade and the absence of comedo necrosis (Bobrow *et al.*, 1995). An increased level of *cyclin D1* mRNA has been found in 76–83% of cases of low- and high-grade DCIS (Weinstat-Saslow *et al.*, 1995). Using a monoclonal antibody, Gillett *et al.* (1998) found cyclin D1 overexpression in 64% of cases of DCIS with no relationship to oestrogen receptor expression or nuclear grade. Others, however, have found that although cyclin D1 may be detected in oestrogen receptor-negative cases, it is more likely to

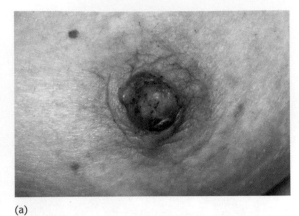

(a)

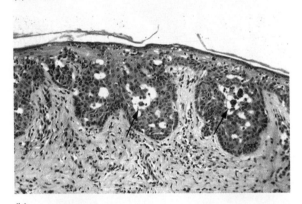

(b)

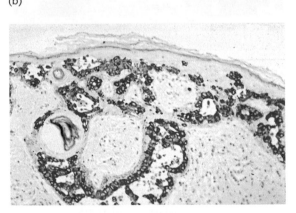

(c)

8.34 Pigmented Paget's disease. (a) The nipple shows erosion, crusting and patchy pigmentation. (b) There are numerous atypical cells within the epidermis, but only a few are identifiable at this power. The rete pegs are markedly distended and contain melanophages, particularly on the right of the illustration (arowed). (c) Immuno-alkaline phosphatase stain for low molecular weight keratins, revealing the epithelial nature of the infiltrating cells. Immunostaining for S100 was negative. An underlying ductal carcinoma *in situ* was later discovered.

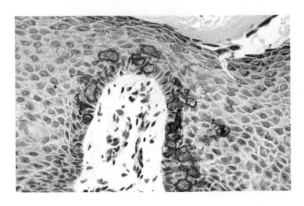

8.35 Paget's disease stained immuno-histochemically with an antibody to c-erbB-2, showing intense positivity of the tumour cells.

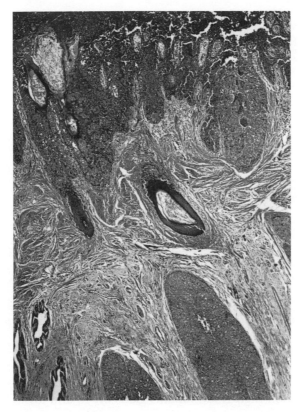

8.36 Paget's disease of the nipple. The epidermis is extensively infiltrated (top). Ductal carcinoma *in situ* is seen at the bottom right. Note the residual normal lactiferous sinuses at the bottom left (H&E).

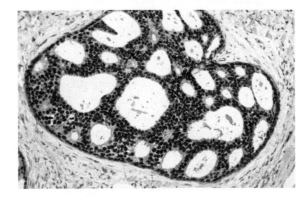

Fig.8.37 Low nuclear grade ductal carcinoma *in situ* stained immuno-histochemically for oestrogen receptors, showing intense and extensive nuclear positivity.

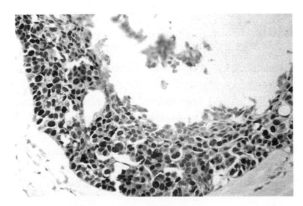

8.38 High nuclear grade ductal carcinoma *in situ* stained immuno-histochemically for p53, showing extensive and intense nuclear positivity.

be found in oestrogen receptor-positive cells (Shoker, in preparation).

c-erbB-2 expression is seen in 40–70% of cases of DCIS, where it is strongly associated with high nuclear grade and mitotic rate, as well as the presence of comedo necrosis and periductal lymphocytic infiltration (Ramachandra *et al.*, 1990). Positivity is almost invariably seen in cases of Paget's disease (*see* Fig. 8.35 above). The incidence of positivity is higher than in invasive carcinomas, in which it is found in only 15–30%. The reasons for this difference are not properly understood but may be related to the fact that a higher proportion of cases of DCIS that are detected clinically or radiologically are of high nuclear grade. Positivity for c-erbB-2 in DCIS has been reported to be related to the extent of spread (De Potter *et al.*, 1995). Amplification of the *c-erbB-2* gene may be detected directly by fluorescence *in situ* hybridization (FISH), increased number of hybridization signals being seen in each nucleus.

Gobbi *et al.* (2000) reported an inverse correlation between DCIS grade and the immunohistochemically detected expression of *transforming growth factor-β type II*.

p53 immunostaining is found in about between a quarter and a third of cases of DCIS (Fig. 8.38) (Poller *et al.*, 1993; Bobrow *et al.*, 1995) and, like that of c-erbB-2, is seen predominantly in lesions of high nuclear grade, although there appears to be only a weak association with c-erbB-2 expression and the lack of steroid receptors. The anti-apoptosis molecule bcl-2, which is consistently expressed in normal breast epithelium, hyperplasia of usual type, atypical ductal hyperplasia and lobular *in situ* neoplasia, is variably expressed in DCIS, mainly in low- and intermediate-grade lesions and in the absence of p53 positivity. High-grade DCIS showing p53 positivity is usually but not invariably negative for bcl-2 (Siziopikou *et al.*, 1996).

Immunostaining for the nm23 gene product was found by Simpson *et al.* (1994) to be surprisingly greater in comedo than in non-comedo types of DCIS. Less surprisingly, however, a greater expression was seen in comedo cases that were purely *in situ* than in those which were associated with invasion.

In contrast to lobular carcinoma *in situ*, immunostaining for *E cadherin* is usually positive in DCIS (Moll *et al.*, 1993).

Immunostaining with *antibodies to endothelial cells* reveals the formation of new stromal vessels in DCIS as well as in invasive carcinoma. As the development of invasive disease depends, *inter alia*, upon the ability of the tumour to stimulate the formation of new blood vessels, it has been argued that neovascularization around *in situ* carcinoma could be one of the first steps in invasion and consequently a prognostic indicator. Using antibodies to factor VIII-related antigen, Engels *et al.* (1997) observed two distinct vascular patterns: a diffuse increase in stromal vascularity between duct lesions and a garland-like rim of microvessels around individual ducts adjacent to the basement membrane. They argued that the first pattern might be caused by angiogenic factors released from stromal cells and the second by the tumour cells themselves.

Teo *et al.* (submitted and in preparation) found that the small blood vessels surrounding ducts involved by DCIS were less likely to be positive for factor VIII-related antigen and more likely to be positive for CD34 than those surrounding normal ducts and acini, indicating a change in phenotype. Vascular density was greatest in cases of intermediate nuclear grade and correlated negatively with duct size and the degree of tumour necrosis, suggesting that angiogenesis increases with the growth rate of DCIS but is unable to keep pace with the most rapidly growing lesions. Cases that subsequently recurred exhibited greater vascular density than those which did not, and among the recurring cases, those accompanied by invasive disease exhibited the greatest vascular density.

Stromelysin-3 protein and mRNA have been detected by immunohistology and by *in situ* hybridization, respectively, in a proportion of *in situ* carcinomas, particularly comedo DCIS. Non-comedo DCIS and lobular carcinoma *in situ* are less frequently positive (Wolf *et al.*, 1993; Basset *et al.*, 1994). Localization is often to fibroblasts immediately surrounding the tumour cells.

Using the microdissection of formalin-fixed, paraffin-embedded sections and the polymerase chain reaction, *loss of heterozygosity* (allelic imbalance, AI) (*see* Fig. 7.4) has been demonstrated at loci on chromosomes 17p, 17q and 16q in DCIS, with a frequency similar to that observed in invasive carcinoma (Stratton *et al.*, 1995). The region of the *BRCA1* gene is frequently involved (Munn *et al.*, 1996). O'Connell *et al.* (1998) studied AI in 137 cases of DCIS at 15 loci and found that it was present in 70–80% of cases. A substantial rate of loss (up to 37%) was observed at loci on chromosomes 16q, 17p and 17q. Where invasive carcinoma was also present, DCIS shared AI at one or more loci with the invasive component in 80% of cases.

Studies using *comparative genomic hybridization* have shown multiple changes involving nearly all the chromosomes, the number increasing with nuclear grade. In the study of Buerger *et al.* (1999), an average of 2.5 abnormalities was found in low, 5.5 in intermediate and 7.1 in high nuclear grade DCIS. In the non-high-grade variants gains on 1q and losses on 11q and 16q were common, whereas in the high-grade cases gains were found on 1q, 5p, 8q and 17q and losses on 8p, 13q, 11q and 14q. The significantly higher frequency of 16q losses in the non-high-grade cases argued strongly against the evolution of high-grade DCIS from lower-grade lesions and in favour of separate histogenetic pathways. In DCIS associated with invasive disease, the changes in the *in situ* and invasive components were generally the same.

FISH studies on formalin-fixed, paraffin-embedded sections using pericentromeric probes have shown aneusomy (an abnormal number) of chromosomes 1, 16, 17, 18 and X, similar to that seen in invasive carcinoma (Micale *et al.*, 1994). Murphy *et al.* (1995) observed frequent gains of chromosomes 3, 10 and 17 and losses of chromosome 18. Amplification of the *c-erbB-2* gene was observed in about 25% of cases. An examination of paired specimens from the same case showed shared genetic alterations and also some unique ones, indicating clonal diversity within tumours. Molecular genetic changes in DCIS thus appear to exhibit the same degree of complexity as those in invasive carcinoma.

REFERENCES

Abati A.D., Kimmel M., Rosen, P.P. (1990) Apocrine mammary carcinoma. A clinico-pathologic study of 72 cases. *Am. J. Clin. Pathol.*, **94**, 371–7.

Ashikari R., Hajdu S.I., Robbins G.F. (1971) Intraductal carcinoma of the breast (1960–1969). *Cancer*, **28**, 1182–7.

Ashworth M.T., Haqqani M.T. (1986) Endocrine variant of ductal carcinoma *in situ* of the breast: ultrastructural and light microscopical study. *J. Clin. Pathol.*, **39**, 1355–9.

Azzopardi A.G. (1979) *Problems in Breast Pathology.* London, W.B. Saunders.

Badve S., A'Hern R., Ward A.M. *et al.* (1998) A long-term comparative study of the ability of 5 classifications of ductal carcinoma *in situ* of breast to predict local recurrence after surgical excision. *Hum. Pathol.*, **29**, 915–23.

Basset P., Wolf C., Rouyer N., Bellocq J.-P., Rio M.-C., Chambon P. (1994) Stromelysin-3 in stromal tissue as a control factor in breast cancer behaviour. *Cancer*, **74**, 1045–9.

Bellamy C.O., McDonald C., Salter D.M., Chetty U., Anderson T.J. (1993) Noninvasive ductal carcinoma of breast: the relevance of histological categorization. *Hum. Pathol.*, **24**, 16–23.

Bethwaite P., Smith N., Delahunt B., Kenwright D. (1998) Reproducibility of new classification schemes for the pathology of ductal carcinoma *in situ* of the breast. *J. Clin. Pathol.*, **51**, 450–4.

Betshill W.L., Rosen P.P., Lieberman P.H., Robbins G.F. (1978) Intraductal carcinoma: long-term follow-up after treatment by biopsy alone. *J. Am. Med. Assoc.*, **239**, 1863–7.

Bobrow L.G., Happerfield L.C., Gregory W.M., Millis R.R. (1995) Ductal carcinoma *in situ*: assessment of necrosis and nuclear morphology and their association with biological markers. *J. Pathol.*, **176**, 333–41.

Brown P.W., Silverman J., Owens E., Tabor D.C., Terz J.J., Lawrence W. (1976) Intraductal 'noninfiltrating' carcinoma of the breast. *Arch. Surg.*, **111**, 1063–7.

Buerger H., Otterbach F., Simon R. *et al.* (1999) Comparative genomic hybridization of ductal carcinoma *in situ* of the breast-evidence of multiple genetic pathways. *J. Pathol.*, **187**, 396–402

Carter D., Orr S.L., Merino M.J. (1983) Intracystic papillary carcinoma of the breast: after mastectomy, radiotherapy or excisional biopsy alone. *Cancer*, **19**, 14–19.

Consensus Conference Committee (1997) Consensus conference on the classification of ductal carcinoma *in situ*. *Cancer*, **80**, 1798–802.

Cross A.S., Azzopardi J.G., Krausz T., Van Norden S., Polak J.M. (1985) A morphological and immunocytochemical study of a distinctive variant of ductal carcinoma *in situ* of the breast. *Histopathology*, **9**, 21–37.

De Potter C.R., Schelfhout A.-M., Verbeeck P. *et al.* (1995) *Neu*-overexpression correlates with extent of disease in large cell ductal carcinoma *in situ* of the breast. *Hum. Pathol.*, **26**, 601–6.

Engels K., Fox S.B., Whitehouse R.M., Gatter K.C., Harris A.L. (1997) Distinct patterns are associated with high-grade *in situ* ductal carcinomas of the breast. *J. Pathol.*, **181**, 207–12.

European Commission (1996) *European Guidelines for Quality Assurance in Mammography Screening*, 2nd edn. Office for Official Publications of the European Communities.

Faverly D.R.G., Burgers L., Bult P., Holland R. (1994) Three dimensional imaging of mammary ductal carcinoma *in situ*: clinical implications. *Semin. Diagn. Pathol.*, **11**, 193–8.

Fisher F.R., Gregorio R.M., Fisher B., Redmond C., Vellios F., Sommers S.C. and co-operating investigators (1975) The pathology of invasive breast cancer: a syllabus derived from findings of the National Surgical Adjuvant Breast Project (Protocol No. 4). *Cancer*, **36**, 1–84.

Fisher E.R., Constantino J., Fisher B., Palakar A.S., Redmond C., Mamounas E. (1995) Pathological findings from the National Adjuvant Breast Project (NSABP) Protocol B-17. Intraductal carcinoma (ductal carcinoma *in situ*). *Cancer*, **75**, 1310–19.

Gatalica Z. (1997) Immunohistochemical analysis of apocrine breast lesions. Consistent over-expression of androgen receptor accompanied by the loss of estrogen and progesterone receptors in apocrine metaplasia and apocrine carcinoma in situ. *Pathol. Res. Pract.*, **193**, 753–8.

Gillett C.E., Lee A.H.S., Millis R.R., Barnes D.M. (1998) Cyclin D1 and associated proteins in mammary ductal carcinoma *in situ* and atypical ductal hyperplasia. *J. Pathol.*, **184**, 396–400

Giri D.D., Dundas S.A.C., Nottingham J.F., Underwood J.C.E. (1989) Oestrogen receptors in benign epithelial lesions and intraduct carcinomas of the breast: an immunohistological study. *Histopathology*, **15**, 575–84.

Gobbi H., Arteaga C.L., Jensen R.A. *et al.* (2000) Loss of expression of transforming growth factor beta type II receptor correlates with high tumour grade in human breast in-situ and invasive carcinomas. *Histopathology*, **36**, 168–77.

Goldstein N.S., Murphy T. (1996) Intraductal carcinoma associated with invasive carcinoma of the breast: a comparison of the two lesions with implications for intraductal carcinoma classification systems. *Am. J. Clin. Pathol.*, **106**, 312–18.

Guerry P., Erlandson R.A., Rosen P.R. (1988) Cystic hypersecretory hyperplasia and cystic hypersecretory duct carcinoma of the breast: pathology, therapy and follow up of 39 patients. *Cancer*, **61**, 1611–20.

Haagensen C.D. (1971) *Diseases of the Breast*, 2nd edn, London, W.B. Saunders.

Harrison M., Coyne J.D., Gorey T., Dervan P.A. (1996) Comparison of cytomorphological and architectural heterogeneity in mammographically-detected ductal carcinoma *in situ*. *Histopathology*, **28**, 445–50.

Holland R., Hendriks J.H.C.L., Verbeek A.L.M., Mravunac M., Schuurmans Stekhoven J.H. (1990) Extent, distribution and mammographic/ histological correlations of breast ductal carcinoma *in situ*. *Lancet*, **335**, 519–22.

Holland R., Peterse J.L., Millis R.R. *et al.* (1994) Ductal carcinoma *in situ*: A proposal for a new classification. *Semin. Diagn. Pathol.*, **11**,167–80.

Kanitakis J., Thivolet J., Claudy A. (1993) p53 expression in mammary and extramammary Paget's disease. *Anticancer Res.*, **13**, 2429–34.

Kramer W.M., Rush B.F. (1973) Mammary duct proliferation in the elderly: a histopathologic study. *Cancer*, **31**, 130–7.

Lagios M.D. (1990) Ductal carcinoma *in situ*: pathology and treatment. *Surg. Clin. North Am.*, **70**, 853–71.

Lagios M.D. (1995) Heterogeneity of ductal carcinoma *in situ* (DCIS): relationship of grade and subtype analysis to local recurrence and risk of invasive transformation. *Cancer Lett.*, **90**, 97–102.

Lagios M.D., Westdahl P.R., Margolin F.R., Rose M.R. (1982) Duct carcinoma *in situ*: relationship of extent of noninvasive disease to the frequency of occult invasion, multicentricity, lymph node metastases, and short-term treatment failures. *Cancer*, **50**, 1309–14.

Lagios M.D., Margolin F.R., Westdahl P.R., Rose M.R. (1989) Mammographically detected duct carcinoma *in situ*. Frequency of local recurrence following tylectomy and prognostic effect of nuclear grade on local recurrence. *Cancer*, **63**, 618–24.

Lefkowitz M., Lefkowitz W., Wargotz E.S. (1994) Intraductal (intracystic) papillary carcinoma of the breast and its variants. *Hum. Pathol.*, **25**, 802–9.

Lennington W.J., Jensen R.A., Dalton L.W., Page D.L. (1994) Ductal carcinoma *in situ* of the breast: heterogeneity of individual lesions. *Cancer*, **73**, 118–24.

Maluf H.M., Koerner F.C. (1995) Solid papillary carcinoma of the breast. A form of intraductal carcinoma with endocrine differentiation frequently associated with mucinous carcinoma. *Am. J. Surg. Pathol.*, **19**, 1237–44.

Micale M.A., Visscher D.W., Gulino S.E., Wolman S.R. (1994) Chromosomal aneuploidy in proliferative breast disease. *Hum. Pathol.*, **25**, 29–35.

Millis R.R., Thynne S.J. (1975) *in situ* intraduct carcinoma of the breast: a long term follow-up study. *Br. J. Surg.*, **62**, 957–62.

Moll R., Mitze M., Frixen H., Birchmeier W. (1993) Differential loss of E-cadherin expression in infiltrating ductal and lobular breast carcinomas. *Am. J. Pathol.*, **143**, 1731–42.

Moss S.M., Michel M., Patnick J., Johns L., Blanks R., Chamberlain J. (1995) Results of the NHS breast screening programme 1990-1993. *J. Med. Screening*, **2**, 186–90.

Munn K.E., Walker R.A., Menasce L., Varley J.M. (1996) Mutation of the TP53 gene and allelic imbalance at chromosome 17p13 in ductal carcinoma *in situ*. *Br. J. Cancer*, **74**, 1578–85

Murphy D.S., Hoare S.F., Going J.J. *et al.* (1995) Characterisation of extensive genetic alterations in ductal carcinoma *in situ* by fluorescence *in situ* hybridisation and molecular analysis. *J. Natl Cancer Inst.*, **87**, 1694–704

National Coordinating Group for Breast Screening Pathology (1995) *Pathology reporting in breast cancer screening*. NHSBSP publication No.3.

O'Connell P.O., Pekkel V., Fuqua A.W., Osborne C.K., Clark G.M., Allred D.C. (1998) Analysis of loss of heterozygosity in 399 premalignant breast lesions at 15 genetic loci. *J. Natl Cancer Inst.*, **90**, 697–703.

Ohtake T., Abe R., Kimijima I. *et al.* (1995) Intraductal extension of primary invasive breast carcinoma treated by breast-conservative surgery: computer graphic three-dimensional reconstruction of the mammary duct-lobular systems. *Cancer*, **76**, 32–45.

Ottesen G.L., Graversen H.P., Blichert-Toft M., Zedeler K., Andersen J.A.. (1992) Ductal carcinoma *in situ* of the female breast. Short-term results of a prospective nation-wide study. *Am. J. Surg. Pathol.*, **16**, 1183–96.

Ozzello L. (1971) Ultrastructure of the human mammary gland. *Pathol. Ann.*, **6**, 1–59.

Page D.L., Dupont W.D., Rogers L.W., Landenberger M. (1982) Intraductal carcinoma of the breast: follow-up after biopsy only. *Cancer*, **49**, 751–8.

Patchefsky A.S., Schwartz G.F., Finkelstein S.D. *et al.* (1989) Heterogeneity of ductal carcinoma of the breast. *Cancer*, **63**, 731–41.

Poller D.N., Snead D.R.J., Roberts E.C. *et al.* (1993) Oestrogen receptor expression in ductal carcinoma *in situ* of the breast: relationship to flow cytometric analysis of DNA and expression of the cerbB2 oncoprotein. *Br. J. Cancer*, **68**, 156–61.

Poller D.N., Silverstein M.J., Galea A. *et al.* (1994) Ductal carcinoma *in situ* of breast: a proposal for a new simplified histological classification association between cellular proliferation and c-erbB2 protein expression. *Mod. Pathol.*, **7**, 257–62.

Quinn C.M., Ostrowski J.L. (1997) Cytological and architectural heterogeneity in ductal carcinoma *in situ* of the breast. *J. Clin. Pathol.*, **50**, 596–9.

Ramachandra S., Machin L., Ashley S. Monaghan P., Gusterson B.A. (1990) Immunohistochemical distrubution of cerbB2 in *in situ* breast carcinoma-a detailed morphological analysis. *J. Pathol.*, **161**, 7–14.

Rayne S.C., Santa Cruz D. (1992) Anaplastic Paget's disease. *Am. J. Surg. Pathol.*, **16**, 1085–91.

Recht A., Rutgers E.J.Th., Fentiman I.S., Kurtz J.M., Mansel R.E., Sloane J.P. (1998) The Fourth EORTC DCIS Consensus Meeting (Chateau Marquette, Heemskerk, The Netherlands, 23–24 January 1998) – Conference Report. *Eur. J. Cancer*, **34**, 1664–9.

Reiff D.B., Cooke J., Griffin M., Given-Wilson R. (1994) Ductal carcinoma *in situ* presenting as a stellate lesion on mammography. *Clin. Radiol.*, **49**, 396–9.

Rosen P.P., Scott M. (1984) Cystic hypersecretory duct carcinoma of the breast. *Am. J. Surg. Pathol.*, **8**, 31–41.

Rosen P.P., Braun D.W., Kinne D.E. (1980) The clinical significance of pre-invasive breast carcinoma. *Cancer*, **46**, 919–25.

Sandison A.T. (1962) An Autopsy Study of the Adult Human Breast. National Cancer Institute Monograph No. 8. Washington, DC, US Department of Health, Education and Welfare.

Schnitt S.J., Silen N., Sadowsky N.L., Connolly J.L., Harris J.R. (1988) Ductal carcinoma in situ (intraductal carcinoma) of the breast. *N. Engl. J. Med.*, **318**, 898–903.

Schwartz G.F., Patchefsky A.S., Finkelstein S.D. et al. (1989) Nonpalpable in situ ductal carcinoma of the breast. Predictors of multicentricity and microinvasion and implications for treatment. *Arch. Surg.*, **124**, 29–32.

Schwartz G.F., Finkel G.C., Garcia J.G., Patchevsky A.S. (1992) Subclinical ductal carcinoma in situ of the breast. Treatment by local excision and surveillance alone. *Cancer*, **70**, 2468–74.

Silverstein M.J., Waisman J.R., Gamagami P. et al. (1990) Intraductal carcinoma of the breast (208 cases). Clinical factors influencing treatment choice. *Cancer*, **66**, 102–8.

Silverstein M.J., Waisman J.R., Colburn W.J. *et al.* (1993) Intraductal breast carcinoma (DCIS) with and without microinvasion (MI): is there a difference in outcome? *Proc. Am. Soc. Clin. Oncol.*, **12**, 56.

Silverstein M.J., Poller D.N., Waisman J.R. *et al.* (1995) Prognostic classification of breast ductal carcinoma in situ. *Lancet*, **345**, 1154–7.

Silverstein M.J., Lagios M.D., Craig P.H. et al. (1996) A prognostic index for ductal carcinoma in situ of the breast. *Cancer*, **77**, 2267–74.

Silverstein M.J., Lagios M.D., Martino S. *et al.* (1998) Outcome after invasive local recurrence in patients with ductal carcinoma in situ of the breast. *J. Clin. Oncol.*, **16**, 1367–73.

Simpson J.F., O'Malley F., Dupont W.D., Page D.L. (1994) Heterogeneous expression of nm23 gene product in noninvasive breast a carcinoma. *Cancer*, **73**, 2352–8.

Siziopikou K.P., Prioleau J.E., Harris J.R., Schnitt S.J. (1996) bcl-2 expression in the spectrum of preinvasive breast lesions. *Cancer*, **77** (3), 499–506.

Sloane J.P. and members of the National Coordinating Group for Breast Screening Pathology (1994) Consistency of histopathological reporting of breast lesions detected by screening: findings of the U.K. National EQA Scheme. *Eur. J. Cancer*, **30A**, 1414–19.

Sloane J.P., Amendoeira I., Apostolikas N. et al. (1998) Consistency achieved by 23 European pathologists in categorising ductal carcinoma in situ of the breast using 5 classifications. *Hum. Pathol.*, **29**, 1056–62.

Sloane J.P. Amendoeira I., Apostolikas N. et al. (1999) Consistency achieved by 23 European pathologists from 12 countries in diagnosing breast disease and reporting prognostic features of carcinomas. *Virchows Archiv*, **434**, 3–10.

Solin L.J., Yeh I.T., Kurtz J. et al. (1993) Ductal carcinoma in situ (intraductal carcinoma) of the breast treated with breast-conserving surgery and definitive irradiation. Correlation of pathologic parameters with outcome of treatment. *Cancer*, **71**, 2532–42.

Soo M.S., Williford M.E., Walsh R., Bentley R.C., Kornguth P.J. (1995) Papillary carcinoma of the breast: imaging findings. *Am. J. Roentgenol.*, **164**, 321–6.

Stratton M.R., Collins N., Lakhani S.R., Sloane J.P. (1995) Loss of heterozygosity in ductal carcinoma in situ of the breast. *J. Pathol.*, **175**, 195–201.

Tavassoli F.A. (1998) Ductal carcinoma in situ: introduction of the concept of ductal in situ neoplasia. *Mod. Pathol.*, **11**, 140–54.

Tsang W.Y.W., Chan J.K.C. (1996) Endocrine ductal carcinoma in situ of the breast. *Am. J. Surg. Pathol.*, **20**, 921–43.

Waldman F.M., DeVries S., Chew K.L., Moore D.H., Kerlikowske K., Ljung B.M. (2000) Chromosomal alterations in ductal carcinomas in situ and their in situ recurrence. *J. Natl Cancer Inst.*, **92**, 313–20.

Weinstat-Saslow D., Merino M.J., Manrow R.E. et al. (1995) *Nature Med.*, **1**, 1257–60.

Welch H.G, Black W.C. (1997) Using autopsy series to estimate the disease 'reservoir' for ductal carcinoma in situ of the breast: how much more breast cancer can we find? *Ann. Intern. Med.*, **127**, 1023–8.

Wellings S.R., Jensen H.M., Marcum R.G. (1975) An atlas of subgross pathology of the human breast with special reference to possible precancerous lesions. *J. Natl Cancer Inst.*, **55**, 231–73.

Westbrook K.C., Gallager H.S. (1975) Intraductal carcinoma of the breast: a comparative study. *Am. J. Surg.*, **130**, 667–70.

Wolf C., Rouyer N., Lutz Y. et al. (1993) Stromelysin 3 belongs to a subgroup of proteinases expressed in breast carcinoma fibroblastic cells and possibly implicated in tumor progression. *Proc. Natl Acad. Sci. USA*, **90**, 1843–7.

9 Lobular *in situ* neoplasia

This chapter is devoted to lobular carcinoma *in situ* (LCIS) and the related disorder of atypical lobular hyperplasia (ALH). These are often collectively known as lobular *in situ* neoplasia because their histological, clinical and molecular features are similar and the difference between them more quantitative than qualitative. Despite the nomenclature these lesions are distinguished from the intraductal proliferations described in Chapters 7 and 8 by cytological and architectural features rather than their site of origin. Most ductal carcinomas *in situ* (DCIS) are now thought to arise in terminal duct–lobular units. Furthermore, ALH and LCIS may also spread into the interlobular ducts. The distinction between LCIS and DCIS is important, however, in view of their different behaviour, particularly with respect to multicentricity. The main histological features distinguishing DCIS and LCIS are summarized in Table 9.1.

TABLE 9.1 Major histological features distinguishing lobular carcinoma *in situ* (LCIS) and low nuclear grade ductal carcinoma *in situ* (DCIS)

Histological features	DCIS	LCIS
Cells	Small and monomorphic with round hyperchromatic nuclei and high nuclear-to-cytoplasmic ratio	Small and monomorphic with round hyperchromatic nuclei and high nuclear-to-cytoplasmic ratio
Intracytoplasmic lumina	Rare	Common
Growth pattern	Variable, usually cribriform or micropapillary. Sometimes solid	Solid with complete obliteration of lumina
Cell cohesion	Usually good	Usually poor
Degree of distension of involved structures	Moderate to great	Slight to moderate
Pagetoid spread along interlobular ducts	Rare	Common
Necrosis	Uncommon	Very rare
Mitoses	Infrequent	Infrequent
Calcification	Fairly common	Uncommon

All the features of a lesion should be taken into account when making a diagnosis. No criterion is reliable on its own.

9.1 (Left) Lobular carcinoma *in situ* accompanied by classic invasive lobular carcinoma. The lobule shows moderate distension but much less than is encountered in ductal carcinoma *in situ*. The proliferating cells are uniform, relatively small and uncohesive, and the growth pattern is solid (H&E).

9.3 (Right) Lobular carcinoma *in situ*. At this higher power view of Fig. 9.2, the cytological features are more easily discerned. The cells are very uniform and the nuclear-to-cytoplasmic ratio very high. The cells are rather uncohesive but less so than in some examples. The growth pattern is solid, the apparent formation of secondary lumina being caused by cell drop-out as a consequence of individual cell necrosis. The neoplastic cells are unaccompanied by myoepithelial-like cells or leucocytes (H&E).

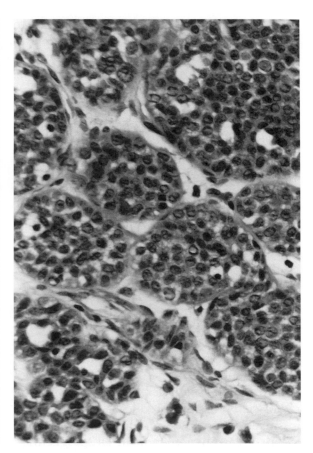

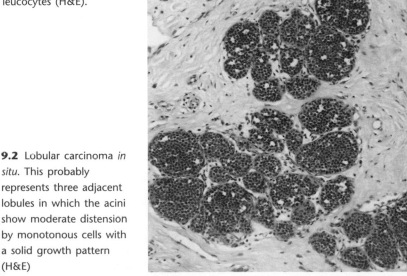

9.2 Lobular carcinoma *in situ*. This probably represents three adjacent lobules in which the acini show moderate distension by monotonous cells with a solid growth pattern (H&E)

LOBULAR CARCINOMA *IN SITU*

Histology

As LCIS is not clinically palpable, detectable by conventional macroscopic examination or generally visible on radiography, it is almost invariably an incidental finding in biopsy or resection specimens removed for other malignant or benign processes.

Histologically, there is lobular enlargement that rarely exceeds two or three times the normal size and is considerably less than is usually seen in DCIS (Figs 9.1 and 9.2). The cells are uniform, small and rounded with dark nuclei, inconspicuous nucleoli and a high nuclear-to-cytoplasmic ratio. The proliferation is monomorphic, with no spindle cells or leucocytes. There is usually complete obliteration of the lumina, the cells appearing loose and uncohesive (Fig. 9.3). Mitoses are infrequent, and necrosis and haemorrhage are not seen.

Haagensen *et al.* (1972) have recognized two forms of the disease based on nuclear appearance. In one (type A) the nuclei have the classic appearance described above, being uniform, small, dark, round and anucleolate. In type B lesions the nuclei are somewhat larger and more pleomorphic, exhibiting a less uniform chromatin pattern, sometimes with a prominent nucleolus (Fig. 9.4). Good-quality sections are needed to distinguish the two types. A mixture of type A and B cells may be seen within the same lobule. Rosen *et al.* (1978) found the type A lesion to be the more common.

In contrast to DCIS, stromal fibrosis and elastosis are not seen, and significant mononuclear cell infiltration is very rare (*see* Fig. 9.2 above).

LCIS may occur in large, atrophic or otherwise normal lobules. Furthermore, it may be superimposed on pre-existing lobular changes, including fibroadenomas (*see* Fig. 13.4). When superimposed on sclerosing adenosis and radial scars, it may produce a picture easily mistaken for invasive carcinoma (*see* Fig. 6.24 for a similar phenomenon in DCIS) (Fechner, 1981).

Interlobular duct involvement is common and may even be seen without lobular changes. The presence of LCIS in the ductal phase only was found by Haagensen *et al.* (1978) to be related to age, accounting for no cases under the age of 40 but more than a fifth in patients aged 55 or over. This phenomenon is presumably related to normal lobular involution.

When the cells extend into the interlobular ducts, they may assume a variety of growth patterns (Fechner, 1972). A pagetoid form of spread is usually seen in which the neoplastic cells extend between the basement membrane and the residual epithelial cells that form a flattened layer over the luminal surface (Fig. 9.5). In smaller ducts there may be solid filling. There may in some cases even be finger-like projections extending into the lumen. Small acinus-like structures packed with neoplastic cells are occasionally seen arising from the walls of larger ducts; Haagensen *et al.* (1972) refer to this as the 'clover leaf' pattern (Fig. 9.6). Necrosis,

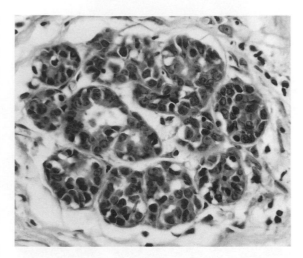

9.4 Lobular carcinoma *in situ* type B. The cells are larger and more pleomorphic than those in Fig. 9.3 and contain discernible nucleoli (H&E).

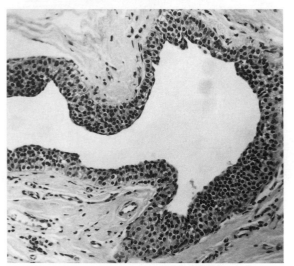

9.5 Lobular carcinoma *in situ* showing pagetoid spread along an interlobular duct. The residual epithelial cells are pushed towards the lumen, where they form a flattened layer covering the neoplastic cells (H&E).

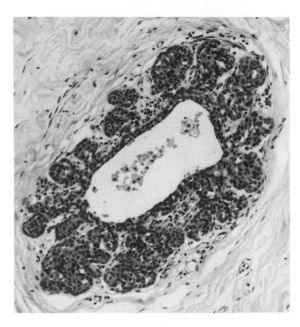

9.6 'Clover leaf' pattern of lobular carcinoma *in situ*. There are numerous acinus-like structures arising from the wall of an interlobular duct (H&E).

haemorrhage, periductal fibrosis, elastosis and inflammation are rarely encountered, even with interlobular duct involvement.

It should be remembered that LCIS and DCIS may co-exist, although the reported frequency with which this occurs varies widely from less than 5% to more than 20% of cases (Ringberg *et al.*, 1982; Page *et al.*, 1991; Ottesen *et al.*, 1993). Reasons for this variation include the extent of sampling of the involved breast and the diagnostic criteria employed, particularly in distinguishing LCIS

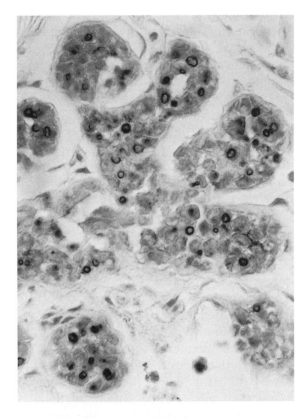

9.7 Formalin-fixed, paraffin-embedded section of lobular carcinoma *in situ* immunostained for epithelial membrane antigen. Note the numerous intracytoplasmic lumina.

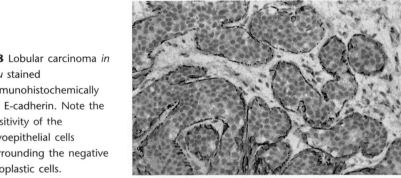

9.8 Lobular carcinoma *in situ* stained immunohistochemically for E-cadherin. Note the positivity of the myoepithelial cells surrounding the negative neoplastic cells.

from low nuclear grade DCIS with a solid growth pattern involving lobules with minimal distension (*see* Table 9.1 above). Fisher *et al.* (1996) used the term ductolobular carcinoma *in situ* to describe those cases in which the histological appearances were entirely equivocal so that it was impossible to categorize a lesion confidently as DCIS or LCIS.

Conventional histochemistry

Mucin stains reveal that a variable proportion of the neoplastic cells contains intracytoplasmic globules of mucin, which may vary in size and number. Sometimes they are barely visible, but on other occasions they may be large, solitary structures occupying half the cell (Gad and Azzopardi, 1975). In alcian blue–periodic acid–Schiff preparations after diastase digestion, they often exhibit a rather characteristic appearance with a red or purple central dot and a blue rim (*see* Fig. 3.1). These structures often appear to correspond to the intracytoplasmic lumina seen on electron microscopy and by immunohistology using antisera to the milk fat globule membrane (epithelial membrane antigen) (see below).

Immunohistochemistry

Immunostaining for epithelial membrane antigen using antibodies raised against the milk fat globule membrane generally gives positive results, demonstrating well the intracytoplasmic lumina seen on mucin staining and by electron microscopy (see below) (Fig. 9.7). This demonstrates that the lining of the lumina is similar to the plasma membrane biochemically as well as ultrastructurally. The epithelial specific cell–cell adhesion molecule E-cadherin is usually reduced or absent in LCIS (Fig. 9.8) (Moll *et al.*, 1993). The significance of this finding is not certain, but it is clear that the loss of this molecule does not necessarily lead to invasion. It may, however, be related to the uncohesive nature of the cells of LCIS. Immunopositivity for oestrogen and progesterone receptors is seen in the great majority of cases, whereas c-erbB-2 is negative (Giri *et al.*, 1989; Fisher *et al.*, 1996).

Molecular genetics

Using microdissection and the polymerase chain reaction, it has been shown that LCIS exhibits allelic imbalance (AI) at several chromosomal loci. Lakhani *et al.* (1995) found AI at a telomeric locus on chromosome 16q with a frequency similar to that seen in DCIS and invasive ductal (nst) carcinomas, whereas AI on chromosome 17p, although common in DCIS and invasive nst carcinomas, was rare in LCIS. The finding of AI by this methodology confirms that LCIS is a monoclonal and hence neoplastic disorder and that patients with truly multicentric or bilateral disease have multiple neoplasms. The occurrence of AI at 16q with more or less equal frequency in LCIS and DCIS suggests that these two disorders may initially develop along a common pathway on which AI at 16q is an early event. As in invasive lobular carcinoma, truncating mutations of the E-cadherin gene have been found in a significant proportion of cases (Vos *et al.*, 1997). Using comparative genomic hybridization, Lu *et al.* (1998) found losses of genetic material on chromosomes 16p, 16q, 17p and 22q and gains on 6q with equal frequency in LCIS and ALH (see below). Fluorescence *in situ* hybridization (FISH) studies on formalin-fixed, paraffin-embedded sections using pericentromeric probes have shown true or borderline aneusomy of chromosomes 1 and X (Micale *et al.*, 1994). These genetic findings provide strong evidence that LCIS is a precursor of invasive carcinoma and not simply a marker of risk.

Electron microscopy

The ultrastructural characteristics of the cells are not dissimilar to those of DCIS despite their cytological dissimilarity (Ozzello, 1971). Surface microvilli are scanty but rough endoplasmic reticulum is often increased and the Golgi apparatus hypertrophic. A striking feature is the presence of intracytoplasmic lumina in a proportion of the cells (*see* Fig. 3.1). A membrane bearing microvilli lines these lumina. Serial sectioning usually reveals that they have contact with the surface membrane and thus represent invaginations.

In a few cases, however, they appear to be separate from the surface. There may be bundles of filaments in the cytoplasm, but these usually lead to desmosomes, and evidence of myoepithelial differentiation is lacking (Tobon and Price, 1972). Residual non-neoplastic myoepithelial cells may, however, be seen around the periphery of acini and ducts. In the stroma, the epithelial stromal junction is often maintained (Ozzello, 1971). The basal lamina may show irregular zones of thickening and thinning, but gaps are less frequent than in DCIS.

Radiology

Calcification is very rare in association with LCIS. It may sometimes be sufficiently dense and extensive to be detectable by mammographic screening, but this is very rare. It exhibits no specific features. Furthermore, on histological examination the calcified deposits are often located in accompanying benign or malignant changes or even in nearby normal ducts and lobules. When calcification is actually present in LCIS, it may be seen between epithelial cells or in the stroma. (Pope *et al.*, 1988; Beute *et al.*, 1991).

Incidence

LCIS is not a common lesion, accounting for only a few per cent of all breast carcinomas. It is found in about 0.5–4.0% of otherwise benign breast biopsies (Page *et al.*, 1991). It is predominantly, but not exclusively, a disease of premenopausal women. This suggests that postmenopausal regression occurs in many cases. Rosen *et al.* (1978) found that only 5 of 83 patients with LCIS were postmenopausal, and only one was more than 60 years old. After the menopause it is more frequently associated with infiltrating tumour. LCIS has, however, been seen in women who have undergone bilateral oophorectomy without hormonal replacement, suggesting that postmenopausal regression is not simply a reflection of ovarian function. The lack of a clear relationship between normal breast involution and ovarian function may be relevant in this context.

It has been suggested that LCIS and invasive lobular carcinoma are associated with a family history of breast cancer (Claus *et al.*, 1993). The International Breast Cancer Linkage Consortium did not, however, find a disproportionate number of lobular carcinomas in patients with familial breast cancer due to *BRCA1* and *BRCA2* mutations (Lakhani *et al.*, 1998).

Multicentricity and bilaterality

The disease is widely reported to be multifocal in the majority of cases. It is, however, difficult or impossible in histological sections to distinguish between true multicentric origin and spread from lobule to lobule along the interlobular ducts. Nevertheless, the involved structures are in many cases so widely dispersed that it is highly unlikely that they would belong to the same duct system.

Bilaterality is, however, indisputable evidence of multicentricity and is encountered with great frequency. The actual incidence of bilateral involvement varies from study to study and largely reflects the extent of sampling. Urban (1967) found that about 35% of patients with LCIS who underwent contralateral breast biopsy had bilateral disease.

In the study of Beute *et al.* (1991), LCIS was found to be bilateral in 50% of cases when the contralateral breast was sampled by either mirror image biopsy or mastectomy. Ringberg *et al.* (1982) examined contralateral mastectomy specimens from patients with *in situ* carcinoma by cutting the breast into 3–5 mm slices that were then embedded and cut in large sections, allowing all the lesions to be mapped. LCIS was found to be bilateral in 63% of cases, in contrast to 17% of cases of DCIS.

In view of the high incidence of multicentricity and bilaterality, there is no need to assess the adequacy of excision of LCIS.

Development of invasive carcinoma

LCIS is associated with an elevated risk of developing invasive breast cancer, although the size of the risk varies from study to study. Major reasons for this variation include the relatively small number of cases studied given the rarity of the lesion and the different diagnostic criteria employed, particularly in distinguishing LCIS from ALH (see below). Page *et al.* (1991) reported 44 cases and reviewed four widely quoted studies by other workers. The number of patients varied from 32 to 211 and the period of follow-up from 14 to 24 years (Andersen, 1974; Wheeler *et al.*, 1974; Haagensen *et al.*, 1978; Rosen *et al.*, 1978). Between 12.5 and 36.4% of patients developed invasive breast carcinoma, giving a relative risk of 7.2–12.0. Invasive tumours developed in the ipsilateral and contralateral breast with similar frequency, some being bilateral.

Fisher *et al.* (1996) studied a large number of pathological characteristics of LCIS and found that the only feature associated with an increased risk of developing invasive disease was a great degree of acinar and lobular distension with obliteration of the interacinar stroma. Other workers have, however, found that no clinical or pathological features, including family history and exogenous hormone usage, are associated with an increased risk of developing invasive carcinoma (Page *et al.*, 1991). The invasive tumour may appear after a very long time interval. In the series of Rosen *et al.* (1978), invasive carcinomas appeared 2–31 years (average 16 years) after the diagnosis of LCIS, which is significantly later than those following DCIS.

Rather surprisingly, the subsequent tumours in most series have been predominantly of the invasive ductal (nst) type. Infiltrative lobular carcinomas do occur, however, with a greater relative frequency. Tubular carcinomas have also been reported (Page *et al.*, 1991). There is some evidence to suggest that the infiltrative ductal (nst) tumours occur somewhat earlier than the infiltrative lobular types.

ATYPICAL LOBULAR HYPERPLASIA

ALH is an intralobular proliferation similar to LCIS for which one or more of the major diagnostic criteria are not met *or* for which all the criteria are fulfilled in less than 50% of the acini within the lobule (Page *et al.*, 1985). The

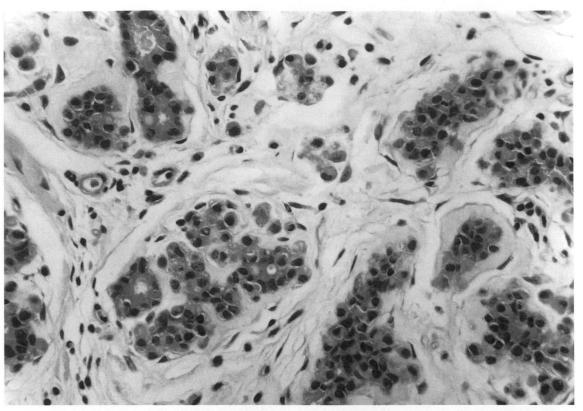

9.9 Atypical lobular hyperplasia. The photograph shows part of a lobule containing cells characteristic of lobular carcinoma *in situ*. The acini are, however, only minimally dilated, many lumina are preserved, and the neoplastic cells are mixed with other cell types (H&E).

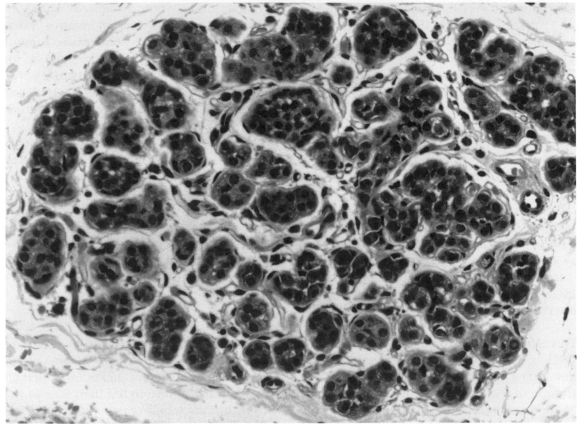

9.10 Atypical lobular hyperplasia. Almost all the normal epithelial cells in this lobule have been replaced by a monomorphic population of cells characteristic of lobular carcinoma *in situ*. There are no discernible residual lumina, but the acini show no or minimal distension (H&E).

TABLE 9.2 Major features distinguishing lobular carcinoma *in situ* (LCIS) and atypical lobular hyperplasia (ALH)

Histological features	LCIS	ALH
Cells	Monomorphic cells with small round hyperchromatic nuclei and high nuclear-to-cytoplasmic ratio	Essentially like LCIS but may show some variation in nuclear pattern, size or shape
Nuclear placement	Regular	May be irregular
Cellular composition	One cell type	May be spindle-shaped cells and leucocytes in addition to proliferating epithelial cells
Cellular cohesion	Usually poor	May be good
Luminal occlusion	Complete	May be partial
Extent of lobular involvement	Complete	May be partial
Acinar distension	Slight to moderate	May be insignificant
Pagetoid extension into interlobular ducts	Common	Common

All the features of a lesion should be taken into account when making a diagnosis. No criterion is reliable on its own.

cells invariably resemble those of LCIS but may lack their striking monotony, exhibiting some variation in nuclear pattern, size or shape. Nuclear placement may be irregular, and the proliferation may include spindle-shaped cells and leucocytes. The degree of acinar distension may be less than in LCIS and may even be insignificant (Figs 9.9 and 9.10). The lumina may be preserved (*see* Fig. 9.9). ALH may occur in large or atrophic lobules and may rarely be superimposed upon pre-existing lobular disorders such as sclerosing adenosis. It is occasionally present within fibroadenomas.

The major points of distinction between ALH and LCIS are summarized in Table 9.2. The criteria for distinguishing ALH from ADH are essentially the same as those employed for the corresponding *in situ* carcinomas.

As defined above ALH is encountered in fewer than 2% of benign biopsies, although the incidence strongly correlates with the extent of sampling (Page *et al.*, 1988). The age incidence is similar to that of LCIS.

The available evidence suggests that ALH is associated with a significantly increased risk of developing carcinoma, albeit less than that accompanying LCIS. In a very small group of seven patients followed for a long period of time, Rosen *et al.* (1978) found that one patient developed invasive carcinoma after 12 years. Toker (1974) found that 12% of patients with milder forms of ALH and 25% of those with severe lesions developed ipsilateral carcinoma within a 15-year follow-up period. This represented respectively about one quarter and one half the incidence of carcinoma occurring after LCIS.

Page *et al.* (1985) studied 126 patients with ALH and found that carcinoma developed in 16 of them between 4.6 and 21.9 years (average 11.9 years) later. This gave a relative risk of 4.2, approximately half that associated with LCIS. The risk for ALH was, however, doubled in the presence of a family history of carcinoma. Ductal involvement was also associated with an increased risk of developing carcinoma intermediate between that of ALH and that of LCIS (Page *et al.*, 1988). In the study of Marshall *et al.* (1997), a greater risk was found for ALH than atypical ductal hyperplasia (ADH). Furthermore ALH was more strongly associated with the risk of premenopausal than postmenopausal breast cancer, whereas the association of risk and ADH varied little by menopausal status.

The invasive carcinomas developing after a diagnosis of ALH are mostly ductal (nst, that is, no specific type), although other types, including invasive lobular carcinomas, have been described.

For a further discussion of the possible precancerous significance of intralobular and intraductal hyperplasia, see Chapter 10.

REFERENCES

Andersen J.A. (1974) Lobular carcinoma *in situ*. A long-term follow-up in 52 cases. *Acta Path. Microbiol. Scand. Sect. A.*, **82**, 519–33.

Beute B.J., Kalisher L., Hutter R.V.P. (1991) Lobular carcinoma *in situ* of the breast: clinical, pathologic, and mammographic features. *Am. J. Roentgenol.*, **157**, 257–65.

Claus E.B., Risch N., Thompson W.D., Carter D. (1993) Relationship between breast histopathology and family history of breast cancer. *Cancer*, **71**, 147–53.

Fechner R.E. (1972) Epithelial alterations in the extralobular ducts of breasts with lobular carcinoma. *Arch. Pathol.*, **93**, 164–71.

Fechner R.E. (1981) Lobular carcinoma *in situ* in sclerosing adenosis: a potential source of confusion with invasive carcinoma. *Am. J. Surg. Pathol.*, **5**, 233–9.

Fisher E.R., Costantino J., Fisher B. *et al.* (1996) Pathologic findings from the National Surgical Adjuvant Breast Project (NSABP) protocol B-17. Five-year observations concerning lobular carcinoma in situ. *Cancer*, **78** (7),1403–16.

Gad A., Azzopardi J.G. (1975) Lobular carcinoma of the breast: a special variant of mucin-secreting carcinoma. *J. Clin. Pathol.*, **28**, 711–16.

Giri D.D., Dundas S.A.C., Nottingham J.F., Underwood J.C.E. (1989) Oestrogen receptors in benign epithelial lesions and intraduct carcinomas of the breast: an immunohistological study. *Histopathology*, **15**, 575–84.

Haagensen C.D., Lane N., Lattes R. (1972) Neoplastic proliferation of the epithelium of the mammary lobules: adenosis, lobular neoplasia, and small cell carcinoma. *Surg. Clin. North Am.*, **52**, 497–524.

Haagensen C.D., Lane N., Lattes R., Bodian C. (1978) Lobular neoplasia (so-called lobular carcinoma *in situ*) of the breast. *Cancer*, **42**, 737–69.

Lakhani S.R., Collins N., Sloane J.P., Stratton M.R. (1995) Loss of heterozygosity in lobular carcinoma *in situ* of the breast. *J. Clin. Pathol. Mol. Pathol.*, **48**, M74–M78.

Lakhani S.R., Jacquemier J., Sloane J.P. *et al.* (1998) Multifactorial analysis of differences between sporadic breast cancer and cancers involving BRCA1 and BRCA2 mutations. *J. Natl Cancer. Inst.*, **90**, 1138–45.

Lu Y.J., Osin P., Lakhani S.R., Di Palma S., Gusterson B.A., Shipley J.M. (1998) Comparative genomic hybridisation analysis of lobular carcinoma *in situ* and atypical lobular hyperplasia and potential roles for gains and losses of genetic material in breast neoplasia. *Cancer Res*, **58**, 4721–7.

Marshall L.M, Hunter D.J., Connolly J.L. *et al.* (1997), Risk of breast cancer associated with atypical hyperplasia of lobular and ductal types. *Cancer Epidemiology, Biomarkers and Prevention*, **6**, 297–301.

Micale M.A., Visscher D.W., Gulino S.E., Wolman S.R. (1994) Chromosomal aneuploidy in proliferative breast disease. *Hum. Pathol.*, **25**, 29–35.

Moll, R., Mitze M., Frixen H., Birchmeier W. (1993) Differential loss of E-cadherin expression in infiltrating ductal and lobular breast carcinomas. *Am. J. Pathol.*, **143**, 1731–42.

Ottesen G.L., Graversen H.P, Blichert-Toft M., Zedeler K., Andersen J.A. (1993) Lobular carcinoma *in situ* of the female breast. Short-term results of a prospective nationwide study. *Am. J. Surg. Pathol.*, **17**, 14–21.

Ozzello L. (1971) Ultrastructure of the human mammary glands. *Pathol. Ann.*, **6**, 1–59.

Page D.L., Dupont W.D., Rogers L.W., Rados M.S. (1985) Atypical hyperplastic lesions of the female breast. A long-term follow-up study. *Cancer*, **55**, 2698–708.

Page D.L., Dupont W.D., Rogers L.W. (1988) Ductal involvement by cells of atypical lobular hyperplasia in the breast: a long-term follow-up study of cancer risk. *Hum. Pathol.*, **19**, 201–7.

Page D.L., Kidd T.E., Dupont W.D., Simpson J.F., Rogers L.W. (1991) Lobular neoplasia of the breast: higher risk for subsequent invasive cancer predicted by more extensive disease. *Hum. Pathol.*, **22**, 1232–9.

Pope T.L., Fechner R.E., Wilhelm M.C., Wanebo H.J., de Paredes E.S. (1988) Lobular carcinoma *in situ* of the breast: mammographic features. *Radiology*, **168**, 63–6.

Ringberg A., Palmer B., Linell F. (1982) The contralateral breast at reconstructive surgery after breast cancer operation – a histopathological study. *Breast Cancer Res. Treat.*, **2**, 151–61.

Rosen P.P., Lieberman P.H., Braun D.W., Kosloff C., Adair F. (1978) Lobular carcinoma *in situ* of the breast: detailed analysis of 99 patients with average follow-up of 24 years. *Am. J. Surg. Pathol.*, **2**, 225–51.

Tobon H., Price H.M. (1972) Lobular carcinoma *in situ*: some ultrastructural observations. *Cancer*, **30**, 1082–91.

Toker C. (1974) Small cell dysplasia and *in situ* carcinoma of the mammary ducts and lobules. *J. Pathol.*, **114**, 47–52.

Urban J.A. (1967) Bilaterality of cancer of the breast: biopsy of the opposite breast. *Cancer*, **20**, 1867–70.

Vos C.B., Cleton-Jansen A.M., Berx G. *et al.* (1997) E-cadherin inactivation in lobular carcinoma *in situ* of the breast: an early event in tumourigenesis. *Br. J. Cancer*, **76**, 1131–3.

Wheeler J.E., Enterline H.T., Roseman J.M. *et al.* (1974) Lobular carcinoma *in situ* of the breast. Long-term follow-up. *Cancer*, **34**, 554–63.

10 Premalignancy in the breast

INTRODUCTION

Breast carcinomas are frequently associated with the epithelial changes described in Chapters 6 and 7. In some cases there may even be a continuous spectrum of change from normality to *in situ* and invasive malignancy through grades of typical and increasingly atypical hyperplasia. There are several possible interpretations of such a picture. First, carcinogenic agents may induce a variety of benign and malignant changes in a one-stage process. Second, some or all the changes may represent carcinomas at an early non-infiltrative stage of their development that will inevitably progress to infiltrating carcinoma given enough time. Third, carcinomas may evolve in a multistage fashion from precursor or precancerous lesions that are not in themselves neoplastic but have a greater probability of becoming so than do normal tissues. Such considerations are of not only fundamental interest, but also practical importance to histopathologists who are increasingly being asked to assess the risk of developing breast cancer associated with the non-malignant lesions they have diagnosed.

ANIMAL EXPERIMENTS

Although there is much indirect evidence that human breast tumours evolve from precursor lesions, the concept of premalignancy cannot be adequately validated as it is unethical to follow the evolution of malignant tumours without therapeutic intervention. In experimental animals, however, morphological changes can be observed at different intervals after the administration of carcinogens, but even these experiments have limitations. The existence of a preneoplastic state can ultimately only be demonstrated satisfactorily if putative precursor lesions can be identified, isolated and transplanted into other sites where their subsequent behaviour can be observed.

Transplantation studies

DeOme *et al.* (1959) showed that hyperplastic alveolar nodules (HANs) removed from the breasts of female mice infected with mouse mammary tumour virus developed into tumours more frequently than did normal breast tissue when transplanted into mammary fat pads cleared of epithelial tissue in new hosts. Transformation was not inevitable, and HANs varied in their potential for tumour development. In addition, transplanted normal tissues could develop into HANs. Transformation was rarely observed when HANs were transplanted into subcutaneous tissue, showing that environmental factors are important in determining progression. More recently, it has been shown that

HANs are immortalized mono- or oligoclonal proliferations rather non-clonal hyperplasias as their name suggests (Morris and Cardiff, 1987). The same appears to be true of human atypical and at least some non-atypical hyperplasias (*see* below and p. 105).

Effect of hormones

Fisher *et al.* (1975a, 1975b), administered carcinogens to rats and found that carcinomas evolved through various stages of mild and advanced hyperplasia. Mild hyperplasia could also be induced by the administration of oestradiol or progesterone, but, although the appearances were morphologically indistinguishable from the early changes induced by carcinogens, they did not progress further. This demonstrates the important point that histologically similar lesions may not have the same capacity to develop into malignant neoplasia. This may also be true for the human, but reliable methods of distinguishing them are not yet available.

Transgenic animals

These animals (usually mice or rats) are produced by microinjecting cloned genes into the embryos of animals so that every cell in the fully developed animal contains the transgene (for a review, see Cardiff and Muller, 1993). A targeted expression of the genes is achieved by linking them to specific promoters. For expression in breast epithelium, mouse mammary tumour virus long terminal repeats or whey acidic protein promoter/ enhancer elements are usually used. These produce different effects: the former are transcriptionally active during all stages of mammary epithelial differentiation and also active in the seminal vesicle, epididymis, prostate and salivary gland, and the latter are expressed at a high level only in mid-pregnant and lactating mammary glands.

Transgenic rodents have been produced expressing many genes, including *c-myc, ras, neu (c-erbB-2), ret, wnt-1, int2, int3, TGFα* and *p9Ka (S100A4)*. Different transgenes are associated with a different rate, incidence and latency of tumour development, as well as a different morphological appearance. In some systems precursor lesions can be identified that can give insight into the morphological and molecular evolution of tumours associated with specific oncogenes, but detailed transplantation and other studies of these precursors have not been extensively undertaken. The fact that tumours and precursor lesions co-exist with normal epithelium in these animals demonstrates that the overexpression of oncogenes is not enough by itself to cause oncogenesis and that other superimposed changes are also needed.

By crossing animals with different transgenes, the effect of combinations of overexpressed genes can be studied, thus giving further insight into multistage carcinogenesis. One example can be found in *c-erbB-2* transgenic rats that produce tumours with a similar histological appearance to that of human c-erbB-2+ breast carcinomas and, like their human counterparts, tend to develop and grow rapidly. Precursor lesions can be found and may thus provide information on the development of this type of human carcinoma. In one system numerous tumours developed rapidly in *c-erbB-2* transgenic rats but did not metastasize. When these animals were crossed with *S100A4* transgenics, metastasizing tumours of similar appearance developed (Barraclough *et al.*, 1998). It is likely that significant insight into the stages of development of human breast carcinomas may be obtained from transgenic animals.

Caution has, however, to be exercised in assessing the relevance of animal experiments to the human. There is no precise human counterpart for the hyperplastic alveolar nodules that resemble the lobuloalveolar units of prelactating mammary glands. Furthermore, they arise in animals infected with an oncogenic virus, and there is no proven viral aetiology for human carcinoma. Although transgenic animals may overexpress human genes, their cells may not respond in the same way as human cells. Apart from species differences, at the age at which carcinomas usually develop, human cells have been exposed to the effects of numerous menstrual cycles and postmenopausal involution. Finally, the tumours that eventually develop in animals, although regarded as carcinoma, are often expansile rather than infiltrative and may have little or no metastasizing potential. These animal experiments nevertheless support premalignancy in the breast as a valid concept.

HUMAN STUDIES

A very large number of studies, extending over a long period of time, have been undertaken to determine the possible preneoplastic significance of common benign epithelial lesions in the human breast. Many of the results have been conflicting, producing a complex picture. The general principles of these investigations apply to all lesions with putative precancerous significance, so an overview is provided here to avoid repetition. The significance of rare lesions is discussed in the appropriate sections of Chapters 6, 7 and 13 in view of the limited data available.

Evidence for a precancerous state in the human breast derives mainly from five indirect sources. First, some lesions resemble carcinoma either cytologically (e.g. intraductal or intralobular hyperplasias) or architecturally (e.g. sclerosing adenosis, radial scar and microglandular adenosis). Second, carcinomas may merge with or apparently arise in certain benign lesions (e.g. radial scar and papilloma). Third, some lesions exhibit a higher incidence in cancerous than non-cancerous breasts (see below). Fourth, epidemiological studies of pathological changes have shown that certain lesions occur more frequently in populations at greater risk of developing breast cancer (see below). Finally, follow-up studies have demonstrated that the risk of developing carcinoma is increased in women in whom certain benign lesions have been identified in otherwise benign biopsies (see below).

Experimental studies have also been undertaken but have so far not been very informative. Improvements in microdissection and molecular technology have in recent years led to many investigations of the molecular changes occurring in putative precancerous lesions. The occurrence in benign lesions of molecular changes that usually characterize carcinomas is, by itself, no greater evidence of a precancerous state than is morphological similarity, although it may give greater insight into the mechanisms involved.

Breast lesions co-existing with carcinoma

There have over the years been many studies in which the histological changes occurring in breasts harbouring carcinomas have been compared with those in non-cancerous breasts. Foote and Stewart (1945a) looked for the presence of 11 lesions often collectively and loosely referred to as chronic cystic mastitis in 300 cancerous and 200 non-cancerous breasts. The lesions examined were cysts, duct papillomatosis (hyperplasia), blunt duct adenosis, apocrine change, stasis and distension of the ducts, periductal mastitis, fat necrosis, hyperplasia of the duct epithelium, fibroadenoma and fibroadenomatoid hyperplasia. If only one of these features was necessary to make a diagnosis of chronic cystic mastitis, the condition was present in 83% of cancer-bearing breasts and 90% of the controls. If the criteria for diagnosis were restricted to any of the first five changes, the incidence dropped in both groups but was still slightly higher in the non-cancer cases. If the diagnostic criteria were made even more rigid by insisting on at least three out of the first five lesions, the overall figure was lowered even further but was still somewhat higher in the non-malignant group, even when corrected for age. Thus there did not appear to be an association between chronic cystic mastitis and carcinoma.

The results have to be interpreted with some caution in view of the nature of the control group, which consisted of surgical biopsy specimens in which the various lesions would be expected to be more frequent than in the general population. Furthermore, the small size of most surgical biopsies can lead to sampling problems. Despite such reservations, Foote and Stewart (1945b) found that, although orderly papillary hyperplasia occurred with similar frequency in cancerous and non-cancerous breasts, papillary hyperplasia with cytologic atypia was about five times more frequent in the malignant group.

Later studies of this type employed autopsy material for controls, thus overcoming the problem of case selection and minimizing sampling error. Ryan and Coady (1962) examined the changes in 100 cancer-bearing breasts and compared them with those occurring in 100 pairs of breasts taken from routine autopsies. Serial 10 mm slices were made through each breast, and blocks were taken from all four quadrants, from the subareolar region, from the axillary tail and from any macroscopically suspicious areas. The study focused on one pathological change, namely epithelial proliferation. The proliferative changes were graded from I to IV, grade I change being merely the multilayering of well-differentiated epithelial cells and grade IV in situ carcinoma. Proliferative changes in general were four times more common in the malignant series and seven times more common if only grade III and IV changes were considered.

Karpas et al (1965) examined 645 consecutive benign and malignant surgical specimens of the breast. As in the studies of Foote and Stewart, the control group consisted of breast tissue that would be expected to contain an increased number of benign lesions. Although the overall incidence of proliferative change was similar in each group, atypical proliferations were 14 times more common in the malignant specimens.

In the study of Gallagher and Martin (1969), 60 radical mastectomy specimens were examined in immense detail, taking 200–300 125 × 175 mm slices from each specimen. Ductal epithelial hyperplasia of variable extent was present in every specimen, ranging from simple hyperplasia to in situ carcinoma. There was no sharp demarcation between the various degrees of change, which merged with one another, suggesting the possibility of progression. A change in the mammary lobules varying from simple hyperplasia to lobular carcinoma in situ were present in 40% of the breasts. Breasts lacking lobular lesions were generally from patients older than 65 years.

Black and Chabon (1969) used a numerical grading system to describe epithelial proliferation in the breast. Grade I was normal and grade V in situ carcinoma. Of 97 benign breast biopsies, only 12% showed changes in excess of grade III and one in excess of grade IV. In 55 breasts containing invasive carcinoma, 77% had changes in excess of grade III.

The most detailed study of this type is perhaps that of Wellings et al. (1975), who adapted the subgross sampling technique used in rodents to human breasts. The whole breast was cut into 50–150 slices 2 mm thick, which were stained with haematoxylin and examined under the dissecting microscope. Lesions were thus selected for conventional histological examination, the procedure considerably reducing sampling problems. Another advantage was that the low-power, three-dimensional view afforded by the dissecting microscope gave a better appreciation of the microanatomy of the lesions under study.

The morphological evidence gained from this study supports the idea that most lesions grouped as fibrocystic disease (including apocrine cysts, sclerosing adenosis and fibroadenomas), ductal carcinoma in situ (DCIS) and lobular carcinoma in situ arise in terminal duct–lobular units. The evidence that ductal carcinomas in situ arise from terminal duct–lobular units is that they had a lobular configuration, were connected to terminal interlobular ducts and occasionally contained residual normal acini. Furthermore, the subgross technique allowed the detection of minute lesions in which the lobular architecture was even more easily recognized.

The study concentrated on two types of atypical lobules: type A and type B. Type A lesions represented the spectrum of hyperplasia of usual type, atypical ductal hyperplasia and DCIS, whereas type B lesions represented the spectrum of atypical lobular hyperplasia and lobular carcinoma in situ. Each type of lobule was graded from I to V in severity, grade I showing little proliferation and grade V being in situ carcinoma of the relevant type.

In breasts taken from routine autopsies, atypical lobules of grades I and II were common at all ages but grades in excess of III were rare. In contrast, in breasts containing clinically evident carcinoma, atypical lobules of grade III or more were frequent. Grade I and II atypical lobules were also more frequent than in autopsy breasts in patients past the fourth decade. Type A atypical lobules (ductal type) were more frequent than type B atypical lobules (lobular type), DCIS occurring in 40% of the cancerous breasts but lobular carcinoma *in situ* occurring in only 20%. Of the autopsy glands 4% contained intraduct carcinoma and none contained intralobular carcinoma. Atypical lobules as a whole occurred almost four times more frequently in cancer-containing breasts than in autopsy glands (Jensen *et al*, 1976).

Epidemiological studies

The incidence of putative precancerous lesions has been studied in populations at different risk of developing breast cancer. In a forensic autopsy study of females more than 14 years old, Bartow *et al*. (1987) determined the prevalence of various benign, atypical and occult malignant lesions in Anglos (non-Hispanic whites), Hispanics and American Indians from New Mexico and Eastern Arizona, USA. The risk of developing breast cancer in these three groups was 89, 46 and 25 per 100 000 per year respectively. Eighteen blocks per case (nine per breast) were examined.

Thirty-four per cent of Anglo women aged 45–54 had moderate-to-severe epithelial hyperplasia compared to 24% of Hispanics and 2% of Indians. Similar ethnic/racial age-specific differences were seen in marked-to-moderate cystic change. Cystic change, epithelial hyperplasia, apocrine metaplasia, sclerosing adenosis and lobular microcalcification, when considered at all degrees of severity in all age groups were not, however, encountered more commonly in Anglo than Hispanic women but were more common in both these groups than in Indians. The explanation for this was not clear but could have been related to the rising incidence of breast cancer in Hispanics. The incidence of fibroadenoma was not greatly different in the three groups, but these lesions were not subdivided into complex and non-complex types. Atypical lobular and ductal hyperplasia, carcinoma *in situ* and occult invasive carcinoma were uncommon but also occurred in ethnic/racial groups in a pattern that paralleled their cancer risk.

Follow-up studies

There have been many studies designed to assess the risk of developing infiltrating breast carcinoma after various non-malignant breast lesions have been diagnosed. Some have been described as prospective but are actually prospective studies carried out in retrospect. A large number of benign biopsies are retrieved from the archives, the histological changes being interpreted without a knowledge of the patients' clinical course and then related to the subsequent development of invasive cancer. Others have been case control studies in which patients with invasive carcinoma who have had previous benign biopsies are identified and matched with a group of control patients with benign biopsies (usually at least twice the size of the reference group) who did not develop cancer over the same period. The histological changes in both groups are then compared.

In some of the early investigations the benign lesions were not characterized histologically, the mere occurrence of a previous benign biopsy being related to the subsequent development of cancer. In others general terms such as chronic cystic mastitis, cystic disease or benign breast disease were employed. Clearly it is difficult to identify lesions as being precancerous in studies of this type simply because the changes present are diverse, and more recent investigations with any credibility have included a detailed histological characterization of all lesions observed.

Many difficulties still arise. First, there is the problem of subjectivity of histopathological interpretation, particularly in defining lesions known to be associated with significant diagnostic inconsistency, such as atypical hyperplasia (Sloane *et al*., 1994, 1999). High-quality illustrations and precise definitions of terminology are thus essential.

Another obvious problem is that the lesions under study have been removed and cannot themselves develop into cancer. Two important assumptions have to be made: (1) that similar lesions were left behind, and (2) that lesions of no greater severity, particularly an occult carcinoma, were present. Even if these assumptions are correct, it cannot be proved that the subsequent cancer developed from lesions similar to those under study, which could simply represent 'markers of risk'. Studies of this type are less suitable for studying the precancerous potential of lesions of a more focal nature, such as radial scars detected by mammographic screening.

Sampling problems exist in the control groups. Proliferative lesions are usually focal and asymptomatic, being discovered incidentally in the course of removing clinically overt lesions such as cysts or fibroadenomas. The breasts of patients in control groups thus contain a proportion of undiscovered premalignant changes, and this tends to minimize their significance.

The evolution of mammary carcinoma in the human may be very slow, and long follow-up periods are necessary. Furthermore, the incidence of breast carcinoma varies between geographical, racial and cultural groups, and the development of cancer in patients with various benign lesions has to be seen in the context of the natural breast cancer incidence in the group of patients from whom they are removed.

Davis *et al.* (1964) followed 284 patients who had had local excisions for cystic breast disease for an average of 13 years. Their term cystic disease covered a variety of lesions as diverse as cysts and papillary hyperplasia. Carcinoma developed in 2.4% of these patients, that is, about 1.7 times the expected incidence. Individuals with ductal hyperplasia developed carcinoma at 2.5 times the expected frequency compared with 1.2 times in those without hyperplastic changes. These authors also reviewed 20 previous studies performed between 1892 and 1960. The results were very variable, the proportion of patients with cystic disease who developed carcinoma varying from 0 to 10.3%. A risk factor was calculated in only four studies, varying from three to four-and-a-half times the expected frequency of cancer development. Much of the variation in these results

can be explained by the problems outlined above.

Black *et al.* (1972) studied a group of patients who had had benign breast biopsies and subsequently developed carcinoma. For each of these so-called 'reference' cases, three controls were chosen who had not subsequently developed carcinoma and who were matched for age and date of biopsy. The Black and Chabon system was used to grade epithelial proliferation. On reviewing the histological sections, some of the breast lesions were reclassified as carcinoma *in situ* (grade V), this being found five times more frequently in the 'reference' than in the control group. Ductal hyperplasia of grades III and IV was found in 30% of the 'reference' group and 8% of the controls. The risk of developing cancer within the test period was five times greater for patients exhibiting grade III and IV changes than in those exhibiting changes of grades I and II. Apocrine metaplasia, intraduct papilloma, fibroadenoma, blunt duct adenosis and sclerosing adenosis were found not to be associated with an increased risk.

In their follow-up study of chronic mastopathy, Kodlin *et al.* (1977) used the Black and Chabon grading system described above. In 2092 patients with scores of I or II, there was an increased risk of cancer development of 2.3. This rose to 2.4 for the 262 patients with grade III changes, to 6.0 for the 49 patients with grade IV changes and to 16.7 for the 8 subjects with carcinoma *in situ* (grade V). The cancer risk thus increased with the degree of atypia in the proliferative lesions. The overall incidence rate for cancer in this series was similar to that which the authors obtained by pooling data from previous studies.

In a critical and detailed study, Page *et al.* (1978) followed 925 patients for up to 24 years after biopsy for a benign lesion. The histological lesions under study were carefully defined and included cysts, duct ectasia, sclerosing adenosis, fibroadenoma, apocrine change, papillary apocrine change, ductal hyperplasia with and without apocrine-like changes, ductal hyperplasia with atypia and atypical lobular hyperplasia. The cancer incidence for

TABLE 10.1 Relative risk of developing breast cancer in relation to histological changes in benign biopsies

Authors	Number		Follow-up	Relative risk				
	Pts	Ca	(years)	NPD	HUT	AH	Other	FH
Dupont and Page (1985)	3303	134	17 (median)	0.89	5.3	5.3	Calcification, Cysts+ FH(2.7)*	2.5
Carter et al. (1988)	16 692	485	8.3 (mean)	1.5	1.9	3.0**	Fibroadenoma (1.7)	1.8
London et al. (1992)	609	121***	9 (median)	1.0	1.6	3.7**		NS
McDivitt et al. (1992)	665	417***	Not stated	1.5	1.8	2.6	Fibroadenoma (1.7)	NS
Bodian et al. (1993)	1799	157	20.6 (mean)	1.6	2.1	Mild 2.3 Moderate to severe 3.0	Adenosis (3.7)	NS
Marshall et al. (1997)	975	214	10 (median)	1.0 (reference group)	1.7	3.4 ALH 5.3 (premen. 9.6 postmen. 3.7) ADH-2.4	Fibroadenoma included with HUT	NI

*Cysts not significant alone; **Risk greater in premenopausal women; ***Nested case control study.

Pt .= patients; Ca = carcinomas; NPD = no proliferative disease; HUT = hyperplasia of usual type; AH = atypical hyperplasia; FH = family history; NS = not significant; NI = not investigated.

each subgroup was compared with that obtained for their group as a whole, with that quoted in the third National Cancer Survey of the United States and with that obtained from a previous study of white women in Atlanta, Georgia. The risk of developing carcinoma was increased six-fold in patients with atypical lobular hyperplasia who were under 45 years of age at the time of biopsy, but this fell to three-fold in patients who were over 45. The increased risk to patients with ductal lesions was different in magnitude and age pattern, being associated with a three-fold increase in risk of invasive cancer over the age of 45 but with no increased risk below this age. Very surprisingly, in this study atypical duct lesions did not exhibit a greater risk than ductal proliferations without atypia. Apocrine change with papillary tufting had an elevated cancer risk, with an age pattern similar to that of ductal hyperplasia.

Dupont and Page (1985) later published a much larger study of 3303 women who had been followed up for a median of 17 years after a benign breast biopsy. The relative risk of subsequently developing invasive carcinoma was 0.89 for women in whom no proliferative lesions were found and 1.9 for those in whom proliferation without atypia was seen. Although the presence of proliferation doubled the risk, this had questionable clinical importance, as the absolute risk remained low. On the other hand, women with atypical proliferations (atypical ductal or lobular hyperplasia) had a risk that was 5.3 times that of the general population, this doubling if there was also a family history (in the mother, sister or daughter) of breast cancer. Surprisingly, calcification also had a significant prognostic effect but only if it occurred with atypical proliferation. Women with atypia and no calcification thus had a four-fold increase in risk compared to one of 6.5 in those with calcification.

Within 15 years of their entry biopsy, 20% of the women in this study who had atypical proliferations and a family history of breast cancer had developed infiltrating carcinoma of the breast compared to 8% of those with atypia and no family history. Only 2% of women with non-proliferative lesions and 4%

of those with proliferative disease without atypia had developed cancer within the same period.

Several large studies with long periods of follow-up have been undertaken since the findings of Dupont and Page were published; the results of six of these are summarized in Table 10.1. Broadly similar findings were obtained, but there were also some important differences. In three of the studies, a slight increase in risk was found in patients whose breasts did not exhibit intraductal or intralobular hyperplasia. This finding would be consistent with the existence of lesions carrying risk other than intraductal and intralobular hyperplasias. There is general agreement that hyperplasia of usual type is associated with a slight increase in relative risk of around 1.5–2.0. There is also an agreement that the risk associated with atypical hyperplasia is greater than that of hyperplasia of usual type, but the size of the risk varies significantly. This can be explained by a number of factors including the age of the patients studied as there is evidence that atypical hyperplasia carries a greater risk in younger women (Carter *et al.*, 1988).

Pathologists' diagnostic criteria are also important. The higher risk in the study of Dupont and Page could be explained by more stringent criteria for making a diagnosis of DCIS of low nuclear grade. Their cases of atypical hyperplasia would thus include some which would have been diagnosed as DCIS by other pathologists. Diagnosing atypical ductal hyperplasia is associated with a low level of diagnostic consistency even using the stringent diagnostic criteria of Page and Rogers (1992) (Sloane *et al.*, 1999). In the study by Carter *et al.* (1988), no central pathology review was undertaken of the histological slides that were derived from 29 centres. Atypical hyperplasia was therefore less precisely defined, and a higher incidence was encountered.

Another possible explanation for the variable risk reported for atypical hyperplasia is suggested by the study of Marshall *et al.* (1997), in which a greater risk was found for the lobular than the ductal variant.

Furthermore, atypical lobular hyperplasia was more strongly associated with the risk of premenopausal than postmenopausal breast cancer, whereas the association of risk and atypical ductal hyperplasia varied little by menopausal status.

Although family history is a well-recognized risk factor for developing breast cancer, there is a lack of agreement in the six studies on the effect of family history on the size of the risk associated with the histological changes.

Various other lesions have been found less consistently to be associated with an increased risk of developing breast cancer. These include calcification, cysts in the presence of a family history of breast cancer, fibroadenoma and adenosis (*see* Table 10.1 above). In addition to the studies listed in the table, fibroadenomas have been found to be associated with an increased risk of developing breast cancer, particularly if they contain cysts, sclerosing adenosis, epithelial proliferation or papillary apocrine changes (complex fibroadenomas), for which a relative risk of 3.1 has been reported (Dupont *et al.*, 1994). In the same study patients in whom benign proliferative disease was identified in the breast adjacent to the fibroadenoma had a relative risk of 3.88. Patients with complex fibroadenomas and a family history of breast cancer had a relative risk of 3.72 compared with controls with a family history. The majority of patients, however, had non-complex fibroadenomas and no family history, and they were not at increased risk.

There is evidence that patients with significant sclerosing adenosis may have an increased risk of developing breast carcinoma. Jensen *et al.* (1989) found an increased relative risk of 2.1, which decreased to 1.7 when patients who also had atypical hyperplasia were excluded and rose to 6.7 when those with both sclerosing adenosis and atypical hyperplasia were analysed. A family history of breast cancer did not increase the risk in those with sclerosing adenosis alone. Sclerosing adenosis was also found to be associated with an increased risk of developing breast cancer in the study of Tavassoli and Norris (1990) but only in the presence of atypical hyperplasia.

From the practical point of view, there is insufficient evidence for taking any clinical action when sclerosing adenosis is discovered.

There were until recently conflicting data on the precancerous significance of radial scars. Some authors (Sloane and Mayers, 1993; Douglas-Jones and Pace, 1997) had found that radial scars detected by mammographic screening contained foci of *in situ* or invasive carcinoma at a frequency much greater than would be expected by chance. This did not, however, apply to smaller scars discovered incidentally in surgical material. Data on the frequency with which radial scars occur in cancerous and non-cancerous breasts have been conflicting, and follow-up studies had not previously revealed an increased risk of developing breast cancer. Recently, however, a large prospective investigation conducted within the Nurses' Health Study in the USA found that women with a radial scar of any size were at increased risk of developing breast cancer (Jacobs *et al.*, 1999). This study had far greater statistical power than any conducted previously.

There thus appear to be two types of risk associated with radial scars. First, carcinomas may be found with disproportionate frequency within them, but only if they are detected by mammography. This is related not only to the age of the patient, but also to the greater size of the scar – a situation similar to that encountered with colorectal adenomas. The smaller, incidentally discovered scars seem to be associated with a slightly increased risk of developing carcinoma in either breast, analogous to the situation encountered in hyperplasia of usual type or sclerosing adenosis.

There is also some evidence that a few other lesions are precancerous, but, because they are uncommon and/or of a more localized nature, the evidence is weaker or more circumstantial. They are discussed in the relevant parts of this book, and include solitary and multiple intraduct papillomata, microglandular adenosis, apocrine adenosis juvenile papillomatosis and adenoma of the nipple.

The chances of patients with ductal and lobular carcinoma *in situ* subsequently developing invasive carcinoma are discussed in Chapters 8 and 9.

Cytogenetic and molecular genetic studies

Early lesions show less complex molecular changes than do established invasive cancers, so the chance of finding those of pathogenetic importance is consequently greater. Furthermore, a greater knowledge of the molecular alterations that take place in the early development of breast cancer could lead to the identification of some changes that could be exploited to improve diagnosis and prognostication, which seems unlikely to be achieved by conventional morphological methods alone. In the longer term, specific molecular changes could provide targets for prophylactic therapeutic intervention.

The rationale for using genetic analysis in studying premalignancy is that it is assumed that the various steps in the development of cancer are characterized by the acquisition of irreversible genetic changes. Consequently, if lesions were precancerous they would share some of the genetic changes with the cancers into which they evolved. If a lesion exhibits genetic changes not found in cancer, it is highly unlikely to be a precursor of that particular type of tumour. The sharing of genetic abnormalities by benign and malignant lesions is not proof of the premalignant status of the former but provides greater evidence than does shared phenotypic or epigenetic changes. Conversely, the failure to detect a genetic change does not exclude precancerous potential. Genetic abnormalities in cancers are highly numerous and variable, and not all can be investigated in benign lesions. Genetic events have proved less useful in placing a lesion at a particular stage in the development of cancer as they are probably acquired in a stochastic fashion.

Genetic abnormalities have been demonstrated in various benign breast lesions, using a variety of techniques. Fisher and Paulson (1978) applied traditional *chromosomal analysis* to human breast lesions in an attempt to identify those with precancerous potential. Fibroadenomas, sclerosing adenosis, blunt duct adenosis, apocrine metaplasia and simple cysts generally contained fewer than 12% aneuploid cells, and the chromosomes appeared normal. In six samples showing notable intraductal hyperplasia and varying cellular atypia but no histological evidence of cancer, 7–40% of cells were aneuploid. Three of these samples showed morphologically aberrant chromosomes. All the cells from invasive carcinomas exhibited aneuploidy and morphologically abnormal chromosomes. The major disadvantages of this type of conventional cytogenetics, however, are that only dividing cells can be studied and that it is generally impossible to know from what part of a heterogeneous piece of breast tissue the cells under investigation are derived.

More recently, *interphase cytogenetic studies* have been undertaken, in which the number of chromosomes in interphase cells can be determined by *in situ* hybridization to tissue sections of probes for chromosome-specific centromeric DNA sequences. In the study of Micale *et al.* (1994), aneuploidy of chromosomes 16, 17, 18 and X was detected in hyperplasia of usual type and atypical lobular hyperplasia as well as in *in situ* and invasive carcinomas. Alternatively, locus-specific probes can be used to detect any change in the number of copies of specific genes, although this approach is technically more demanding and has not at the time of writing generated any significant data in precancerous lesions of the human breast.

At the time of writing, *comparative genomic hybridization* has been used mainly to study *in situ* and invasive carcinomas. Buerger *et al.* (1999) demonstrated that certain chromosomal losses and gains were found more frequently in low- than in high-grade DCIS, suggesting that the latter does not arise from the former but along a separate histogenetic lineage.

Improvements in *microdissection* techniques and the ability of the *polymerase chain reaction* to amplify a very small amount of DNA, even from formalin-fixed, paraffin-embedded sections, have greatly increased the scope for undertaking molecular genetic investigations on putative precursor lesions. Despite their frequently small size, poor circumscription and difficult histological appearances, it has become possible to detect phenomena such as mutations and allelic imbalance.

Allelic imbalance (AI) is a very common change in *in situ* and invasive carcinomas and may involve numerous chromosomal loci. It has also been demonstrated in hyperplasia of usual type and atypical ductal hyperplasia, occurring at a much higher frequency in the latter than the former (Lakhani *et al.*, 1995, 1996). Hyperplasias from cancerous breasts often share AI with the accompanying cancer, further supporting their precursor status (O'Connell *et al.*, 1998). These observations show that AI can be a very early change in the development of breast cancer and support the notion that hyperplasias are actually precursors of carcinomas rather than simply markers of risk. The finding of AI also argues in favour of hyperplasias actually being neoplastic. One recent study has shown that patients with proliferative lesions exhibiting AI do not necessarily develop malignancy over the long term (Kasami *et al.*, 1997). It is not yet known, however, whether the presence, extent or distribution of AI within the genome could provide a more precise and reproducible assessment of risk than can be obtained by morphological methods alone.

Mutation of the E-cadherin gene has been found in atypical lobular hyperplasia and lobular carcinoma *in situ* but not in atypical ductal hyperplasia or hyperplasia of usual type (Vos *et al.*, 1997). Similar mutations are encountered in invasive lobular carcinomas. So far, mutations of the *TP53* gene have not been found in hyperplasias (Done *et al.*, 1998).

Immunohistochemical studies

These have been more numerous than those concerned with genetics, many being discussed in the appropriate sections of this book. At the time of writing, immunohistochemical investigations have not become part of the routine assessment of patients with potentially precancerous lesions, although there have been some promising observations.

Shoker *et al.* (1999a, 1999b) have shown evidence of a progressively abnormal regulation of the oestrogen receptor in non-atypical and atypical hyperplasias. An abnormal expression of the cell cycle proteins cyclins D1 and B1 has been described in DCIS and hyperplasias (Weinstat-Saslow *et al.* 1995; Kawamoto *et al.*, 1997; Gillett *et al.*, 1998; Shoker *et al.*, in preparation). A reduced expression of transforming growth factor-β type II receptor has been found to be related to the risk of developing breast cancer (Gobbi *et al.*, 1999). Increased immunostaining for p53 has been described in hyperplasia of usual type and to a greater extent in atypical ductal hyperplasia, although the significance of this is unclear in view of the failure to detect *TP53* gene mutations. (Done *et al.*, 1998; Schmitt *et al.*, 1995a; *see* above). A loss of expression of the E-cadherin protein has been found in atypical lobular hyperplasia and lobular carcinoma *in situ* but not in atypical ductal hyperplasia or hyperplasia of usual type (Vos *et al.*, 1997).

Interestingly, some changes fairly commonly observed in invasive carcinomas, usually of high grade, have not been seen in atypical or non-atypical hyperplasias. They include the overexpression of c-erbB-2 (Schmitt *et al.*, 1995b) and increased telomerase activity (Poremba *et al.*, 1998). There are several possible explanations for this. First, these changes may occur very late in the development of breast cancer. Second, in evolving from precursor lesions, breast cancers can radically change their differentiation characteristics. Third, not all cancers arise from known precancerous lesions: recognizable precursor stages for high-grade carcinomas may not exist or may be so transient that the chance of detecting them is extremely small.

Transplantation studies

Jensen *et al.* (1976) identified individual lobules in breast biopsies and mastectomy specimens and transplanted them into the cleared fat pad of athymic nude mice. Sometimes the epithelium did not survive, but in other cases there was a variable degree of epithelial disorganization and immaturity within enlarged ductular units. The latter phenomenon was seen in 20 of 61 normal lobules removed from breasts containing cancer and in 11 of 48 lobules removed from breasts without cancer. The data obtained from the transplantation of atypical lobules were too scanty for analysis. None of the transplants filled the fat pads as do the HANs of mice, and none underwent malignant change.

Although transplantation techniques of this kind could be useful in assessing the malignant potential of human lesions, the identification and dissection of individual lesions is immensely time consuming and the chance of finding and accurately characterizing appropriate lesions low. Even if malignant change could be induced, the process might be exceedingly slow, perhaps even longer than the life of the animal. Either some way of accelerating the process, or a reliable endpoint short of actual malignancy, is needed. Furthermore, factors operating in the host may be necessary for progression, and these would not be taken into account.

CONCLUSIONS

Animal experiments have established that at least some breast neoplasms may evolve in a multistage fashion from precursor lesions, which, although not themselves cancerous, have a higher probability of developing into malignant tumours than do normal tissues. Although the existence of precancer cannot be directly established in humans, many studies have shown that certain lesions are associated with a higher risk than others of subsequent malignancy and are therefore likely to have precancerous potential. These lesions include various forms of intraductal and intralobular hyperplasia, sclerosing adenosis and more localized lesions such as radial scar, intraduct papilloma and fibroadenoma, but do not appear to include other benign lesions, such as cysts, blunt duct adenosis, duct ectasia or lactational foci.

Recent molecular studies support the notion that those changes associated with an increased risk of developing cancer are actually precursor lesions rather than simply markers of risk, and there is a prospect that molecular changes may soon be identified that can help in histological diagnosis and prognostication. There is as yet insufficient information on rare lesions like microglandular adenosis, juvenile papillomatosis and adenoma of the nipple to draw any firm conclusions.

The risk associated with the less extensive, cytologically non-atypical forms of intralobular and intraductal proliferation appears to be small, their very common occurrence making detailed patient follow-up an impractical proposition. At the other extreme, DCIS, although not invariably progressing to infiltrative carcinoma, has a high probability of doing so, generally over a relatively short period, which consequently justifies therapeutic intervention.

Multifocal lesions associated with significantly increased risk, such as lobular carcinoma *in situ* and the atypical hyperplasias, present a major problem of patient management. It has been suggested by some that it would be better for pathologists not to report them as the clinical dilemmas they create are insuperable. It would, however, be a dangerous precedent for pathologists to withhold information from clinicians about lesions they have detected, albeit incidentally, in breast biopsy or resection specimens. Patients have a right to know what abnormalities are present in their breasts and what risks these carry. Furthermore, the problems will not be solved if they are ignored.

The options chosen by patients have ranged from bilateral mastectomy at one extreme to doing nothing at the other. In between lie the choices of close surveillance (usually annual mammography) and prophylactic treatment with tamoxifen. The results of the tamoxifen prevention trials have been inconclusive, but heterogeneous groups of patients have been entered in them, including those with inherited gene mutations who usually develop oestrogen receptor-negative carcinomas. The efficacy of prophylactic treatment with tamoxifen for patients with strongly oestrogen receptor-positive precancerous lesions remains to be determined but offers some hope for the future.

REFERENCES

Barraclough R., Chen H., Davies B.R. *et al.* (1998) Use of DNA transfer in the induction of metastasis in experimental mammary systems. *Biochem. Soc. Symp.*, 63, 273–94.

Bartow S.A., Pathak D.R., Black W.C., Key C.R., Teaf S.R. (1987) Prevalence of benign, atypical, and malignant lesions in populations at different risk for breast cancer. *Cancer*, 60, 2751–60.

Black M.M., Chabon A.B. (1969) *In situ* carcinoma of the breast. *Pathol. Ann.*, 4, 185–210.

Black M.M., Barclay T.H.C., Cutler S.J. Hankey, F., Asire A.J. (1972) Association of atypical characteristics of benign breast lesions with subsequent risk of breast cancer. *Cancer*, 29, 338–43.

Bodian C.A., Perzin K.H., Lattes R., Hoffman P., Abernathy T.G. (1993) Prognostic significance of benign proliferative breast disease. *Cancer*, 71, 3896–907.

Buerger H., Otterbach F., Simon R. *et al.* (1999) Comparative genomic hybridization of ductal carcinoma *in situ* of the breast-evidence of multiple genetic pathways. *J. Pathol.*, 187, 396–402

Cardiff R D., Muller W.J. (1993) Transgenic models of mammary tumorigenesis. *Cancer Surv.*, 16, 97–113.

Carter C.L., Corle D.K., Micozzi M.S., Schatzkin A., Taylor P.R. (1988) A prospective study of the development of breast cancer in 16,692 women with benign breast disease. *Am. J. Epidemiol.*, 128, 467–77.

Davis H.H., Simons M., Davis J.B. (1964) Cystic disease of the breast: relationship to carcinoma. *Cancer*, 17, 957–78.

DeOme K.B., Faulkin L.J., Bern H.A., Blair P.B. (1959) Development of mammary tumours from hyperplastic alveolar nodules transplanted into the gland free mammary fat pads of female C3H mice. *Cancer Res.*, 19, 515–20.

Done S.J., Arneson N.C., Ozcelik H., Redston M., Andrulis I.L. (1998) p53 mutations in mammary ductal carcinoma *in situ* but not in epithelial hyperplasias. *Cancer Res.*, 58, 785–9.

Douglas-Jones A.G., Pace D.P. (1997) Pathology of R4 spiculated lesions in the breast screening programme. *Histopathology*, 30, 214–20.

Dupont W.D., Page D.L. (1985) Risk factors in women with proliferative breast disease. *N. Engl. J. Med.*, **312**, 146–51.

Dupont W.D., Page D.L., Parl F.F. *et al.* (1994) Long-term risk of breast cancer in women with fibroadenoma. *N. Engl. J. Med.*, **331**, 10–15.

Fisher E.R., Paulson J.D. (1978) Karyotypic abnormalities in precursor lesions of human cancer of the breast. *Am. J. Clin. Pathol.*, **69**, 284–8.

Fisher E.R., Shoemaker R.H., Sabnis A. (1975a) Relationship of hyperplasia to cancer in 3-methyl-cholanthrene-induced mammary tumorogenesis. *Lab. Invest.*, **33**, 33–42.

Fisher E.R., Shoemaker R.H., Palekar A.S. (1975b) Identification of premalignant hyperplasia in methylcholanthrene-induced mammary tumorogenesis. *Lab. Invest.*, **33**, 446–50.

Foote F.W., Stewart F.W. (1945a) Comparative studies of cancerous versus noncancerous breasts. *Ann. Surg.*, **121**, 6–53.

Foote F.W., Stewart F.W. (1945b) Comparative studies of cancerous versus noncancerous breasts. *Ann. Surg.*, **121**, 197–222.

Gallagher H.S., Martin J.E. (1969) Early phases in the development of breast cancer. *Cancer*, **24**, 1170–8.

Gillett C.E., Lee A.H.S., Millis R.R., Barnes D.M. (1998) Cyclin D1 and associated proteins in mammary ductal carcinoma *in situ* and atypical ductal hyperplasia. *J. Pathol.*, **184**, 396–400

Gobbi H., Dupont W.D., Simpson J.F. *et al.* (1999) Transforming growth factor-beta and breast cancer risk in women with mammary epithelial hyperplasia. *J Natl Cancer Inst.*, **91**, 2096–101.

Jacobs T.W., Byrne C., Colditz G., Connolly J.L., Schnitt S.J. (1999) Radial scars in benign biopsy specimens and the risk of breast cancer. *N. Engl. J. Med.*, **340**, 430–6.

Jensen H.M., Rice J.R., Wellings S.R. (1976) Preneoplastic lesions in the human breast. *Science*, **191**, 295–7.

Jensen R.A., Page D.L., Dupont W.D., Rogers L.W. (1989) Invasive breast cancer risk in women with sclerosing adenosis. *Cancer*, **64**, 1977–83.

Karpas C.M., Leis H.P., Oppenheim A., Mersheimer W.L. (1965) Relationship of fibrocystic disease to carcinoma of the breast. *Ann. Surg.*, **162**, 1–8.

Kasami M., Vnencak-Jones C.L., Manning S., Dupont W.D., Page D.L. (1997) Loss of heterozygosity and microsatellite instability in breast hyperplasia: no obligate correlation of these genetic alterations with subsequent malignancy. *Am. J. Pathol.*, **150**, 1925–32.

Kawamoto H., Koizumi H., Uchikoshi T. (1997) Expression of the G2-M checkpoint regulators cyclin B1 and cdc2 in nonmalignant and malignant human breast lesions. *Am. J. Pathol.*, **150**, 15–23.

Kodlin D., Winger E.E., Morgenstern N.L., Chen U. (1977) Chronic mastopathy and breast cancer: a follow-up study. *Cancer*, **39**, 2603–7.

Lakhani S.R., Collins N., Stratton M.R., Sloane J.P.(1995) Atypical ductal hyperplasia of the breast: a clonal proliferation with loss of heterozygosity on chromosomes 16q and 17p. *J. Clin. Pathol.*, **48**, 611–15.

Lakhani S.R., Slack D.N., Hamoudi R.A., Collins N., Stratton M.R., Sloane J.P. (1996) Detection of allelic imbalance indicates that a proportion of mammary hyperplasia of usual type are clonal, neoplastic proliferations. *Lab. Invest.*, **74**:129–35.

London S.J., Connolly J.L., Schnitt S.J., Colditz G.A. (1992) A prospective study of benign breast disease and the risk of breast cancer. *JAMA*, **267**, 941–4.

Marshall L.M., Hunter D.J., Connolly J.L. *et al.* (1997) Risk of breast cancer associated with atypical hyperplasia of lobular and ductal types. *Cancer Epidemiology, Biomarkers and Prevention*, **6**, 297–301.

McDivitt R.W., Stevens J.A., Lee N.C., Wingo P.A., Rubin G.L., Gersell D. (1992) Histologic types of benign breast disease and the risk for breast cancer. The Cancer and Steroid Hormone Study Group. *Cancer*, **69**, 1408–14.

Micale M.A., Visscher D.W., Gulino S.E., Wolman S.R. (1994) Chromosomal aneuploidy in proliferative breast disease. *Hum. Pathol.*, **25**, 29–35.

Morris D.W., Cardiff R.D. (1987) Multistep model of mouse mammary tumor development. *Adv. Viral Oncol.*, **7**, 123–40.

O'Connell P.O., Pekkel V., Fuqua A.W., Osborne C.K., Clark G.M., Allred D.C. (1998) Analysis of loss of heterozygosity in 399 premalignant breast lesions at 15 genetic loci. *J. Natl Cancer Inst.*, **90**, 697–703.

Page D.L., Rogers L.W. (1992) Combined histologic and cytologic criteria for the diagnosis of mammary atypical ductal hyperplasia. *Hum. Pathol.*, **23**, 1095–7.

Page D.L., Vander Zwaag R., Rogers L.W., Williams L.T., Walker W.E., Hartmann W.H. (1978) Relation between component parts of fibrocystic disease complex and breast cancer. *J. Natl Cancer Inst.*, **61**, 1055–63.

Poremba C., Boecker W., Willenbring H. *et al.* (1998) Telomerase activity in proliferative breast lesions. *Int. J. Oncol.*, **12**, 641–8.

Ryan J.A., Coady C.J. (1962) Intraductal epithelial proliferation in the human breast-a comparative study. *Can. J. Surg.*, **5**, 12–18.

Schmitt F.C., Leal C., Lopes C. (1995a) p53 protein expression and nuclear DNA content in breast intraductal proliferations. *J. Pathol.*, **176**, 233–41.

Schmitt F.C., Figueiredo P., Lacerda M. (1995b) Expression of c-erbB-2 protein and DNA ploidy in breast carcinogenesis. *Arch. Pathol. Lab. Med.*, **119**, 815–20.

Shoker B.S., Jarvis C., Sibson R., Walker C., Sloane J.P. (1999a) Oestrogen receptor expression in the normal and pre-cancerous breast. *J. Pathol.*, **188**, 237–44.

Shoker B.S., Jarvis C., Clarke R.B. *et al.* (1999b) Estrogen receptor positive proliferating cells in the normal and precancerous breast. *Am. J. Pathol.*, **155**, 1811–15.

Sloane J.P., Mayers M.M. (1993) Carcinoma and atypical hyperplasia in radial scars and complex sclerosing lesions: importance of lesion size and patient age. *Histopathology*, **23**, 225–31.

Sloane J.P. and members of the National Coordinating Group for Breast Screening Pathology (1994) Consistency of histopathological reporting of breast lesions detected by screening: findings of the UK National EQA Scheme. *Eur. J. Cancer.*, **30A**, 1414–19.

Sloane J.P. Amendoeira I., Apostolikas N. *et al.* (1999) Consistency achieved by 23 European pathologists from 12 countries in diagnosing breast disease and reporting prognostic features of carcinomas. *Virchows Archiv.*, **434**, 3–10.

Tavassoli F.A., Norris H.J. (1990) A comparison of the results of long-term follow-up for atypical introductal hyperplasia and intraductal hyperplasia of the breast. *Cancer*, **65**, 518–29.

Vos C.B., Cleton-Jansen A.M., Berx G. *et al.* (1997) E-cadherin inactivation in lobular carcinoma *in situ* of the breast: an early event in carcinogenesis. *Br. J. Cancer*, **76**, 1131–3.

Weinstat-Saslow D., Merino M.J., Manrow R.E. *et al.* (1995) *Nature Med.*, **1**, 1257–60.

Wellings S.R., Jensen H.N., Marcum R.C. (1975) An atlas of subgross pathology of the human breast with special reference to possible precancerous lesions. *J. Natl Cancer Inst.*, **55**, 231–73.

11 Infiltrating carcinoma – pathological types

HISTOLOGICAL TYPES

There are many histological types of breast carcinoma; a few are common, most are uncommon, and others are very rare. The correct classification of many of the subtypes depends on adequate sampling as the special histological features may sometimes comprise only part of what is otherwise an ordinary infiltrative ductal, no special type (nst) carcinoma. In these circumstances a carcinoma is generally classified as invasive ductal (nst) if the histological features of the special subtype comprise less than 10% of the tumour, and as mixed (specifying the types present) if the special features form between 10 and 90%. Carcinomas are classified as one of the special subtypes if the special histological features form more than 90% of the area of the tumour in the histological sections examined.

The identification of specific histological subtypes is of value for a number of reasons. Some of the more common variants are known to exhibit different behaviours. Although the prognostic significance of some of the less common types is difficult to assess in view of their rarity, their identification makes it possible to obtain more information on them. Finally, some types of breast carcinoma may, because of their unusual appearance, be mistaken for carcinomas of non-mammary origin or even for non-epithelial tumours if their appearance is not recognized correctly.

Infiltrative ductal carcinoma, no special type (nst)

Most invasive breast carcinomas fall into this category. They include all those that lack specific features and do not fall into any of the special groups listed below. They are thus of very variable appearance and may even exhibit significant structural and cytological heterogeneity within the same tumour.

Since it is now generally recognized that most breast carcinomas arise in the terminal duct–lobular units, the terms infiltrative ductal and infiltrative lobular carcinoma have come to indicate the cytological and structural appearances of breast carcinomas rather than their presumed sites of origin. As the designation is based upon the histological features of the infiltrative tumour itself, it is not necessary to identify a particular type of *in situ* component in order to make a diagnosis. *In situ* carcinoma co-existing with similar invasive tumour does not necessarily mean that it gave rise to it. Conversely, morphological dissimilarity of co-existent *in situ* and invasive carcinoma does not necessarily

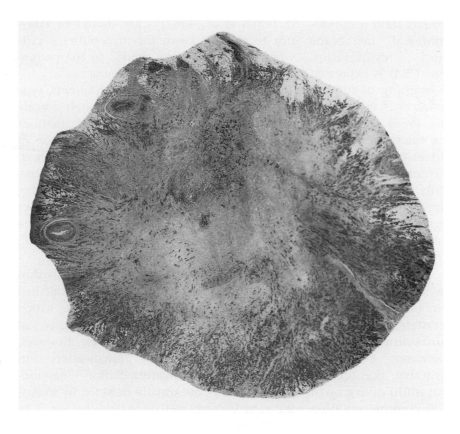

11.1 Infiltrative ductal (nst) carcinoma. This low-power view shows the irregular stellate outline of the tumour and the extensive fibrous stroma (H&E).

exclude the origin of the latter from the former.

Macroscopically, most tumours are of the so-called scirrhous type, having an irregular stellate outline (Fig. 11.1) and a hard, grey, gritty cut surface, often exhibiting yellow flecks of elastin. Less commonly, they are soft and/or circumscribed.

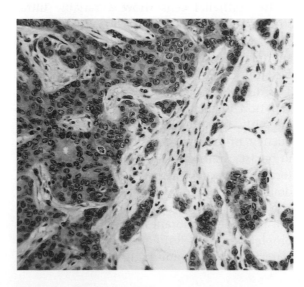

11.2 Infiltrative ductal (nst) carcinoma. The epithelial cells form a large mass on the left of the picture and smaller nests and cords on the right. Stromal fibrosis and mononuclear cell infiltration are not marked in this example. There is an infiltration of fat at the bottom right. Note the formation of a glandular lumen at the centre left (H&E).

Histologically, the neoplastic cells grow in nests, cords or large masses (Fig. 11.2). There is often some tubule formation. In comparison with carcinomas in many other organs, the cells are usually fairly uniform in size, shape and staining intensity, hence the old terms of spheroidal or polygonal cell carcinoma and carcinoma simplex. Some tumours, however, exhibit a more anaplastic appearance with marked pleomorphism.

Necrosis is not a prominent feature in most ductal (nst) carcinomas but may be seen in the more cellular tumours. Very rarely, rapidly growing, densely cellular lesions may undergo extensive central cystic necrosis with only a thin rim of residual tumour cells, simulating a large cyst.

Most tumours contain mucin-secreting cells, but their number is very variable. The mucin may be acid, neutral or both; it may be located within tubular lumina or diffusely within the cytoplasm. Mucin-containing vacuoles are more usually seen in tumours of the infiltrative lobular type (*see* Fig. 3.1).

Nearly all breast carcinomas stain immuno-histochemically for epithelial membrane antigen (EMA) and cytokeratins. Carcinoembryonic antigen (CEA) is expressed less consistently. Immunostaining of tumour cells for myoepithelial markers is very rarely observed (Gusterson et al., 1982) and significant positivity should raise the possibility of a myoepithelial tumour. Invasive ductal (nst) carcinomas generally express a detectable amount of the cell–cell adhesion molecule E-cadherin, although immunostaining intensity is often reduced in higher-grade tumours. Although antibodies to E-cadherin may disrupt cell adhesion in monolayer cultures of MCF-7 cells (Oka et al., 1993), there is no evidence that it plays a significant role in invasion and metastasis in breast carcinomas in vivo. Lymph node metastases may exhibit strongly positive immunostaining, and there is no correlation between E-cadherin immunopositivity and whether the tumour exhibits an expansile or an infiltrative growth pattern (Moll et al., 1993). Immunostaining for the associated molecules α and β catenins (see Chapter 3) is usually also positive (Hashizume et al., 1996).

The stroma is usually abundant and contains a large quantity of collagen (see Fig. 11.1 above). Immunohistological and biochemical studies have shown that breast carcinomas differ from benign lesions and normal breast in containing a very much larger amount of type V collagen, which can be identified as fibrillar and linear deposits in the stroma (Barsky et al., 1982). Stromal elastosis is present in many invasive ductal (nst) carcinomas, particularly those of the scirrhous type, in which the incidence is about 90% (Azzopardi and Laurini, 1974). Elastosis is seen mainly around ducts and blood vessels (see Fig. 3.2), but it may also be distributed diffusely.

Immunohistological stains for the contractile proteins myosin and smooth muscle actin reveal myofibroblasts in the stroma, particularly in the more cellular portions. Myofibroblasts are not usually seen in the normal breast, in benign disorders or even around ductal carcinoma in situ (DCIS) (Schurch et al., 1982). Care should be taken not to mistake them for myoepithelial cells when they are closely applied to the periphery of nests of infiltrating tumour.

The basement membrane components, type IV collagen and laminin, although readily identifiable by immunohistological methods in the normal breast (see Fig. 3.11) or in benign alterations, are rarely demonstrable in infiltrating carcinomas. Occasionally, however, groups of infiltrating cells may show focal cytoplasmic positivity or a complete or partial investment by basement membrane material (Barsky et al., 1982; Gusterson et al., 1982).

Many tumours exhibit calcification within the epithelium or the stroma, the calcified material being mainly hydroxyapatite, which is haematoxyphilic. The radiodensity of invasive ductal (nst) carcinomas, however, often obscures the calcification in radiographs, particularly clinical mammograms, so they are usually detected in screening as radiodense stellate masses (see Fig. 2.7).

Variable numbers of lymphocytes, histiocytes and plasma cells are seen in the stroma, but the density of lymphocytes within the epithelium itself is usually considerably lower than in the normal breast. Nearly all the lymphocytes are T cells, consisting of a mixture of CD4+ and CD8+ cells. This is also in contrast to the normal breast, where they are almost exclusively of the latter type (Lwin et al., 1985).

The epithelial cells show a variable ultrastructural appearance (Ozzello, 1971; Fisher, 1976), with some cells exhibiting a prominent endoplasmic reticulum and Golgi apparatus next to others with inconspicuous organelles. This difference may simply reflect a temporary variation in metabolic activity. Myofilaments are only rarely seen, confirming the infrequency of true myoepithelial differentiation in breast carcinoma. Secretory granules in the form of lysosomes, dense bodies or sometimes double membrane-bound, dense-core granules may be seen in the cytoplasm, especially near the luminal membranes. Glycogen and lipid droplets are not infrequent. There may be intracytoplasmic lumina lined by microvilli (*see* Fig. 3.14) but much less commonly than in lobular carcinomas. The epithelial–stromal junction is badly deranged, and the vessels (particularly venules) often contain endothelium with numerous fenestrations. The presence of stromal myofibroblasts is confirmed.

The prognosis associated with invasive ductal (nst) carcinomas depends very heavily on the pathological prognostic features that they exhibit (see Chapter 12), but the outlook is overall poorer than for the other, more common types of invasive breast carcinoma. In the large series of Ellis *et al.* (1992), 47% of tumours were assigned to this category, and 47% of the patients from whom they were removed survived 10 years.

Infiltrative carcinoma with extensive intraduct component

Infiltrative carcinomas with extensive intraduct components (EICs) should be distinguished from microinvasive carcinomas, which are predominantly intraductal and in which none of the invasive foci exceeds 1 mm in diameter. Invasive carcinomas with EIC can in theory be of any size, but the accompanying intraduct component forms at least 25% of the tumour area in the histological sections (Schnitt *et al.*, 1984). In a publication from the Joint Center for Radiation Therapy, Harvard, the 5-year recurrence rate for 584 stage I–II breast cancer patients treated by local excision and radiotherapy was 23% for those whose tumours showed EIC compared to only 5% for those that did not (Boyages *et al.*, 1990). This difference was highly significant. Bulman *et al.* (1988) also found a higher local recurrence rate in tumours in which more than 25% comprised intraductal carcinoma, particularly if the latter was accompanied by necrosis. In the study of Jacquemier *et al.* (1990), the risk of local recurrence was markedly higher, increasing with the extent of the intraductal component. The presence of EIC, however, had no influence on overall survival, median time to local recurrence or short-term survival after local treatment failure.

The reason for the greater recurrence rate of tumours with EIC could be the greater difficulty of achieving complete excision or the relative insensitivity of DCIS to irradiation. Support for the former explanation comes from the study of Holland *et al.* (1990), who used a very detailed pathological and radiological mapping technique to study mastectomy specimens containing tumours less than 50 mm in diameter. Overall, 30% of the carcinomas were classified as having EIC, intraductal carcinoma being prominently present within the invasive component as well as extending significantly beyond it. They found that intraductal carcinoma was more likely to be found in the remainder of the breast, up to a distance of 80 mm, in carcinomas with EIC than those without. Invasive carcinoma was also more likely to be found but only up to 20 mm from the main lesion. The incidence of vascular invasion was similar in both groups. Schnitt *et al.* (1987) also found that residual tumour was more likely to be present in re-excision specimens from patients whose tumours showed EIC.

In the guidance issued in association with European Breast Screening Programmes (National Coordinating Group for Breast Screening Pathology, 1995; European Commission, 1996), it is recommended that two measurements are given for invasive breast carcinomas:

1. the size of the invasive component alone;
2. the whole size of the tumour to include any intraductal carcinoma extending more than 1 mm beyond the invasive tumour margin (*see* Fig. 2.9).

This enables easy recognition of an EIC that extends beyond the invasive tumour and which may thus contribute significantly to the risk of local recurrence.

Inflammatory carcinoma

Clinically, this type of breast carcinoma is characterized by a variety of features usually associated with inflammation, namely redness, swelling, oedema, pain, tenderness and heat. The onset may be sudden. Cases have been divided by some into primary and secondary depending on whether there are inflammatory symptoms and signs at presentation or whether they develop later in the course of the disease. The characteristic histological change is the presence of carcinoma within the dermal lymphatics, but this is not associated with any morphological evidence of acute or chronic inflammation. The majority of patients have axillary lymph node involvement, and the prognosis is usually poor.

The underlying carcinoma does not exhibit any specific histological features; it is usually of the invasive ductal (nst) type, although other variants may be seen. The radiological features are similar to those of non-inflammatory carcinomas of similar histology and stage. There are problems of definition as not all patients with the clinical features have dermal lymphatic involvement, and vice versa. In the Surveillance, Epidemiology and End Results (SEER) study of 51 030 white women with breast cancer, three groups were recognized (Levine *et al.*, 1985):

1. 153 patients with the clinical and pathological features of inflammatory carcinoma;
2. 2937 women with only clinical signs consistent with the diagnosis;
3. 81 women with histological evidence of dermal lymphatic invasion without clinical evidence of the disease.

It is thus not clear whether there is a causative relationship between the dermal lymphatic involvement and the clinical inflammatory features. The presence of clinical features without dermal lymphatic invasion could be explained by undersampling and the reverse situation by insufficient involvement to produce the clinical changes. It is likely, however, that other factors are important, perhaps involving the release of cytokines by the tumour. The prognosis is poor. The 3-year survival rates for the three groups above in the SEER study were 34%, 60% and 52% respectively, compared with 90% for patients with all other forms of breast cancer.

Infiltrating lobular carcinoma

This tumour is composed of small, round uniform cells that are cytologically indistin-

guishable from those seen in lobular carcinoma *in situ* (LCIS) (*see* Chapter 9). The diagnosis is made on the appearance of the infiltrative component alone, and it is not necessary to identify co-existent LCIS; extensive sampling, however, usually reveals the presence of the *in situ* lesion. DCIS may occasionally be associated with infiltrating lobular carcinoma, but it is generally assumed that the two processes simply co-exist.

The reported incidence of infiltrating lobular carcinoma has varied from 1% to 15% of all infiltrating breast carcinomas (Wheeler and Enterline, 1976; Martinez and Azzopardi, 1979; Ellis *et al.*, 1992). This difference in incidence is largely the result of varying diagnostic criteria, but demographic and racial differences may be important. There have been suggestions that the tumour is more common in the UK than in the USA and that it occurs more frequently in Negroes than Caucasians (Ashikari *et al.*, 1973; Martinez and Azzopardi, 1979).

Macroscopically, most tumours appear as ill-defined scirrhous carcinomas. In the *classic* form the neoplastic cells are usually widely dispersed as single cells or in columns one cell wide, often known as Indian files (Fig. 11.3). There is thus a considerable amount of intervening stroma, which can give rise to diagnostic problems, especially in small biopsies or frozen sections, where the neoplastic nature of the cells may not be appreciated. The uncohesive growth pattern is associated with less tissue destruction than occurs in ductal (nst)

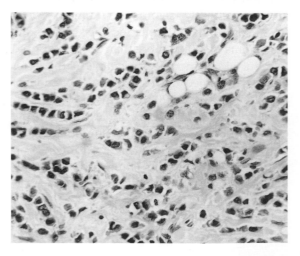

11.3 Infiltrating lobular carcinoma, classic type. The tumour cells are small, uniform, rounded and exhibit a high nuclear-to-cytoplasmic ratio as in lobular carcinoma *in situ*. They infiltrate singly or in single files (left). Note the infiltration of fat at the top right of the picture (H&E).

11.4 (Left) Infiltrating lobular carcinoma. Note the target-like appearance formed by rings of dissociated tumour cells around an atrophic duct (H&E).

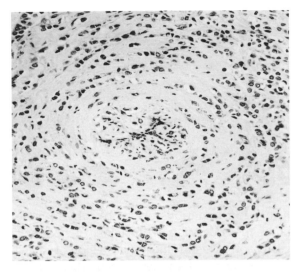

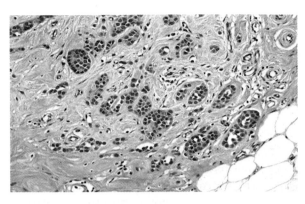

11.5 (Right) Alveolar lobular carcinoma. Cells with the characteristic cytological appearances invade in rounded groups (H&E).

11.6 (Left) Infiltrating lobular carcinoma exhibiting a solid growth pattern. At higher powers the cells have the characteristic appearance. Despite the cohesive nature of the lesion, large clusters of adipocytes and occasional interlobular ducts (arrow) are preserved within the tumour mass. The uniformity and lack of stroma may sometimes give rise to a mistaken diagnosis of lymphoma (H&E).

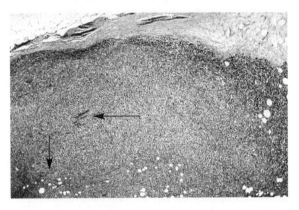

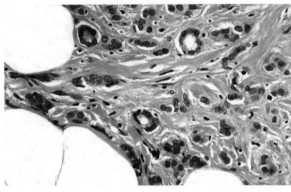

11.7 (Right) Tubulolobular variant of invasive lobular carcinoma. In addition to being arranged singly and in files, some of the cells in this illustration form small tubules (H&E).

carcinomas, and many normal structures may be retained, sometimes surrounded by dispersed neoplastic cells that have been likened to showers of rain. A target-like appearance produced by concentric rings of dissociated neoplastic cells around residual normal ducts is a characteristic feature (Fig. 11.4). The stroma is densely fibrotic and exhibits elastosis in about 90% of cases (Azzopardi and Laurini, 1974). The features of the stroma are essentially similar to those in ductal (nst) carcinomas.

Not all tumours conform to this classic growth pattern, although the cytological features are the same. The *alveolar* variant (Fig. 11.5) (Martinez and Azzopardi, 1979) exhibits small aggregates of 20 or more cells. It is clearly important to distinguish this form from LCIS. In the *solid* variety (Fechner, 1975) the cells grow in much larger solid masses

with little intervening stroma (Fig. 11.6). The uniformity of the cells could lead to an erroneous diagnosis of malignant lymphoma. It is rare for a primary tumour to exhibit this appearance exclusively.

The *tubulolobular* type (Fisher *et al.*, 1977) shows microtubule formation alongside the classic pattern (Fig. 11.7). It is distinguishable from tubular carcinoma by the smaller size and rounder, less angulated appearance of the tubules as well as the accompanying overall infiltrative pattern of a classic lobular carcinoma. An *in situ* component of lobular or ductal type is identified in about one quarter of cases. The lesion is thought to represent a tubular variant of lobular carcinoma rather than vice versa, as the features are more like the latter than the former.

The *pleomorphic* variant is uncommon; it has the growth pattern of classic lobular carcinoma throughout but is composed of cells exhibiting significant pleomorphism (Fig. 11.8). There has been debate about whether this tumour should be included with lobular carcinomas given its cytological deviancy, but Eusebi *et al.* (1992) found that it is frequently associated with LCIS, that the nodal metastases are typically sinusoidal and that intracytoplasmic lumina are present in half the cases. Tumours exhibiting combinations of these patterns are classified as *mixed* lobular carcinomas.

Carcinomas that are composed of mixed lobular and ductal (nst) elements are classified as lobular if this component comprises more than 90% of the tumour, as mixed lobular and ductal (nst) if it makes up 10–90% and as ductal (nst) if it accounts for less than 10%. The whole tumour may sometimes exhibit an appearance intermediate between ductal and lobular carcinoma, consequently being very difficult to classify. Such tumours are best regarded as ductal (nst), although it is advisable to state on reports that classification was difficult.

Infiltrating lobular carcinoma cells resemble those of the *in situ* form histochemically as well as morphologically. Intracytoplasmic mucin vacuoles are common and may exhibit the target-like appearance, with a central magenta dot and a blue peripheral rim on alcian blue–periodic acid–Schiff (AB–PAS) stains (*see* Fig. 3.1). A proportion of cells may assume a signet-ring appearance in H&E stained sections.

Immunohistochemical staining for EMA, cytokeratin and CEA is similar to that of infiltrative ductal (nst) carcinomas. These markers (particularly keratins) may thus be of value in distinguishing the solid form from malignant lymphoma, as well as in identifying the dissociated cells as epithelial in suboptimal biopsy material or in minimally involved regional lymph nodes. Immunostaining for EMA can also reveal the intracytoplasmic lumina, a useful diagnostic feature (*see* Fig. 9.7).

Invasive lobular carcinomas usually fail to show immunostaining for E-cadherin and the catenins (Gamallo *et al.*, 1993; Moll *et al.*, 1993; Hashisumi *et al.*, 1996). E-cadherin-negative tumours frequently exhibit protein

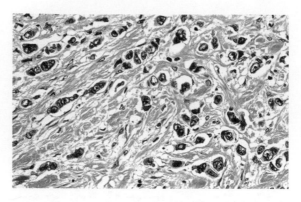

11.8 Pleomorphic lobular carcinoma. The cells infiltrate singly and in lines but exhibit gross nuclear pleomorphism (H&E).

truncation mutations of the E-cadherin gene, often in association with a loss of heterozygosity of the chromosomal region 16q22.1 containing the E-cadherin locus (Berx *et al.*, 1995). It is tempting to conclude that this is causally related to invasion and/or the characteristic dissociated cell growth pattern of invasive lobular carcinomas. Reduced or absent expression is, however, also seen in LCIS, and normal expression is seen in a minority of invasive lobular carcinomas. Moll *et al.* (1993) concluded that the lack of E-cadherin immunopositivity signifies a partial loss of epithelial differentiation and may be related to the extended spread of the tumour, but other factors are clearly involved in the tumour's ability to invade and metastasize.

The incidence of oestrogen receptor positivity is higher in lobular than in ductal (nst) carcinomas. This may have some therapeutic value if oestrogen receptor status cannot be determined (Rosen *et al.*, 1975; Eusebi *et al.*, 1977).

At the ultrastructural level, intracytoplasmic lumina (*see* Fig. 3.14) are seen more commonly than in ductal carcinomas. Rough endoplasmic reticulum is usually prominent, and mitochondria are generally large and unevenly distributed in the cytoplasm. Glycogen deposits are often prominent. There are occasional cytoplasmic filaments, but myofilaments are not seen. The cells are only rarely surrounded by basal lamina. Some of the cells may exhibit very prominent surface microvilli, sometimes arising from one pole of the cell extending into the surrounding stroma (Eusebi *et al.*, 1977).

Invasive lobular carcinomas exhibit a variable appearance on mammograms, ranging from ill-defined architectural distortions and densities to denser, more confluent tumour masses. In the latter case, however, the tumour borders are often indistinct and wispy in appearance. The false-negative rate for detecting invasive lobular carcinoma by mammography has been reported by some workers to be higher than that for ductal (nst) carcinomas (Krecke and Gisvold, 1993). Others, however, have found no significant difference in the mammographic appearances of the two tumours (Cornford et al., 1995).

Although some authors have reported that there is no significant difference in prognosis between infiltrating lobular and ductal (nst) carcinomas (Ashikari et al., 1973; Wheeler and Enterline, 1976), the larger studies show a small but significantly better survival in the former. In a study of 1621 patients with invasive breast carcinoma, Ellis et al. (1992) found that the 10-year survival for those with lobular carcinoma was 54%, compared to 47% for those with invasive ductal (nst) tumours. DiConstanzo et al. (1990) also found that lobular carcinomas were associated with an improved prognosis but that this only applied to stage I patients. Stage II patients exhibited a prognosis similar to that of those with ductal (nst) carcinoma of similar stage.

The different subtypes of invasive lobular carcinoma also seem to differ in prognosis. DuToit et al. (1989) found that the 12-year actuarial survival rate was 100% for the tubulolobular subtype but only 47% for the solid variant. Similar differences were found in disease-free interval and the incidence of regional and distant metastases. The tubulolobular type was more likely to be of low histological grade and node negative. The other subtypes did not differ in their histological parameters or clinical behaviour. In the study of Fisher et al. (1977), the short-term treatment failure rate for tubulolobular carcinoma was intermediate between those of pure tubular and pure lobular carcinoma. DiConstanzo et al. (1990) compared patients with classic lobular carcinoma with those with variant types and found that the former were younger and more likely to have multifocal disease but that there was no difference in

tumour size, lymph node status, overall or disease-free survival. The variants did not, however, include tubulolobular carcinoma, and any adverse prognosis associated with the solid type could have been masked by its inclusion with the alveolar and mixed variants that also comprised this group. It is difficult to determine the outlook for patients with the pleomorphic type in view of its rarity, but it appears to be a very aggressive tumour, 6 of 10 patients reported by Eusebi et al. (1992) dying within 42 months of diagnosis.

Grading is of prognostic significance; in the study of Pereira et al. (1995), lobular carcinomas spanned all three grades, with 10-year survival ranging from less than 50% for those with grade 3 to 80% for those with grade 1 tumours.

Classic invasive lobular carcinomas can be diagnosed with a high level of consistency by histopathologists; in a recent study by the EC Working Group on Breast Screening Pathology, a κ statistic of 0.76 was achieved (Sloane et al., 1999).

Histiocytoid carcinoma

Hood et al. (1973) drew attention to this uncommon variant of breast carcinoma in a study of metastatic carcinoma in the eyelid. Although rare, the breast proved to be the most common primary site, and furthermore the secondaries in the lid were sometimes found before the primary tumour. In more than half the tumours of breast origin, the cells exhibited a histiocytoid appearance with bland, round or oval nuclei, inconspicuous nucleoli and abundant ground-glass cytoplasm containing vacuoles of hyaluronidase-resistant mucin (Fig. 11.9). Stains for lipid were negative. The tumour cells infiltrated singly, in small groups or larger masses. Single files were present in nearly all cases and, together with the mucin vacuoles, which sometimes assumed a targetoid appearance, suggested that histiocytoid carcinoma might be a variant of infiltrating lobular carcinoma.

This view was supported by a later study by Walford and Ten Velden (1989), who reported two cases of primary histiocytoid carcinoma

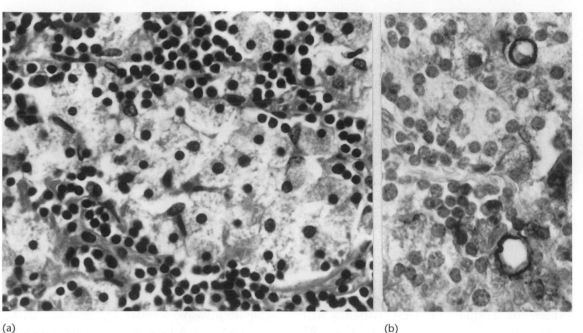

(a)   (b)

11.9 Lymph node metastasis of histiocytoid breast carcinoma. (a) The small uniform nuclei and copious vacuolated cytoplasm of the tumour cells give them a strong resemblance to histiocytes (H&E). (b) The same tumour stained by alcian blue–periodic acid–Schiff after diastase, which reveals the presence of several lumina, some containing secretion. The intracytoplasmic mucin does not show well in this illustration.

in the breast, both of which showed cytological and architectural features similar to those of invasive lobular carcinoma and were accompanied by LCIS. One of the tumours metastasized to the eyelid; in this case, the appearances of the primary and secondary tumours were initially misinterpreted as a fibrosing inflammatory process. They considered that histiocytoid carcinoma represents an apocrine variant of lobular carcinoma, a view supporting that of Eusebi *et al.* (1984), who observed immunopositivity with an antibody against gross cystic disease fluid protein-15, a protein present in apocrine cysts. Many of the eyelid lesions in Hood *et al*'s (1973) study were mistaken for benign histiocytic proliferations. Histiocytoid carcinomas exhibit positive immunostaining for EMA and cytokeratins.

Mucinous carcinoma

This tumour is also known as colloid, mucoid or gelatinous carcinoma and represents about 5% of all breast carcinomas. Macroscopically, it is well circumscribed but not encapsulated, exhibiting a pale, grey, soft, gelatinous cut surface. The tumour is often large, and Silverberg *et al.* (1971) found that 30% exceeded 55 mm in diameter. This seems to

reflect late presentation and long duration rather than a rapid growth rate.

Histologically, the tumour is composed of nests, cords and even isolated cells lying in

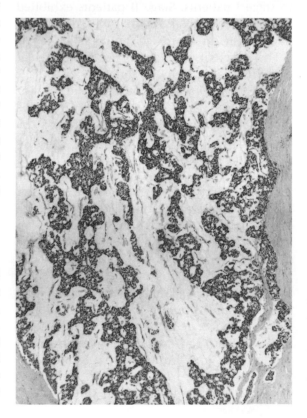

11.10 Mucinous carcinoma. Nests and cords of epithelial cells lie in lakes of mucin. Fibrous septa are seen at the right and bottom left of the illustration (H&E, × 35).

178

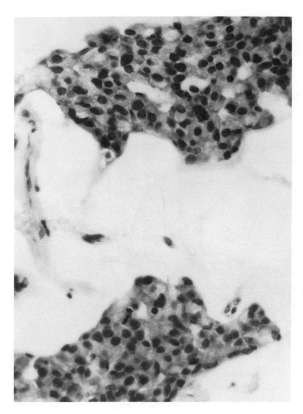

11.11 Detail of Fig. 11.10 showing relatively small uniform tumour cell nuclei (H&E).

lakes of mucin, which often account for more than half the volume of the tumour (Fig. 11.10). In between these lakes is a small amount of fibrous stroma that contains little or no elastin or infiltrating lymphoid cells. Invasion of the lymphatic vessels is rarely seen.

The neoplastic cells usually have relatively small uniform nuclei and exhibit only mild to moderate cytological atypia (Fig. 11.11). Mitoses are not usually conspicuous, and necrosis is absent. Histological grade does, however, vary (see below). The cytoplasm is brightly eosinophilic and only rarely contains granules of mucin. It thus appears that, although these cells produce large quantities of mucin, they have little capacity for storing it. Histochemically, the mucin is a mixture of neutral and non-sulphated sialidase-susceptible acid types (Cooper, 1974). DCIS may be seen around the tumour but is not usually conspicuous. It is usually of the mucinous variant and is occasionally associated with mucocoele-like changes.

Ultrastructurally, the nuclei show only modest chromatin clumping and contain occasional small nucleoli (Fisher, 1976). Desmosomes are infrequent, and the cell surfaces exhibit blunt microvillous processes. Intracytoplasmic filaments may be seen, but myoepithelial cells are not identified. Basal lamina cannot be seen around the neoplastic cells. Mitochondria are small and compact but slightly more numerous than in the normal breast. Rough and smooth endoplasmic reticulum and the Golgi apparatus are very prominent, however, presumably related to the amount of mucin synthesis. Intracytoplasmic lumina (see Fig. 3.14) may be seen in some cells.

Capella *et al.* (1980) recognized three forms of mucinous carcinoma, which they designated A, B and AB. Types A and B each represented about 40% of tumours and AB about 20%. In type A the extracellular mucin accounted for 60–90% of the tumour mass. The neoplastic cells tended to be arranged in trabeculae and ribbons rather than sheets, clumps or nests and contained inconspicuous intracellular mucin. The cytoplasm was hyaline rather than granular and was very occasionally rather foamy. The cells exhibited more pleomorphism than those of type B lesions, but this was not marked. Ultrastructurally, these tumours contained secretory granules but only of an exocrine mucous type.

In type B the extracellular mucin content was somewhat less, accounting for 33–75% of the tumour mass. The epithelial cells were more uniform and grew in solid masses and clumps rather than trabeculae. Their cytoplasm was more granular and, in about 70% of the tumours, contained argyrophil granules that were shown to be true dense-core granules on electron microscopy. Type AB tumours exhibited characteristics of both A and B.

The clinical and histogenetic significance of these subdivisions is not clear, although Capella *et al.* (1980) found type B lesions to occur in older patients. Specific polypeptides or amines have not so far been identified in the dense-core, granule-containing tumours.

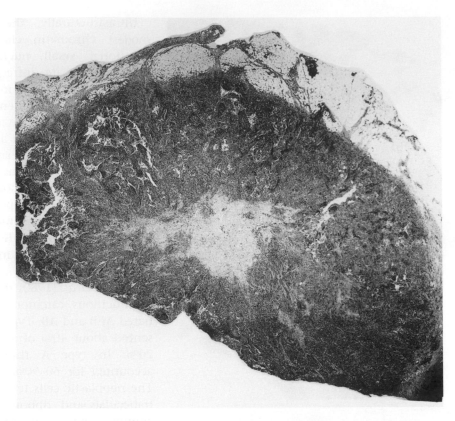

11.12 Medullary carcinoma. This low-power view shows the circumscription and dense cellularity of the tumour. Note the central necrosis (H&E).

Mucinous carcinomas are associated with a better prognosis than infiltrative ductal or lobular carcinomas; in Ellis *et al.*'s (1992) series, the overall 10-year survival was 80%, and in that of Toikanen and Kujari (1989) the 20-year cumulative corrected survival rate was 79%. Clinical outcome is dependent on histological grade, which is almost invariably 1 or 2 using the Nottingham system (Elston and Ellis, 1991). Pereira *et al.* (1995) found that the 10-year survival for grade 1 tumours was over 80%, and that for grade 2 60–80%. The prognosis of the pure form is better than that of the mixed forms, in which only part of the tumour exhibits the classic appearance (Norris and Taylor, 1965; Silverberg *et al.*, 1971; Toikanen and Kujari, 1989).

A carcinoma should be diagnosed as mucinous when at least 90% of the tumour exhibits the appearance described above and as mixed when the mucinous component comprises 10–90%. The other component in mixed tumours is usually ductal (nst). Tumours that are less than 10% mucinous should be classified according the dominant component. Adequate sampling is thus important to ensure accurate classification. Silverberg *et al.* (1971) found that regional lymph node spread occurred less commonly than in infiltrative lobular or ductal (nst) carcinomas and tended to involve fewer nodes. In the pure form the metastases were mucinous in type, whereas in mixed tumours they were usually non-mucinous in appearance.

Mucinous carcinomas are diagnosed by histopathologists with a very high level of consistency, probably because of their very striking appearance; in a recent study by the EC Working Group on Breast Screening Pathology, a κ statistic of 0.92 was achieved, representing almost perfect agreement (Sloane *et al.*, 1999). Mammographically, mucinous carcinomas usually appear as well circumscribed masses without calcification.

Mucinous carcinomas are usually oestrogen receptor positive. Cytogenetic studies have shown that they exhibit little chromosomal derangement and have a relatively simple karyotype compared to other subtypes of breast carcinoma (Pandis *et al.*, 1995).

11.13 Medullary carcinoma. This high-power view shows large pleomorphic tumour cell nuclei containing prominent nucleoli. The cell borders are indistinct, giving the appearance of a syncytium. The masses of epithelial cells are well circumscribed and separated by stroma densely infiltrated by lymphocytes and plasma cells (H&E).

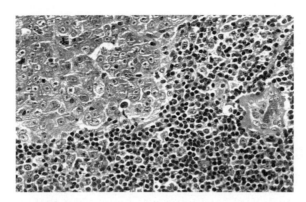

Medullary carcinoma

This is a circumscribed (Fig. 11.12), often large tumour that appears radiologically as a well-circumscribed, often lobulated, round or oval mass of homogeneous density, sometimes surrounded partially or totally by a radiolucent 'halo' (Swann et al., 1987). Calcification is usually lacking. The cells are large with highly pleomorphic vesicular nuclei and prominent nucleoli (Fig. 11.13). They form syncytium-like masses and grow in broad anastomosing cords without evidence of glandular differentiation. Necrosis is common and may be extensive. The mitotic rate is often high. Using the Nottingham system (Elston and Ellis, 1991), medullary carcinomas are thus almost invariably graded as 3, although the mitotic count may rarely be low enough for a grade of 2. Squamous metaplasia and giant cell formation are occasionally seen. The stroma exhibits scant fibrous tissue, and elastosis is absent or minor. There is very extensive stromal infiltration by lymphocytes, plasma cells and macrophages. This and the undifferentiated nature of the neoplastic cells may rarely lead to an erroneous diagnosis of malignant lymphoma. An intraductal component is only occasionally seen and is rarely extensive. Vascular invasion is not usually observed.

In the stroma the lymphocytes are almost exclusively T cells (Schoorl et al., 1976) and may form aggregates with dendritic cells similar to those seen in the paracortex of normal lymph nodes. There appears to be little morphological evidence of the destruction of tumour cells by the lymphoid infil-

trate, although Tanaka et al. (1992) provided evidence from immunohistological staining that the infiltrating lymphocytes were activated and could be capable of killing tumour cells.

Ultrastructurally, mitochondria are few but large and irregular (Fisher, 1976; Ahmed, 1980), secretory granules, filaments and Golgi apparatus being inconspicuous. Polyribosomal aggregates are abundant, however, and a moderate number of lipid droplets may be seen. Desmosomes are few, and basal lamina is not identified around the neoplastic cells. Intracytoplasmic lumina are not usually seen, but true lumina that cannot be identified at light level are very occasionally observed.

Typical medullary carcinomas are almost invariably oestrogen receptor negative, although positivity is occasionally seen in atypical variants (Jensen et al., 1996). Cytogenetic studies have shown considerable chromosomal derangement with complex karyotypes (Lu et al., 1993).

Ridolfi et al. (1977) designated tumours as typical medullary carcinomas if the following criteria were met:

1. a syncytial growth pattern (broad sheets of cells with indistinct borders) comprising over 75% of the tumour area;
2. complete circumscription;
3. moderate-to-marked mononuclear infiltrate of the stroma;
4. severely or moderately pleomorphic nuclei;
5. no intraduct component;
6. no tubular differentiation.

They categorized tumours as being atypical medullary if they exhibited no more than two of the following four atypical features:

1. margins with focal or prominent infiltrative pattern;
2. mononuclear infiltrate mild or at the tumour margins only;
3. benign-appearing nuclei;
4. the presence of microglandular features.

A syncytial growth pattern in at least 75% of the tumour was a prerequisite for both typical and atypical medullary carcinomas. If a tumour exhibited some of the features of a medullary carcinoma but more than two of the above atypical features, it was classified as a non-medullary infiltrating duct carcinoma. As thus defined typical medullary carcinoma is, in the author's experience, very rare, accounting for fewer than 1% of breast carcinomas. McDivitt *et al.* (1968), however, reported an incidence of 5% and Ellis *et al.* (1992) one of 2.7%. In the latter study atypical medullary carcinomas were not surprisingly more frequent, at 4.6%.

A simpler classification of medullary carcinoma was proposed by Pedersen *et al.* (1991) based on only two criteria: (1) syncytial growth pattern involving over 75% of the tumour, and (2) a moderate-to-marked mononuclear stromal infiltrate. This was stimulated by a previous study (Pedersen *et al.*, 1989) in which the authors found an unacceptable level of diagnostic consistency using the Ridolfi criteria (see below).

Typical medullary carcinomas in the study of Ridolfi *et al.* (1977) were associated with a significantly better 10-year survival than non-medullary infiltrating duct carcinomas, which themselves had a prognosis similar to that of ordinary infiltrating duct carcinomas. Atypical medullary carcinomas were associated with an intermediate 10-year survival, but this was not significantly different from that of infiltrative ductal (nst) carcinoma. Interestingly, most patients who died of medullary carcinoma did so in the first 5 years. Although the infiltration of lymphatic vessels is rarely seen around medullary carcinomas, regional lymph node metastases appear to occur about as frequently as in infiltrative ductal (nst) carcinomas. It has, however, been reported that this does not seem to have the same adverse prognostic significance as in other forms of breast cancer, especially if fewer than three nodes are involved (Gorski *et al.*, 1968; Ridolfi *et al.*, 1977).

The favourable prognosis of patients with medullary carcinoma was broadly confirmed by Wargotz and Silverberg (1988), who reported 5-year survival rates of 95% and 80% for typical and atypical medullary carcinomas respectively. In this paper, however, the 5-year survival for carcinomas originally diagnosed as medullary but reclassified as invasive ductal (nst) carcinoma during the study was 70%. In the contemporaneous study of Rapin *et al.* (1988), a 92% disease-free survival rate was found for patients with medullary carcinoma compared to 53% for atypical medullary and 51% for non-medullary carcinomas. Fisher *et al.* (1990) found that the survival of both node-positive and node-negative patients with medullary carcinoma was better than that of those with ductal (nst) tumours. The magnitude of the difference (6% at 5 years and 16% at 10 years) was not, however, as great as was generally perceived.

Some other subsequent studies have failed to confirm that medullary carcinomas are associated with a good prognosis at all, and the tendency not to report negative findings may have led to a significant publication bias. In their study of 1621 invasive breast carcinomas, Ellis *et al.* (1992) found that the overall 10-year survival for patients with medullary carcinomas was 51% and for those with atypical medullary tumours 55%. In neither case was the prognosis significantly different from that associated with invasive ductal (nst) carcinomas. In a later study from the same centre, however, women with medullary carcinomas were found to have a better outcome than those with other grade 3 carcinomas (Pereira *et al.*, 1995). Jensen *et al.* (1997) found an improved survival for patients with typical medullary carcinomas diagnosed using the Ridolfi criteria but not for those with atypical medullary carcinomas. An improved survival was also found for patients with medullary carcinoma diagnosed using the simplified criteria of Pedersen *et al.* (1991), but this just failed to reach statistical significance at the 5% level.

Perhaps surprisingly, given the tumour's striking appearance and the attention that has been given to diagnostic criteria, it is classified rather inconsistently. In the study of Rigaud *et al.* (1993), nine pathologists examined 16 cases originally diagnosed as medullary carcinoma, using the criteria of Ridolfi *et al.* and a data form for entering microscopic findings.

Both inter- and intraobserver agreement were fairly low, with a κ value of less than 0.5. The only histological criterion on which there was more than 50% agreement was the presence or absence of *in situ* carcinoma. The authors concluded that, although the criteria of Ridolfi *et al.* are clear and detailed, they are not easy to apply and that medullary, atypical medullary and invasive ductal (nst) carcinomas form a continuous spectrum rather than discrete entities. Pedersen *et al.* (1989) found that diagnostic interobserver agreement was associated with only a moderate κ statistic of 0.55 and concluded that the criteria of Ridolfi *et al.* (1977) needed to be sharpened and simplified in order to reduce observer variability. In the study of the European Commission Working Group on Breast Screening Pathology, which comprises over 20 histopathologists from different European countries, the overall κ statistic for diagnosing medullary carcinoma was 0.56 (Sloane *et al.*, 1999).

The variable diagnostic criteria and rather low level of diagnostic consistency probably explains much of the difference in incidence and prognosis of medullary carcinoma in different centres. At present there seems to be sufficient evidence in the literature to recommend that pathologists should continue to recognize medullary carcinoma as a histopathological entity, although strict criteria as outlined above should be used in making the diagnosis. It would, however, seem unwise to assume that all patients on whom the diagnosis is made have an excellent prognosis despite the fact that the outlook is probably better than for patients with other grade 3 carcinomas. Caution should thus be exercised in managing patients with medullary carcinoma, and other prognostic features should be taken into account (see Chapter 12). Diagnosing atypical medullary carcinomas appears to have little value in view of the diagnostic inconsistency and dubious prognostic significance.

Tubular and tubular mixed carcinoma

Tubular carcinomas are highly differentiated infiltrating carcinomas composed of uniform cells arranged in well-developed tubules (Figs 11.14 and 11.15). They are encountered more frequently by histopathologists since the introduction of mammographic screening (Rajakariar and Walker, 1995; Cowan *et al.*, 1997). In mammograms they appear as small stellate densities, often with microcalcification (Fig. 11.16).

Macroscopically, they are firm gritty tumours with irregular stellate outlines and often thin

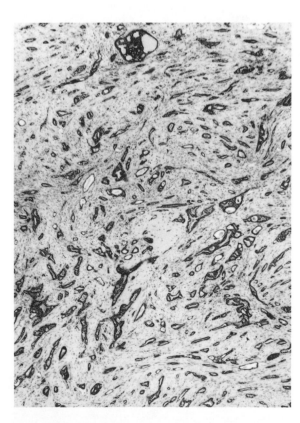

11.14 (Left) Tubular carcinoma. The tumour is composed entirely of well-differentiated tubules embedded in a dense fibrous stroma. A cribriform intraduct component is seen at the top of the picture. A cribriform pattern is also seen, particularly in the lower half of the picture (H&E).

11.15 (Right) Tubular carcinoma. The cells are arranged in single-layered, well-differentiated angulated tubules that exhibit apocrine secretion, especially on the right of the picture. Note the dense fibrous stroma (H&E).

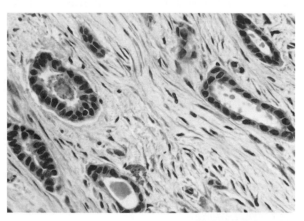

yellow streaks of elastosis. They are usually small, the mean size in two large series being less than 10 mm, with a range of 2–25 mm (Deos and Norris, 1982; McDivitt *et al.*, 1982).

Histologically, tubular carcinomas are composed of highly differentiated tubules lined by a single layer of cells that often exhibit apocrine snouts along the luminal membrane (Fig. 11.17). The tubules are small, angulated, widely patent and show little branching or anastomosis. They do not exhibit intraluminal proliferation, except when there is an accompanying cribriform carcinoma (see below). Mitotic figures are uncommon, perineural invasion is rare, and evidence of vascular invasion is almost always absent. Necrosis is uncommon and mononuclear cell infiltration scanty. There is abundant fibrous stroma that often exhibits significant elastosis. There may also be a moderate degree of microcalcification. An intraduct component is identified in two thirds of cases and is usually of low nuclear grade, often being of cribriform architecture (*see* Fig. 11.14).

The classic appearance is often mixed with invasive ductal (nst) elements. This latter component is usually of low grade and frequently occurs at the periphery of the tumour. This has led some authors to speculate that tubular carcinomas eventually evolve into infiltrative ductal carcinomas given enough time; this would explain the small size of the lesions which, presumably, change in histological appearance as they grow larger. Some workers have referred to this phenomenon as 'phenotypic drift'.

McDivitt *et al.* (1982) defined tubular carcinoma as a tumour in which at least 75% of the tissue exhibited the classic appearance with no more than 25% resembling infiltrative ductal (nst) carcinoma. Deos and Norris (1982), on the other hand, recognized two forms: a pure form in which the whole lesion exhibited the typical appearance and a mixed form in which up to 50% of the tumour resembled an infiltrative ductal carcinoma. Ellis *et al.* (1992) defined a tubular carcinoma as one in which the classic tubular morphology was present in at least 90% of the tumour, a definition that has been adopted by

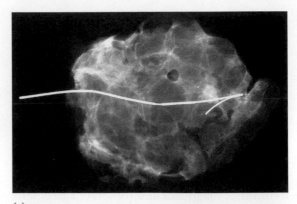
(a)

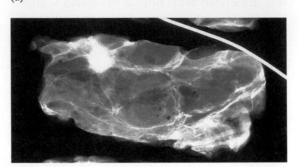
(b)

11.16 (a) Unsliced specimen radiograph showing a small tubular carcinoma near the tip of the guidewire. Note how the tumour appears well clear of the excision margin in this view. (b) Radiograph of a slice of the same specimen, cut along the direction of the guidewire. Note that in this plane the lesion is much closer to the excision margin. The tumour is small and well circumscribed, with a slightly spiculated border.

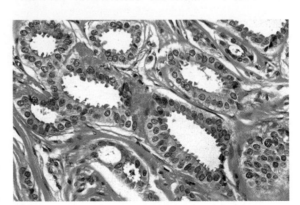

11.17 High-power view of a tubular carcinoma showing apocrine 'snouts' on the luminal border of the cells lining the tubules.

European Breast Screening Programmes. Ellis *et al.*, however, had a broader definition of tubular mixed carcinoma. They required a stellate mass with a central area containing tubules identical to those seen in tubular carcinoma, usually embedded in dense fibroelastotic stroma. The surrounding ductal (nst) carcinoma can be of variable proportion, a tumour being assigned to the tubular mixed category even if only a few tubular structures are found in the centre of the lesion.

In McDivitt et al's (1982) study, only 4% of patients with tubular carcinoma had recurrent or metastatic disease after a follow-up period averaging more than 7 years. In the series of Deos and Norris (1982), none of the patients with the pure form of the tumour had died, but 2% had recurrent disease. With the mixed form 10% had died and 4% were still alive with recurrent tumour. The follow-up period was in excess of 5 years in each case. In the study of Ellis et al. (1992), the overall 10-year survival for patients with tubular carcinoma was 90% and for those with tubular mixed tumours 69%, despite the relatively unrestrictive definition of the latter.

Tubular carcinomas are invariably grade 1 using the Nottingham system (Elston and Ellis, 1991), but tubular mixed tumours may be grade 1 or 2. The former are associated with an overall 10-year survival of over 80% and the latter with one of 60–80% (Pereira et al., 1995). The less restrictive definition of tubular mixed carcinoma of Ellis et al. thus seems to be vindicated, particularly if combined with grading.

Regional lymph node metastases are uncommon and occur with about 6% of pure tumours and 19% of mixed tumours as defined by Deos and Norris (1982). Metastases from pure tumours are usually tubular in type, whereas those from mixed forms resemble either mixed tubular carcinoma or infiltrative ductal carcinoma.

AB–PAS staining after diastase usually reveals the presence of acid mucin within the tubular lumina and occasionally demonstrates target-like intracytoplasmic vacuoles similar to those seen in lobular carcinomas (Eusebi et al., 1979). A relationship with lobular carcinoma is also supported by the high incidence of co-existing LCIS in mastectomy specimens containing tubular carcinomas (Eusebi et al., 1979; Deos and Norris, 1982). Furthermore, like lobular carcinomas, tubular carcinomas are almost invariably oestrogen receptor positive. Basement membrane cannot be demonstrated around the infiltrating tubules either by PAS staining (Flotte et al., 1980) or by immunohistological staining for basement membrane components such as type IV colla-gen and laminin (Ekblom et al., 1984). Immunohistochemical stains for actin fail to reveal myoepithelial cells (Eusebi et al., 1979).

Tubular carcinomas are almost invariably negative for epidermal growth factor receptor (EGFR), c-erbB-2 and p53 on immunostaining. Chromosomal analysis reveals less derangement than in ductal (nst) carcinomas, with relatively simple karotypic patterns (Pandis et al., 1995).

Ultrastructural studies (Jao et al., 1976; Eusebi et al., 1979; Ahmed, 1980) confirm the lack of myoepithelial cells and basal lamina. The cells exhibit prominent microvilli on the luminal surface, but desmosomal attachments are rare. Intracytoplasmic lumina are commonly observed, consistent with the histochemical identification of target-like mucin vacuoles. Myofibroblasts are commonly seen in the stroma. Tubular carcinoma may be difficult to distinguish from benign pseudo-infiltrative lesions (see p. 88).

Sclerosing adenosis can be distinguished on low power by its lobular architecture and on high power by the compression and obliteration of tubular lumina (see Figs. 6.19–6.21). Myoepithelial cells can be identified, especially if immunohistological stains for smooth muscle actin or cytokeratin are used (see Fig. 6.22). Basement membrane material can be seen either in PAS stains (Flotte et al., 1980) or in immunohistological stains for basement membrane components (Ekblom et al., 1984; see Fig. 6.23).

Microglandular adenosis (see Figs 6.27 and 6.28) may prove more difficult. The cytological features are benign. The glands are randomly distributed and do not produce the cohesive stellate appearance of tubular carcinoma. The lumina are more rounded and punched out than in the more angulated and infiltrative tubules of tubular carcinoma. Furthermore, the luminal membranes are flatter and lack the apical snouts. The presence of neighbouring DCIS favours a diagnosis of tubular carcinoma.

Radial scar exhibits a characteristic growth pattern with the central mass of fibroelastosis (see Figs 6.29–6.31). Furthermore, there is usually extensive intraluminal proliferation and/or ductal dilatation (Fig. 6.30), both of which are lacking in tubular carcinoma. Myoepithelial cells and basement membrane can be identified around the infiltrative-looking tubules, which often occupy the centre of the lesion (Figs. 6.31–6.32). Radial scars may contain foci of carcinoma, particularly if detected by mammographic screening.

The small size of the tumour, the single layer of cells lining the tubules, the cytologically uniform appearance and the presence of apocrine snouts should serve to distinguish tubular carcinoma from the more well-differentiated forms of infiltrative ductal (nst) carcinoma exhibiting extensive tubular formation.

Invasive cribriform carcinoma

In this tumour the infiltrating component is identical in growth pattern and cytological features to cribriform intraduct carcinoma, which is usually co-existent (Fig. 11.18). The cells are uniform with only minor or moderate nuclear pleomorphism, and mitoses are rare. Many tumours contain tubular elements, indicating a relationship with tubular carcinoma.

Invasive cribriform carcinoma is not common. Page *et al.* (1983) found 51 examples out of 1003 invasive breast carcinomas and divided them into classic and mixed forms. The former were either exclusively cribriform or contained elements resembling tubular carcinoma. The mixed form also contained zones of infiltrating ductal (nst) carcinoma. In all the lesions the cribriform elements accounted for more than 50% of the tumour. The definition adopted for European Breast Screening Programmes is that of Ellis *et al.* (1992), namely that a tumour is regarded as pure invasive cribriform if over 90% of the tumour exhibits the classic appearance, or when 50% does if the remainder consists only of classic tubular carcinoma.

Of the 35 classic tumours in Page's series, none exhibited blood or lymphatic vascular invasion, but regional lymph node metastases were present in five, all cribriform in type. Three of the 16 mixed tumours exhibited blood or lymphatic vascular invasion, and

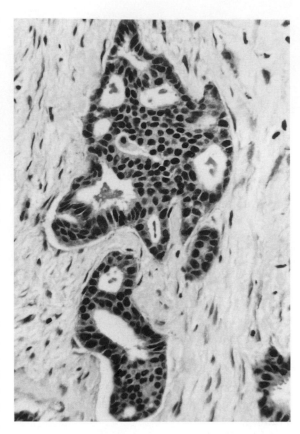

11.18 Invasive cribriform carcinoma. Note the uniformity of the tumour cells and the dense fibrous stroma (H&E).

four had regional nodal deposits that resembled ordinary ductal (nst) carcinoma. None of the patients with a classic tumour died of carcinoma over an average follow-up period of 14.5 years, whereas six of the women with mixed tumours died of breast carcinoma within an average follow-up of 12.5 years. Three of these patients died more than 10 years after diagnosis. Ellis *et al.* (1992) found an overall 10-year survival of 91% for patients with pure invasive cribriform carcinoma.

The outlook thus appears to be similar to that of tubular carcinoma, the pure form being associated with an excellent prognosis. Patients with the mixed form fare less well but better than subjects with ordinary invasive ductal (nst) carcinoma. Venable *et al.* (1990) found oestrogen receptor positivity in 100% of cases and progesterone receptor positivity in 69%.

Invasive cribriform carcinoma may resemble adenoid cystic carcinoma in both growth pattern and cytological features, but it can be

11.19 (Left) Clinical mammogram of an adenoid cystic carcinoma showing a very well delineated outline. This tumour was thought to be a fibroadenoma.

11.20 (Right) Low-power view of an adenoid cystic carcinoma showing rounded masses of infiltrating cells, many of which exhibit a cribriform growth pattern (H&E).

11.21 (Left) High-power view of an adenoid cystic carcinoma showing the typical basaloid cells. There is a biphasic growth pattern with stromal pseudocysts containing haematoxyphilic mucin, and larger glandular spaces lined by epithelial cells (arrows) (H&E).

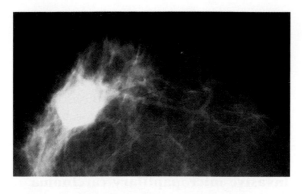

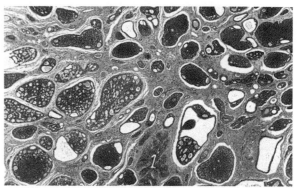

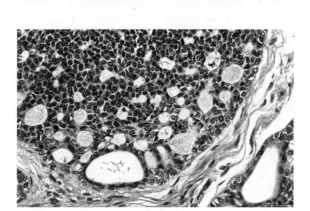

distinguished by the lack of the characteristic biphasic staining for mucin and epithelial membrane antigen. Immunostaining for oestrogen receptors, myoepithelial cells and basement membrane components may also be useful (see below).

Adenoid cystic carcinoma

This tumour, which has also been termed adenocystic carcinoma, basaloid carcinoma and cylindroma, usually arises in the salivary glands but rarely occurs in the breast and other organs. It accounts for well under 1% of all breast cancers: Anthony and James (1975) found only three cases out of 2686 breast carcinomas.

About half the tumours arise in the central part of the breast (Ro *et al.*, 1987). Macroscopically and radiologically, they are usually well demarcated (Fig. 11.19), but on histological examination nearly all tumours exhibit some infiltration at the border. They generally exhibit a lobulated cribriform growth pattern (Fig. 11.20). The neoplastic

cells are small, uniform, darkly staining and basaloid in appearance (Fig. 11.21), rarely exhibiting mitotic activity. Some of the ductal structures are true epithelial lumina lined by microvilli, whereas others are stromal pseudocysts containing collagen fibres and lined by basal lamina (Lawrence and Mazur, 1982).

AB–PAS stains reveal the biphasic appearance. The stromal pseudocysts contain hyaluronidase-sensitive, AB-positive acid mucin, whereas the epithelial lumina usually (but not always) contain PAS-positive material. Immunohistochemical staining for epithelial membrane antigen shows positivity of the epithelial lumina but not of the stromal pseudocysts. The latter are positive for basement components such as type IV collagen and laminin. Immunostaining for smooth muscle actin and cytokeratin 14 usually reveals some positive tumour cells, suggesting myoepithelial differentiation, although a rim of normal myoepithelial cells is not seen around the periphery of the cell masses as in DCIS. Oestrogen and progesterone receptors are not detectable (Ro *et al.*, 1987).

Ro *et al.* (1987) applied a grading system used for adenoid cystic carcinoma in the salivary gland in which grade 1 tumours are completely glandular and cystic with no solid component, grade 2 tumours contain solid regions comprising no more than 30% of the area, and grade 3 tumours have a solid component accounting for more than 30% of this. No patients with grade 1 tumours experienced recurrent disease, whereas one third with grade 2 tumours eventually developed metastases and the one patient with a grade 3 tumour had regional lymph node involvement at presentation. This type of grading may have some clinical value but requires further evaluation. The natural history of adenoid cystic carcinoma of the breast may, however, as in other sites, be very long, and the 5- or even 10-year survival figures can give an erroneous impression of the ultimate prognosis.

Adenoid cystic carcinoma may mimic low-grade *in situ* and invasive cribriform carcinomas but can be distinguished from them by its biphasic pattern, which stains for mucin and EMA may help to reveal. Immunostaining for oestrogen receptors may be useful, being almost invariably negative in adenoid cystic carcinoma and frequently positive in cribriform carcinoma. Distinguishing adenoid cystic carcinomas from adenomyoepitheliomas is usually straightforward on cytological grounds, but the latter may occasionally be composed of basaloid cells, making the distinction very difficult, particularly as both tumours show myoepithelial differentiation. Indeed, certain rare cases seem to indicate a genuine overlap between these two tumour types.

Invasive papillary carcinoma

This is a very rare tumour in which the invasive component forms papillary structures (Fig. 11.22). Fibrovascular stalks are usually seen in at least part of the lesions, but in some areas they may be inconspicuous or lacking. The papillae project into dilated spaces, which may contain necrotic debris. The tumours are often circumscribed and appear as solitary or multiple nodules on mammography, sometimes with calcification (Mitnick *et al.*, 1990). Stromal fibrosis is usually slight. Foci of papillary DCIS are often seen nearby.

There is some dispute about the prognosis associated with this tumour, presumably because of its rarity. Some (McDivitt *et al.*, 1968) have reported a slow growth rate and a low incidence of regional lymph node metastases, whereas others (Kraus and Neubecker, 1962) have found behaviour essentially similar to that of ductal (nst) carcinomas.

Assessing the usual prognostic features (see Chapter 12) is therefore important.

It is clearly essential to distinguish truly infiltrative papillary carcinomas from the encysted papillary form of DCIS, particularly that in which periductal fibrosis obscures the ductal outlines. Stains for basement membrane and myoepithelial cells may be of value in this context.

Invasive micropapillary carcinoma

This is a rare tumour, accounting for fewer than 3% of all breast carcinomas (Luna-More *et al.*, 1994). It is different from the invasive papillary carcinoma described above, having a very distinctive growth pattern characterized by the formation of micropapillary clumps of cells within clear spaces lined by attenuated spindle cells and separated by a delicate fibrovascular stroma (Peterse, 1993; Siriaunkgul and Tavassoli, 1993) (Fig. 11.23). The neoplastic cells are rounded, with variable amounts of finely granular eosinophilic cytoplasm, sometimes containing mucin in

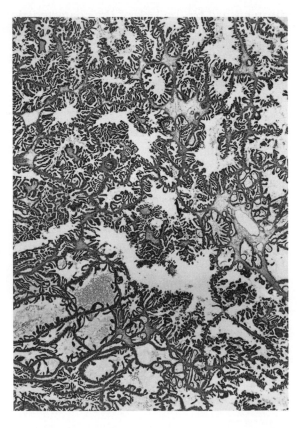

11.22 Invasive papillary carcinoma. Numerous papillary processes project into multiple cystic spaces. Some of the papillae have a fibrovascular core, but most do not (H&E).

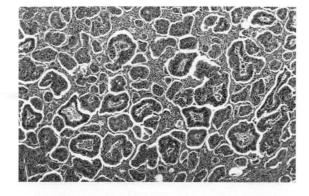

11.23 Invasive micropapillary carcinoma. There are numerous micropapillary structures within clear spaces separated by delicate stroma (H&E).

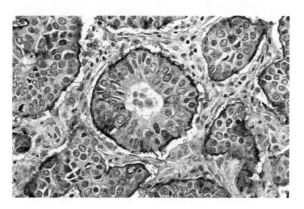

11.24 Same case as illustrated in Fig. 11.23 stained immuno-histochemically for epithelial membrane antigen. Note the positivity of the surface of the papilla rather than of the luminal membrane in the centre.

the form of fine intracytoplasmic vacuoles. The cell clumps often exhibit a small central space but usually lack a stromal core. Myoepithelial cells are absent, the cell clumps thus appearing to form hollow spherules (Peterse, 1993). Immunostaining for EMA reveals membrane positivity around the periphery of the cell masses but not in the centre (Fig. 11.24). This 'inside out' appearance is a useful diagnostic feature, distinguishing the central spaces from the glandular lumina. The EMA positivity corresponds on ultrastructural examination to the presence of microvilli (Luna-More *et al.*, 1994). From these studies it is not clear what the central spaces represent.

The growth pattern is strongly suggestive of extensive vascular invasion, but the spaces lack an endothelial lining on either close morphological examination or immunostaining for endothelial markers such as factor VIII rag, CD34 or CD31. They sometimes contain neutral or acidic mucin. It should be noted, however, that true vascular invasion does

occur in a significant proportion of cases. Pure and mixed forms occur, the latter usually in association with ductal (nst) carcinoma. The unusual morphology may lead to misdiagnosis as a metastatic papillary carcinoma (most probably of ovarian origin) or extensive vascular invasion by primary or secondary breast carcinoma. The characteristic growth pattern is retained in metastases and recurrences.

In a study of 27 cases, Luna-More *et al.* compared the characteristics of invasive micropapillary carcinomas with those of the usual ductal (nst) type and found that they were, on average, larger, of lower grade and more likely to exhibit vascular invasion and axillary lymph node involvement. At present, however, there is no evidence that when the usual prognostic features are taken into account, invasive micropapillary carcinomas are associated with a prognosis significantly different from that of ductal (nst) carcinomas.

Accompanying DCIS is usually of micropapillary or mixed micropapillary and cribriform type.

Secretory (juvenile) carcinoma

This is the most common type of breast carcinoma in children and adolescents, although it occurs more commonly in adults. In a review of the literature by Rosen and Cranor (1991), about one third of patients were under 20, one third between 20 and 30 and the remainder over 30, the oldest being 87 years old. It is a rare tumour, and there are approximately 100 documented cases. A few have occurred in males.

The lesion usually presents with a palpable mass, often near the areola. The mean size is around 25 mm, the range varying from less than 10 mm to over 70 mm. The tumour generally forms a well-circumscribed firm nodule, although less well-delineated examples occur. Rarely it is multicentric with multiple nodules scattered throughout the breast. Histologically, there are often numerous tubular spaces filled with PAS-positive mucinous secretion, sometimes giving a follicular appearance (Fig. 11.25). In some areas there may be more solid areas or large irregular ductal structures. The cells exhibit a rather bland appearance with little variation in nuclear size, shape or staining intensity (Fig. 11.26). Mitoses are infrequent and necrosis and haemorrhage rare. The abundant cytoplasm usually stains palely with eosin but may be vacuolated or even clear cell and hypernephroid in appearance. It usually contains homogeneous PAS-positive secretory material. Not infrequently, there is associated DCIS of identical appearance, sometimes extending significantly beyond the invasive component (*see* Figs 8.23 and 8.24). Inadequate excision of an extensive *in situ* component appears to be a common cause of recurrence after local excision.

The tumour exhibits indolent behaviour, especially in children and even in the presence of axillary metastases. McDivitt and Stewart (1966) reported a 100% 5-year survival rate in seven children aged 3 to 15 years. Tavassoli and Norris (1980) studied 19 patients. Five were aged less than 17 and had no evidence of metastases; of the 14 older than 17 years, 4 had axillary node metastases and 1 died with disseminated disease. Axillary metastases are usually small and rarely involve more than three nodes. Recurrences often occur many years after the initial treatment (Krausz *et al.*, 1989).

This tumour is not associated with any abnormal secretory activity in the remaining breast or any known endocrine dysfunction or abnormal sexual development. There is usually immunohistological positivity for the milk protein α-lactalbumin (*see* Fig. 8.24). This protein is, in the author's experience, hardly ever expressed by other breast carcinomas, and its presence reflects the highly differentiated and lactational phenotype of the tumour. Oestrogen receptor positivity is rare and often seen on scattered cells, as in the normal lactating breast. Progesterone receptors are frequently demonstrable (Rosen and Cranor, 1991). The case reported by Mies (1993) was diploid on flow cytometry. Allelic imbalance has been found at several chromosomal loci with a frequency similar to that seen in ductal (nst) carcinoma, except for 17p13 (the *p53* gene locus), at which it appears to be less common (Maitra *et al.*, 1999).

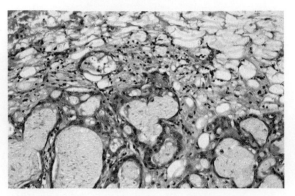

11.25 Secretory carcinoma infiltrating adipose tissue. Note the large tubular structures distended with mucinous secretion and the cellular uniformity.

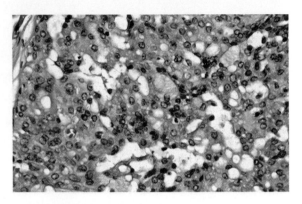

11.26 Secretory carcinoma. Note the bland cytological appearance, cytoplasmic vacuolation and abundant secretion (H&E).

Apocrine carcinoma

This tumour is also known as oncocytic or sweat gland carcinoma. In its pure form it is very rare, accounting for well under 1% of breast carcinomas in most series (Azzopardi, 1979). In studies in which a high incidence has been quoted, apocrine differentiation has been detected in only some of the tumour cells or has been questioned altogether. In the author's experience partial apocrine change is not uncommon in invasive breast carcinomas, but pure tumours are very rare.

Histologically, the cells have copious, variably granular, eosinophilic cytoplasm with large, rounded nuclei, often possessing prominent nucleoli (Fig. 11.27). Eosinophilic inclusions like those seen in benign apocrine metaplasia may be present, and sparse PAS-positive intracytoplasmic granules are common. Any lumina are ill defined, and the lining cells often exhibit apical blebs. In view of these features, apocrine carcinomas are usually graded as 2 or 3 using the Nottingham system (Elston and Ellis, 1991). Steroid receptor expression does not always

11.27 Apocrine carcinoma. There are irregular masses of invasive cells with copious eosinophilic cytoplasm, large vesicular nuclei and prominent nucleoli, forming lumina in places. The size of the cells can be appreciated by comparing them with the lymphocytes in the stroma (H&E).

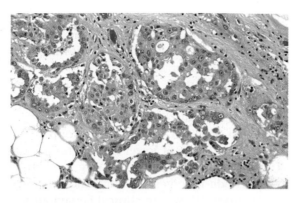

follow the same pattern as that seen in apocrine cysts. Androgen receptor positivity in not always encountered (Gatalica, 1997), and oestrogen receptor positivity may be seen in a significant proportion of cases (Abati *et al.*, 1990). Euscbi *et al.* (1986) found that pure apocrine carcinomas show extensive immunopositivity for gross cystic disease fluid protein-15. Patchy positivity has also been seen in a small number of invasive ductal (nst) carcinomas, perhaps indicating partial apocrine differentiation. Ultrastructurally, the cytoplasm contains numerous mitochondria and scattered osmiophilic granules like the cells of apocrine cysts.

There appears to be general agreement that tumours of this type are associated with a prognosis similar to that of infiltrative ductal (nst) carcinomas. Patient management is thus based on the usual grading and staging criteria. In the study of Abati *et al.* (1990), the disease-free and overall survival rates were similar to those of invasive ductal (nst) carcinomas of comparable stage. The main value of being aware of this variant is that it can be correctly identified as a primary breast carcinoma despite its unusual appearance. Furthermore, it serves to illustrate that apocrine differentiation is not invariably associated with benign lesions.

Neuroendocrine carcinoma (argyrophilic carcinoma)

Some breast carcinomas exhibit histological, histochemical, immunohistological and ultrastructural features in keeping with neuroendocrine tumours (Azzopardi *et al.*, 1982; Cubilla and Woodruff, 1977). They are distinct from (but possibly related to) the argyrophil mucinous carcinomas described on p. 179, the fibroadenomas exhibiting lobular endocrine neoplasia and the occasional

11.28 Argyrophil carcinoma. (a) H&E stain showing uniform tumour cells with inconspicuous nucleoli and clear cytoplasm. There is palisading at the periphery of the cell masses (bottom) and around blood vessels. The stroma is scanty (bottom) (H&E). (b) Grimelius stain revealing numerous intracytoplasmic granules. The inset shows an electron micrograph of the same lesion, exhibiting classic double membrane-bound dense-core vesicles (× 35 100).

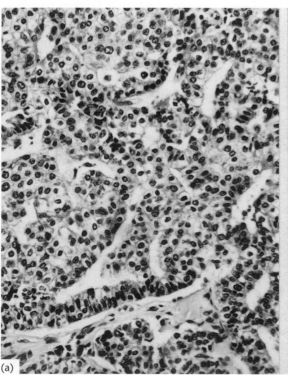

(a)

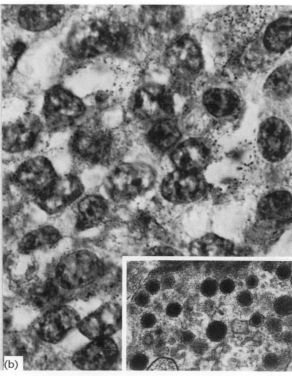

(b)

ordinary infiltrative ductal (nst) carcinomas exhibiting argyrophilia.

The tumours are often fairly well circumscribed and vary in size from about 10 to 50 mm, although they may rarely be extremely large (McKay *et al.*, 1992). For reasons not understood a significant proportion occur in the subareolar region, some being associated with a blood-stained discharge from the nipple. Histologically, they are very variable but are composed to some extent of uniform cells with round or ovoid nuclei, inconspicuous nucleoli and granular or rather clear cytoplasm (Fig. 11.28). Mitoses are not usually numerous, and necrosis is uncommon. Two unusual cases of neuroendocrine carcinoma composed of spindle cells and argyrophilic signet-ring cells were described by Maluf *et al.* (1991). Both occurred in the subareolar area of women aged over 70, were predominantly intraductal and were associated with a bloody nipple discharge.

In a series of 1628 consecutive primary breast carcinomas, Scopsi *et al.* (1992) identified 91 (5.6%) containing argyrophil cells. Three groups could be identified on histological examination, the first and second probably representing pure forms and the third a mixed type. The salient feature of group I was the presence of uniform, bland-looking cells arranged in broad cellular nests and cords with prominent peripheral palisading. The nests were rounded and closely packed with little intervening stroma and contained sharply defined acinar or rosette-like structures. No alcianophilic cells were seen. The great majority of tumours (87.5%) were grade 1 or 2.

The group II tumours were less well differentiated, the cells exhibiting greater pleomorphism and a less orderly arrangement within the cell nests. Peripheral palisading was less evident. Most of the tumours were grade 1 or 2, but the proportion (66%) was lower than in group 1. In group III the neuroendocrine-like features described above were seen in less than half the tumour mass, the remainder exhibiting the appearance of an ordinary invasive ductal (nst) carcinoma. In 9 of the 44 cases belonging to this group, AB staining revealed the presence of intracytoplasmic mucin, sometimes in the same cells as the neuroendocrine granules. Only 48% of cases in group III were grade 1 or 2.

The proportion of cells exhibiting argyrophilia was greater in group I than in group III; their distribution was mostly diffuse in groups I and II but focal in group III. In addition to being of lower grade, group I and II tumours were also less likely to exhibit lymph node involvement than those belonging to group III, whose clinical behaviour was similar to that of ordinary invasive ductal (nst) carcinomas.

Neuroendocrine carcinomas of the breast are thus a diverse group of neoplasms with respect to their appearance and clinical behaviour. The presence of argyrophilia does not, by itself, appear to have any prognostic significance, and it is thus important to provide the same prognostic information, particularly on size, grade and regional lymph node involvement, for these tumours as for other breast carcinomas.

An intraductal component is identifiable in many tumours and resembles the infiltrative component histologically, histochemically and immunohistologically, although it is occasionally papillary in architecture. In the absence of an *in situ* carcinoma, the possibility of metastasis from another site has to be considered. The presence of stromal elastosis is a useful feature in these circumstances, although it is not usually prominent.

In the study of Scopsi *et al.* (1992) immunohistochemistry revealed positivity for chromogranin A or B in 86% of tumours and neurone-specific enolase in 100%. Other groups have found immunopositivity for other products, including gastrin, insulin and bombesin (Andreola *et al.*, 1988). Papotti *et al.* (1989) concluded that Grimelius staining and the immunohistological demonstration of chromogranins A and B and synaptophysin are the most reliable histochemical features, correlating well with the ultrastructural demonstration of dense-core granules. To the author's knowledge no patients have been reported with clinical syndromes attributable

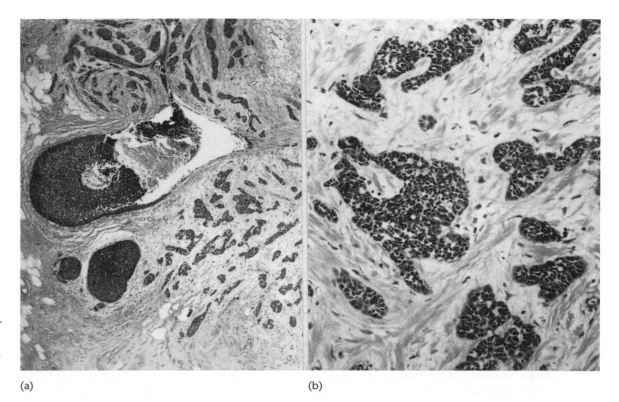

11.29 Small (oat) cell carcinoma of the breast. (a) Low-power view to show large intraduct component in the centre of the picture. (b) Higher-power view to show the classic cytological features (H&E).

(a)

(b)

to the production of polypeptide hormones by argyrophil breast carcinomas. Argyrophilia or immunopositivity for these markers is not usually seen in the neighbouring normal breast tissue but was observed in foci of ductal hyperplasia and in a papilloma by Scopsi *et al.* (1992).

Ultrastructural examination reveals the presence of double-membrane, dense-core granules, but immunoelectron microscopy using antibodies to chromogranin does not always show a localization of the immunopositivity to these structures (Battersby *et al.*, 1992).

Small-cell anaplastic (oat cell) carcinoma

This is an extremely rare variant of breast carcinoma (Fig. 11.29). Papotti *et al.* (1992) reported four cases, each with an *in situ* component and with no evidence of an alternative primary site after extensive clinical investigations. The tumours showed no specific macroscopic features and were histologically identical to small-cell anaplastic carcinomas arising in the lung and elsewhere. The neoplastic cells exhibited small, round, ovoid hyperchromatic nuclei and formed clusters, large sheets and trabeculae. Mitoses were numerous, and necrosis and vascular invasion were prominent. Three of the cases were pure, whereas in the fourth, the small-cell component comprised only 40% of the neoplastic population.

Immunostaining of the three pure tumours revealed the presence of neurone-specific enolase and bombesin/gastrin-releasing peptide in all three, with chromogranins A and B, synaptophysin, serotonin and Leu-7 in two. Grimelius was positive in two cases. Electron microscopy revealed the presence of dense-core granules in the tumour cytoplasm. One of the cases was positive for oestrogen and progesterone receptors.

All three patients with pure tumours had axillary lymph node metastases at presentation, and all died within 15 months of diagnosis. The patient with the mixed tumour had no regional lymph node involvement and died of cerebral haemorrhage after 44 months.

Wade *et al.* (1983) also reported a case of an oat cell-type carcinoma in the breast. Although not argyrophilic, the tumour contained dense-core granules on electron microscopy. No *in situ* component was identified, but the distribution of disease strongly suggested an origin in the breast.

Melanin-containing breast carcinomas

Melanin within breast carcinomas usually results from colonization by melanocytes of tumours that infiltrate the skin (Azzopardi and Eusebi, 1977). It appears to be a relatively common phenomenon in the superficial portions of such tumours. As the carcinoma cells may take up the pigment, there may be confusion with malignant melanoma. The mixture of dendritic melanocytes with tumour cells and the restriction of pigmentation to the zones of cutaneous involvement should enable the distinction to be made.

Lipid-rich carcinoma

This tumour was first described by Aboumrad *et al.* (1963) and later studied in more detail by Ramos and Taylor (1974). It accounts for fewer than 1% of all breast carcinomas. The tumours are usually poorly circumscribed and firm, and their size has ranged from 15 to 40 mm.

Histologically, the cells are large and exhibit abundant foamy cytoplasm that stains strongly for neutral lipid but weakly or negatively for mucin. The nuclei are fairly regular and may contain prominent nucleoli. Mitotic figures are usually moderate. Either intraduct or intralobular carcinoma may accompany the lesion.

At the ultrastructural level the cytoplasm contains numerous lipid vesicles that in some cases occupy most of the cell, leaving only a thin rim of cytoplasm. Glycogen granules are usually prominent, as are tonofilaments, rough endoplasmic reticulum and Golgi apparatus. The mitochondria may contain dark needle-like crystals 125–200 μm in length. The secretory activity of the tumour cells has been likened to that seen in pregnancy.

The cytological appearances may lead to an erroneous diagnosis of a histiocytic or xanthomatous tumour, especially in lymph node metastases, where a sinusoidal pattern of infiltration may be observed. Immunohistochemical stains for epithelial markers are of value in making the correct diagnosis. The identification of *in situ* carcinoma is also useful in establishing the origin from the breast. Both cases reported by Kurebayashi *et al.*(1988) were oestrogen and progesterone receptor negative. It should be noted that a high proportion of breast carcinomas contains lipid in small or moderate amounts, but lipid-rich carcinoma should only be diagnosed in the presence of the fully developed histological picture.

The case described by Aboumrad *et al.* (1963) was associated with Paget's disease of the nipple. The Paget cells, however, exhibited the usual appearance and stained with PAS after diastase digestion.

The limited information available suggests that this is an aggressive tumour. Eleven of the 12 patients studied by Ramos and Taylor (1974) had extensive involvement of their regional lymph nodes, and almost half had died within a year of diagnosis.

Glycogen-rich clear cell carcinoma

This is a very rare form of breast carcinoma composed of columnar polygonal cells with darkly staining nuclei and abundant water-clear cytoplasm staining strongly for glycogen but negatively for fat and mucin (Azzopardi, 1979; Hull *et al.*, 1981). The stroma is modest and elastosis inconspicuous. The tumours are often bulky and may exhibit extensive necrosis.

Toikkanen and Joensuu (1991) reported six cases of this condition. Five had axillary node involvement at presentation, and all five died of their tumour within 7 years. These authors concluded that glycogen-rich carcinomas might be more aggressive than breast carcinomas in general. They were, however, able to find only 14 previous well-documented cases. Statements about prognosis should thus be very guarded, and it is advisable to take into account the usual features of prognostic significance, such as grade, size and nodal involvement, when deciding how to manage an individual patient. Hull *et al.* (1981)

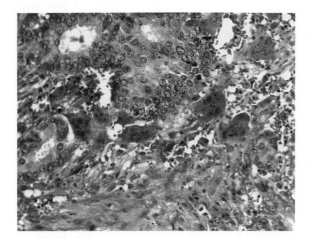

11.30 Mammary carcinoma with osteoclast-type giant cells. Infiltrating ductal (nst) carcinoma is seen on the left of the picture. On the right there are numerous osteoclast-type giant cells embedded in cellular stroma (H&E).

remarked on the ultrastructural resemblance of the cells to those of the breast of a 13-week fetus. Their one case was oestrogen receptor positive but negative for progesterone receptors.

Mucoepidermoid carcinoma

There are very few cases of primary mucoepidermoid carcinoma of the breast in the literature (Patchcfsky *et al.*, 1979; Kovi *et al.*, 1981). Some cases, like those arising in the salivary glands, have been low grade and slowly growing. The case of Kovi *et al.* (1981), however, was a highly malignant tumour composed of pleomorphic squamous elements and smaller mucous cells that metastasized extensively to the regional lymph nodes. An intraduct component was identified.

Acinic cell-like carcinoma

Roncaroli *et al.* (1996) described a single case of an invasive breast carcinoma with salivary-type features, which they called acinic cell-like carcinoma. Mammographically, the tumour showed well-defined margins and scattered granular calcifications. On histological examination the cells had large nuclei with clumped chromatin and one or two nucleoli, and copious granular cytoplasm. They were arranged in large nests, some of which exhibited central, comedo-like necrosis. The stroma consisted of a thin network of connective tissue rich in capillaries. Immunohistologically, the cells were positive for lysozyme

and amylase and ultrastructural examination revealed electron-dense cytoplasmic globules similar to those seen in acinic carcinoma of the salivary glands. One of 18 lymph nodes contained metastatic carcinoma, but follow-up was for only 1 year.

Mammary carcinomas with stromal giant cells

Breast carcinomas may rarely contain histologically benign stromal *osteoclast-type giant cells* (Agnantis and Rosen, 1979) (Fig. 11.30) similar to those found in the variant of metaplastic carcinoma described below, except that the stroma is otherwise unremarkable. The giant cells exhibit no evidence of phagocytosis and occur in limited zones. They may be associated with marked vascularity, and there may be evidence of recent and old haemorrhage. The tumours are otherwise of the infiltrative ductal or lobular type. In the series of eight cases described by Agnantis and Rosen, foci of spindle cell metaplasia were seen in three and osseous metaplasia in one and would probably now be classified as metaplastic carcinomas (see below). The limited data available suggest that the prognosis is not significantly different from that of infiltrative ductal (nst) carcinoma of a comparable grade and stage. The stromal giant cells may be present in metastases (Tavassoli and Norris, 1986).

A stromal granulomatous reaction with *Langerhans'-type giant cells* has also rarely been reported in breast carcinomas. Oberman (1987) described three patients who had an invasive ductal (nst) carcinoma associated with non-caseating granulomata. The granulomata were restricted to the carcinoma, and no granulomatous response was seen in the neighbouring breast or regional lymph nodes. Asteroid or Schaumann bodies were not observed, and stains for acid-fast bacilli and fungi were negative. None had evidence of systemic granulomatous disease, although one patient was found to have granulomata in the porta hepatis at the time of cholecystectomy. In the case subsequently reported by Santini *et al.* (1992), the granulomata were present in both the primary tumour and the regional lymph nodes and were associated with the deposition of an unusual amyloid. This patient also exhibited no evidence of systemic granulomatous disease. Coyne and Haboubi (1992) reported two patients with microinvasive carcinoma in which granulomata containing giant cells were seen in association with the microinvasive foci.

Giant cells of uncertain histogenesis with hyperchromatic multiple nuclei were found by Rosen (1979) in 4.5% of 200 consecutive mastectomy specimens, occurring in localized groups within the mammary stroma. The cells were usually visible at low magnification and were invariably limited to a low-power field, although multiple separate foci could be seen. There was no accompanying evidence of inflammation or foreign material. The multinucleated cells did not usually lie adjacent to the malignant neoplasm and could be seen with a similar frequency in patients with no evidence of malignant neoplasia (*see* p. 272). There was a striking clustering of cases within the 40–50-year age group, suggesting some relationship to an impending menopause. There was no relationship to parity, hormone usage or family history of breast carcinoma. The cells are probably derived from stromal fibroblasts and are similar to those seen in some fibroadenomas (*see* Fig. 13.5) and at other sites in the body, for example nasal polyps.

Giant cell carcinoma

Carcinomas containing pleomorphic, multinucleate epithelial giant cells are very rare: Ravichandran *et al.* (1996) described two cases and identified another five in the literature. Both patients presented symptomatically, and in one the tumour was not visualized by mammography. Both tumours were large and partly cystic on macroscopic examination. Histologically, they were composed of highly pleomorphic bizarre mono- and multinucleated cells exhibiting frequent mitotic figures. A distinctive feature was a heavy infiltrate of inflammatory cells, mainly granulocytes, many of which appeared to have been phagocytosed by the tumour cells. One lesion showed areas of spindle cell metaplasia.

Despite the aggressive-looking histological appearance, both patients were disease free 2–3 years after presentation. The prognosis associated with these tumours is, however, uncertain in view of their rarity. Ravichandran *et al.* considered them to be analogous to similar giant cell tumours occurring in other organs, such as the thyroid, lung, pancreas, gallbladder and intestine.

Adenomyoepithelioma

These low-grade biphasic tumours are included here among the special types of breast carcinoma because they are prone to recurrence and may contain foci of unequivocal carcinoma. Furthermore, they are closely related to the myoepithelial carcinoma (malignant myoepithelioma), which is described in the next section.

Adenomyoepithelioma of the breast appears to have been first described by Hamperl (1970). Subsequent cases were reported by Kiaer *et al.* (1984) and Eusebi *et al.* (1987), who identified two structurally different components that merged together: a distinctly glandular one and a solid one composed of masses of myoepithelial-like cells containing glandular lumina in their centres (Fig. 11.31). Both groups of authors regarded the tumours as being of low-grade malignancy, the former because of multiple local recurrences and the latter because of the histological features: nuclear atypia, a high mitotic rate and infiltrative solid masses of cells.

Tavassoli (1991) reported 27 cases that ranged in size from 10 to 70 mm with a mean of 25 mm. All were solitary. She divided them into three categories based on their growth pattern or cell type: spindle cell, tubular and lobulated. The *spindle cell* type was composed of solid masses of spindle cells that often distended and almost occluded duct-like structures. The cells were usually mixed with a few spaces lined by epithelium that often exhibited apocrine metaplasia and rarely atypical hyperplasia. In some fields there was a monomorphic appearance strongly reminiscent of leiomyoma. The cells were positive for actin and cytokeratin.

The *tubular* type was characterized by the proliferation of numerous rounded tubules

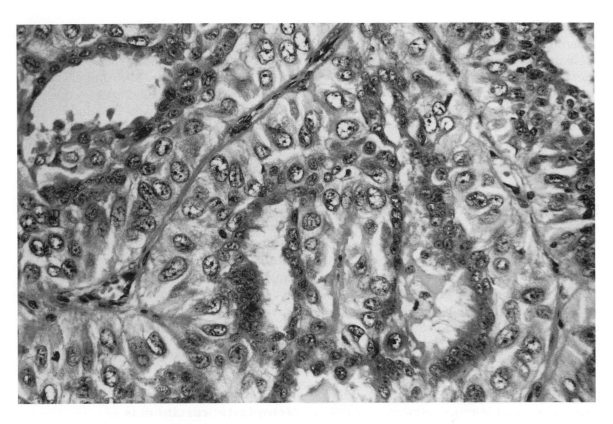

11.31

Adenomyoepithelioma. This high-power view shows several glandular spaces lined by atypical epithelial cells and surrounded by several layers of myoepithelial cells showing even greater cytological atypia, with large pleomorphic vesicular nuclei and prominent nucleoli. These cells showed immunopositivity for smooth muscle actin and cytokeratin 14. A mitosis is seen at the bottom left of the picture (H&E).

lined by epithelial and myoepithelial cells, the latter showing irregular multilayering sometimes obliterating the lumen. The growth pattern was similar to that of tubular or ductal adenomas, although not all cases were well circumscribed and some exhibited extension of the tubules into the surrounding breast, where they blended with the normal breast structures. Rarely, there was also proliferation of the epithelial cells.

The *lobulated* variant was composed of solid nests of myoepithelial cells with clear or eosinophilic cytoplasm around compressed epithelial-lined spaces. In some cases the cells exhibited a plasmacytoid appearance with peripheral displacement of the nucleus. Most tumours were completely or partly surrounded by a thick fibrous capsule, which in one third of cases was penetrated by tumour cells. Fibrous septa of varying thickness divided the lesions into smaller nests and sometimes were so prominent as to replace the neoplastic cells. The mitotic count was usually low but exceeded 10 per 10 high-power fields in one quarter of cases. Central infarction was present in almost half.

Combinations of growth pattern sometimes co-existed. Mucinous, apocrine and squamous metaplasia was not infrequent and sebaceous differentiation less common.

Two of the 27 cases reported by Tavassoli harboured a carcinoma, one an ordinary invasive ductal (nst) carcinoma and the other a myoepithelial carcinoma (see below). One of these patients developed a recurrence after 2.3 years. Recurrence also occurred in 2 of the 27 patients with adenomyoepithelioma without carcinoma, 1 of the tubular and 1 of the lobulated type. Loose *et al.* (1992) described 6 cases of adenomyoepithelioma, of which 2 (1 tubular and 1 lobulated) recurred locally and a third (lobulated) metastasized to the brain and lungs after repeated local recurrences. This tumour exhibited brisk mitotic activity, at 11 per 10 high-power fields. The biphasic appearance was retained in the metastases. Michal *et al.* (1994) reported a patient with an adenomyoepithelioma containing a component of undifferentiated spindle cell carcinoma that reacted negatively with myoepithelial markers on immunostaining. She died 5 months after surgical treatment.

The carcinoma with ductal, myoepithelial, squamous and sebaceous elements reported by Prescott *et al.* (1992) seems to be related to the adenomyoepithelioma, given the range of metaplastic changes described by Tavassoli. This lesion presented as a 50 mm, well-circumscribed mass in a 74-year-old woman without lymph node involvement. At the time of reporting she was free of disease, but the follow-up was only 6 months.

Myoepithelial carcinoma (malignant myoepithelioma)

Myoepithelial carcinomas are very rare tumours that are difficult to recognize. Unlike adenomyoepithelomas, which exhibit a characteristic biphasic growth pattern, they are composed purely of malignant myoepithelial cells, which are usually spindle-shaped (Fig. 11.32) but may occasionally be polygonal. A clear cell variant of the latter containing abundant glycogen has been reported (Kuwubara and Uda, 1997). A combination of morphology and immunohistological staining is thus required to distinguish them from other malignant tumours, mainly spindle cell and clear cell carcinomas and sarcomas. They exhibit immunopositivity for low molecular weight keratins using the antibody Cam 5.2, cytokeratin 14, smooth muscle actin, vimentin and sometimes S100 and glial fibrillary acidic protein. They are negative for cytokeratins 18 and 19 and desmin. Electron microscopy reveals desmosomes, hemidesmosomes, pinocytotic vesicles, plentiful rough endoplasmic reticulum and microfilaments (Lakhani *et al.*, 1995).

These tumours are malignant and usually give rise to metastases, although one purely intraductal case has been described (Tamai, 1992). Diamiani *et al.* (1997) reported three unusual malignant tumours comprising haphazardly intermingled epithelial and myoepithelial cells, which they termed poorly differentiated myoepithelial cell rich carcinoma. None of the patients developed recurrent tumour, but the mean follow-up time was only 32 months and two had regional lymph node metastases at presentation.

Metaplastic carcinomas

The term metaplastic carcinoma has been used to describe a heterogeneous group of tumours in which the malignant epithelial

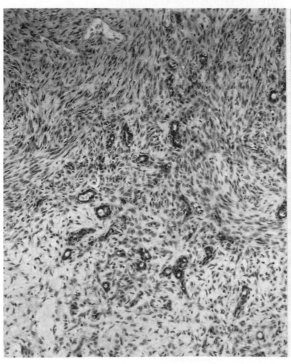

(a)

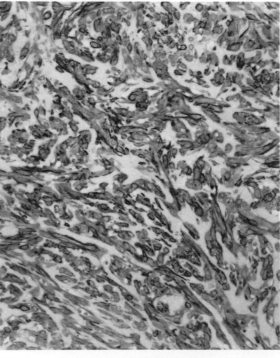

(b)

11.32 Myoepithelial carcinoma (malignant myoepithelioma).
(a) Proliferation of rather bland spindle cells replacing the stroma of the breast but sparing and separating the acini of a lobule in the centre of the field (H&E).
(b) Higher-power view of the same tumour showing immunopositivity for smooth muscle actin. This tumour gave rise to widespread metastases and caused the death of the patient.

cells show evidence of metaplasia to mesenchymal cells or epithelial cells not normally found in the breast. Some tumours show evidence of myoepithelial cell differentiation, but adenomyoepithelioma and myoepithelial carcinomas are excluded because they are derived from cells normally found in the breast. It is possible that some of the sarcomas discussed in Chapter 14 are metaplastic carcinomas in which the epithelial component has not been recognized because immunostaining for epithelial markers was not available (Guarino *et al.*, 1993). In a series of publications Wargotz and Norris described five subtypes:

1. matrix-producing carcinoma (Wargotz and Norris, 1989a);
2. spindle cell carcinoma (Wargotz *et al.*, 1989);
3. carcinosarcoma (Wargotz and Norris, 1989b);
4. squamous cell carcinoma (Wargotz and Norris, 1990a);
5. metaplastic carcinoma with osteoclast-like giant cells (Wargotz and Norris, 1990b).

It will be seen from the descriptions below that there is some overlap among these groups and that some tumours exhibit features of more than one category. This provides a good argument for the use of the all-embracing term metaplastic carcinoma, although in their classic forms the various types differ significantly.

Matrix-producing carcinoma

Matrix-producing carcinoma is a term coined by Wargotz and Norris (1989a), who described 26 cases of a distinct form of metaplastic carcinoma in which there was a direct transition between zones of straightforward invasive carcinoma and cartilaginous and/or osseous stromal matrix without intervening spindle cell or sarcomatoid areas (Fig. 11.33). The tumours were often large (mean 40 mm), usually nodular and well circumscribed. Calcification, central necrosis and haemorrhage were common.

Histologically, most were ductal (nst) carcinomas with occasional foci of squamous or apocrine metaplasia. Mucinous carcinoma predominated in one tumour and another exhibited a medullary-like appearance. All three grades were represented. The carcinomatous areas sometimes comprised the minority of the tumour. In the transitional areas the carcinoma cells appeared to be less cohesive, and individual cells were surrounded by

11.33 (Left) Matrix-producing carcinoma. Invasive carcinoma cells with rather clear cytoplasm merge with wispy masses of osteoid (H&E).

11.34 (Right) Breast carcinoma with osseous metaplasia. There is an extensive formation of histologically benign osteoid in the upper part of the picture. Ductal carcinoma *in situ* of the comedo type is seen at the bottom (H&E).

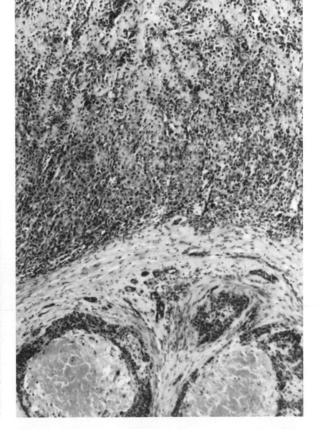

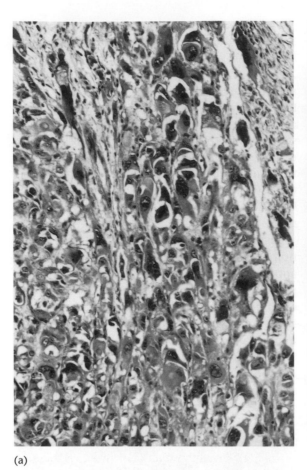

(a)

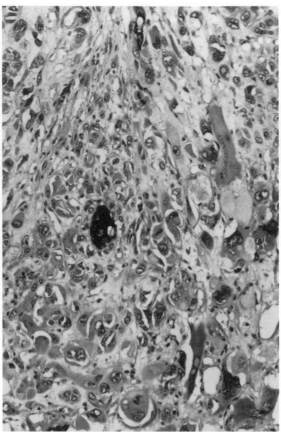

(b)

11.35 Spindle cell carcinoma. (a) The appearance resembles a pleomorphic soft tissue sarcoma (H&E). (b) The same tumour stained immunohistochemically for epithelial membrane antigen reveals a strongly positive cell in the centre of the picture and many less strongly positive cells, especially at the bottom right.

matrix, which comprised cartilage and/or bone in varying proportions. In some cases the cartilaginous component exhibited atypical features. DCIS was present around the periphery in about one third of cases (Fig. 11.34).

Immunostaining revealed positivity for keratins, EMA, S100 and occasionally vimentin. Actin was positive in the transitional areas, suggesting myoepithelial differentiation, an interpretation that was confirmed by ultrastructural examination. The three tumours investigated were oestrogen receptor negative. The cumulative 5-year survival rate was 68%; only 1 of 17 patients had positive axillary lymph nodes. Radiation and chemotherapy had a limited effect.

Spindle cell carcinoma

Spindle cell carcinomas are composed of sheets and interlacing bundles of spindle cells that tend to be plump and pleomorphic near the centre of the lesion (Fig. 11.35a) and less cellular towards the periphery. Some tumours are composed entirely of spindle cells (Gersell and Katzenstein, 1981), whereas others contain zones resembling the more usual forms of breast carcinoma (Huvos *et al.*, 1973). In the study of 100 patients by Wargotz *et al.* (1989), patient age ranged from 29 to 95 years, with a mean of 63. All patients presented with a solitary mass. Tumour size ranged from 6 to 210 mm, the mean being 44 mm. Seventy-two of the 100 neoplasms had areas of invasive ductal (nst) carcinoma or DCIS and 11 had zones of squamous carcinoma. Squamous differentiation often occurred in the form of solid islands or cystic spaces lined by squamous epithelium. The remaining 17 carcinomas were entirely spindle celled and were identified as epithelial by their immunopositivity for cytokeratins,

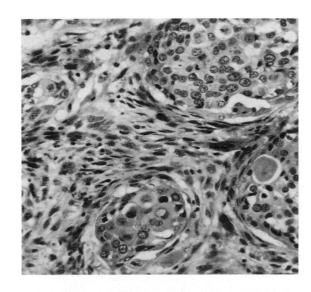

11.36 Carcinosarcoma. The spindle-celled sarcomatous component and the epithelial component are both cytologically malignant, and there is no transition between the two in this illustration (H&E).

which was also detected in the spindle component of 98% of cases overall.

Immunoreactivity was also seen with antibodies against EMA (Fig. 11.35b) in 23%, vimentin in 91%, S100 in 51% and actin in 96%. Stromal myofibroblasts were responsible for at least some of the actin and vimentin positivity, but the authors considered that many cases showed evidence of myoepithelial differentiation, a contention supported by electron microscopy in three cases. Some of these tumours might now be regarded as myoepithelial carcinomas.

Ultrastructurally, the spindle cells may exhibit evidence of squamous differentiation with coarse bundles of tonofilaments and numerous desmosomes. Cytoplasmic organelles are otherwise sparse, and intracytoplasmic lumina are lacking. Premelanosomes and Langerhans' cell granules have been observed in some cases (Gersell and Katzenstein, 1981).

Wargotz *et al.* (1989) found that the cumulative 5-year survival rate for patients with spindle cell carcinoma was 64%. Of the 47 patients who had axillary sampling, only 6% had nodal involvement. Twenty-nine of 30 patients who developed metastases died of their tumour. Local recurrence was, however, not as ominous as only 29% with locally recurrent tumour died. Tumour size was found to be a significant prognostic factor, the mean size of tumours from the patients who died

being 50 mm compared to 37 mm from those who survived. Complete microscopic circumscription was a good prognostic sign.

Carcinosarcoma

Carcinosarcoma is characterized by mixed malignant epithelial and mesenchymal elements (Fig. 11.36). The 70 patients reported by Wargotz and Norris (1989b) all presented with a single palpable mass and ranged in age from 29 to 95 years, with a mean and median of 56. Tumour size ranged from 9 to 190 mm with a mean of 63 mm. Fifteen tumours were regarded as being well circumscribed, although none was encapsulated. Vascular invasion by the sarcomatous component was seen in two of the tumours. Intraductal carcinoma was present in half the neoplasms, but *in situ* sarcoma was not observed. Squamous carcinoma was seen in 15 and was the only epithelial component in two. The sarcomatous element resembled malignant fibrous histiocytoma in 40 cases and fibrosarcoma in 28. The stroma of 4 neoplasms contained foci of osteoid and/or bone, 8 cartilage and 1 bone and cartilage. Two neoplasms contained foci of rhabdomyosarcoma, and in two the stroma showed angiomyxoid change. The stroma contained a significant infiltrate of chronic inflammatory cells in over half the cases, but granulomatous inflammation was not seen. Necrosis and haemorrhage were common.

Although the carcinomatous and sarcomatous components appeared distinct at low power, at high magnification transitional zones were seen where there was subtle merging of the two elements. The sarcomatous component showed varying degrees of positivity for cytokeratin in just over half and for vimentin in nearly all the cases that were studied immunohistologically. A majority were also immunoreactive for actin and S100 protein, although it was not clear to what extent the former represented myoepithelial, myofibroblastic or muscle differentiation. One of the 11 tumours tested was oestrogen receptor positive. The same lesion was also positive for progesterone receptors.

The cumulative 5-year survival rate was 49%, worse than for other forms of metaplastic carcinoma, and, not surprisingly, varied according to stage, being 100% for stage I, 63% for stage II and 35% for stage III. Of patients who underwent axillary sampling, 26% had nodal secondaries, mostly in the form of carcinoma. All but one of the patients who developed metastases eventually died of their disease. Local recurrence was less ominous, only 40% subsequently dying of tumour. Size and circumscription were also prognostically significant.

Some carcinosarcomas are thought to arise in fibroadenomas or phyllodes tumours.

Squamous cell carcinoma

Squamous carcinomas are rare; Eggers and Chesney (1984), for example, found only seven examples in 4351 malignant breast lesions. Some appear to be pure squamous carcinomas, but in the author's experience most reveal foci of adenocarcinoma on extensive sampling. The latter is usually of the ordinary infiltrative ductal (nst) type (Fig. 11.37), but other varieties, such as medullary carcinoma, may be less commonly seen. Occasional cases exhibit prominent myxoid stroma (Foschini *et al.*, 1990). Occasional squamous carcinomas have been reported to arise in phyllodes tumours or fibroadenomas (Geschickter, 1945; Cornog *et al.*, 1971).

Tumours in which squamous differentiation is prominent are often large, some containing cysts lined by squamous epithelium. Spindle cell metaplasia may also be observed, and Wargotz and Norris (1990b) provided immunohistological and ultrastructural evidence of myoepithelial differentiation. The cumulative 5-year disease-specific survival rate of the 22 patients in their series was 63%. Three of 19 women had lymph node metastases at presentation. Squamous differentiation usually persists in metastases.

Drudis *et al.* (1994), reported 23 patients with low-grade adenosquamous carcinoma of the breast. They covered a wide age range, from 33 to 88 years, with a mean of 54. The tumours were stellate, frequently large lesions composed of a varying proportion of squamous and glandular elements, often widely separated by abundant stroma contain-

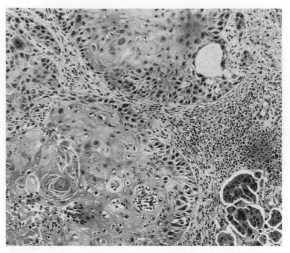

11.37 Squamous carcinoma. Most of the tumour in this field has the appearance of a well-differentiated squamous carcinoma, but a small portion at the bottom right of the photograph resembles an ordinary invasive ductal (nst) carcinoma (H&E).

ing a conspicuous dispersed lymphocytic infiltrate. The stroma frequently showed a swirling arrangement around the epithelial structures, with which it appeared to merge. Cystic degeneration occasionally occurred in the squamous foci, sometimes accompanied by calcification of the keratotic debris. The glandular elements were sometimes so well formed that they were difficult to distinguish from non-neoplastic glands. Osteocartilaginous foci were present in the stroma of two of the tumours. In several cases the tumour was associated with a papilloma or adenomyoepithelioma, suggesting that it might have arisen from it. On immunostaining none of the lesions was positive for oestrogen or progesterone receptors, 46% being positive for c-erbB-2, 13% for p53 and 39% for cathepsin D, the last mainly in areas of squamous differentiation.

Twenty of the 23 patients were disease-free after treatment by excision or mastectomy, but the follow-up time was not stated. Interestingly, all three patients with recurrent disease were alive at the time of the study, including one with lung secondaries, reflecting the slow growth rate of the tumour despite the marker profile, which would usually be associated with aggressive behaviour. The authors used this observation to stress the primary importance of morphology in predicting prognosis.

Some breast neoplasms in which the nuclei are prominent and the cytoplasm abundant and eosinophilic may appear squamoid; squamous differentiation should not be reported, however, unless prickles and/or keratin formation can be seen. It is clearly important to exclude the possibilities of cutaneous origin and spread from distant sites.

Metastatic carcinoma with osteoclast-like giant cells

Metaplastic carcinoma with osteoclast-like giant cells differs from the other carcinomas containing osteoclast-like cells described above in that they exhibit dominant metaplastic stromal components. In the series of 29 patients reported by Wargotz and Norris (1990a), the patients' ages ranged from 28 to 81 years, with a mean of 56. The tumour size was 13–150 mm with a mean of 55 mm. Ten of the carcinomas were well circumscribed, but none was encapsulated. All tumours had carcinomatous elements, mostly of ductal (nst) type of variable grade, but squamous differentiation was present in 3, apocrine differentiation in 2 and an adenoid cystic pattern in 1. The carcinoma was usually invasive but sometimes exclusively intraductal. The stroma contained osteoclast-like giant cells in all cases, often intimately associated with prominent thin-walled blood vessels and evidence of recent and old haemorrhage. They exhibited no evidence of phagocytosis. The remainder of the stroma comprised bland spindle cells in 7 cases, resembled fibrosarcoma in 4 and malignant fibrous histiocytoma in 18. Nineteen contained zones of osteoid, bone or cartilage, which were prominent in only 5, the osteoclast-like giant cells not being confined to these areas.

The giant cells were immunoreactive for vimentin and to a lesser extent actin but uniformly negative for keratins, confirming their mesenchymal nature. In contrast, the spindle cell component of the stroma was positive for cytokeratin in 63% of cases and epithelial membrane antigen in 54%. The disease-specific 5-year survival rate was 68%, comparable to other types of metaplastic carcinoma except carcinosarcomas, for which the outlook was worse (see above). Seventeen women had axillary dissection, but nodal involvement was detected in only two. Eleven of the 29 women developed metastases, mostly to the lungs. Tumour size and circumscription were significant prognostic factors. Steroid receptor analysis was not performed in any of the cases.

MULTICENTRIC BREAST CARCINOMA

The incidence of multicentric breast cancer varies greatly in the literature because of problems of definition and differences in sampling technique. In a review of 11 studies Carter (1986) found that the reported incidence of multifocality varied from 9 to 75% with a mean of 32%.

Multicentricity may result from multiple sites of origin or intramammary spread, and the two processes may be very difficult or impossible to distinguish. Multiple foci of *in situ* carcinoma may, for example, represent spread along the duct system and from one glandular system to another through ductal anastomoses, which are said to be more common near the nipple (Ohtake *et al.*, 1995). It may also be difficult to establish that an apparently separate focus of tumour is not merely an irregular outgrowth from the main tumour mass. Many workers, therefore, define multicentricity as multiple tumours separated by a minimum distance (usually 50 mm).

Fisher *et al.* (1975) found microscopic foci of multicentric carcinoma in about 13% of surgically resected breasts. They acknowledged this to be a conservative estimate as only one block per quadrant was taken and not every quadrant was always available for study. About two thirds of the additional foci of carcinoma were non-infiltrative. Multicentricity was more likely to be encountered with large tumours and with lobular invasive carcinomas.

Lagios *et al.* (1981), using a serial subgross and radiographic method on 286 mastectomy specimens, found multicentric carcinoma in 28%. Multicentricity was defined as two or more separate foci of carcinoma, at least 50 mm apart, in the same breast. Tumour was seen in the nipple or lactiferous ducts in over half the multifocal cases. Lagios *et al.* (1980) found an even higher incidence (56%) of multicentricity in tubular carcinomas using a serial subgross technique on mastectomy specimens. A history of bilateral mammary cancer was obtained in 38%. Gallager and Martin (1969) used whole organ sectioning and found multiple invasive sites in almost half the breasts examined, although these were often in the immediate vicinity of the main tumour.

Multicentricity is thus common at the histological level even where tumours are thought to be unicentric on clinical and radiological examination. This has obvious surgical implications. Rosen *et al.* (1975) set out to answer the important practical question of how often carcinoma was left behind in the breast after wide local excision. Simulated partial mastectomy was performed on 203 mastectomy specimens. The entire quadrant containing the tumour was excised, representing 25–30% of the breast tissue. Central tumours were excised with a 20 mm margin of normal tissue. Two or three sections were then taken from each of the remaining quadrants and the nipple after macroscopic inspection.

Residual carcinoma was found in 26% of breasts where the main tumour was less than 20 mm and in 39% where it was greater than 20 mm. Half the residual foci associated with the smaller tumours were invasive compared with about three quarters with the larger lesions. Multicentricity was more common with subareolar tumours and less common with medullary and colloid carcinomas. Surprisingly, there was no correlation between multicentricity and axillary nodal involvement.

Holland *et al.* (1985) addressed the same question by studying 282 mastectomy specimens from patients who were comparable to those eligible for breast-conserving surgery, using combined specimen radiography and histological techniques. Thirty-seven per cent showed no tumour in the mastectomy specimen around the reference mass. In 20% tumour foci were present within 20 mm of the reference tumour and in 43% more than 20 mm from it. In the latter case 27% of the

foci were non-invasive and 16% invasive. The authors calculated that if the cancers that were 40 mm or less had been removed with a margin of 30–40 mm, 7–9% would have had residual foci of invasive and 4–9% residual foci of non-invasive cancer.

The precise clinical significance of multicentricity, detected only by pathological methods, is not well understood. Egan (1982) found that multicentric tumours detected by specimen radiography and detailed histological assessment were associated with a poorer prognosis than unicentric lesions. There is still no clear evidence that total mastectomy actually prolongs survival, although it is generally accepted that it is associated with a lower risk of local recurrence. Local recurrence following local excision is greatly reduced by adjuvant radiotherapy.

BILATERAL BREAST CARCINOMA

The incidence of bilaterality also depends on how it is demonstrated. A small percentage of patients present with synchronous bilateral breast cancers detectable by clinical examination and/or mammography, the number being higher in patients who have inherited gene mutations predisposing to breast cancer (see below). Urban (1970) biopsied the contralateral breasts of patients undergoing surgery for breast carcinoma and found that 14% contained carcinoma, of which two thirds were non-infiltrating. In their study of patients with invasive lobular carcinoma, Simokovich *et al.* (1993) found that 10% had infiltrating carcinoma, 10% LCIS and 6% DCIS in the contralateral breast on random biopsy. Multicentric invasive tumour in the ipsilateral breast was predictive of bilateral disease.

Concerning metachronous cancers Robbins and Berg (1964) found that patients treated for primary breast carcinoma developed a new *clinically* apparent carcinoma in the opposite breast at a rate of about 1% per year. In studies that have estimated relative risk, it has been found that women with breast cancer develop subsequent contralateral invasive breast cancer at a rate 4–5 times that of the incidence of

11.38 Low-power view of a carcinoma treated primarily by combination chemotherapy before excision. There has been a good response. The tumour is poorly cellular and consists mainly of fibrous tissue. Occasional minute clumps of residual carcinoma cells remain, however, the largest being in the centre of the illustration (arrow) (H&E).

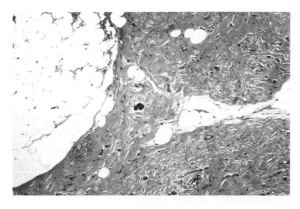

11.39 Higher-power view of a carcinoma treated by primary chemotherapy. A focus of residual carcinoma cells is seen at the right edge of the illustration. The remainder of the field shows fibrous tissue, scattered lymphocytes and ill-defined clusters of foamy macrophages, presumably marking the site of pre-existing tumour cells (H&E).

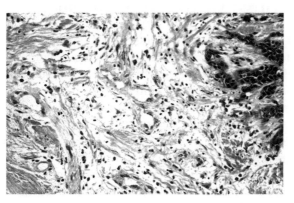

invasive cancer in age-matched women in the general population (Robbins and Berg, 1964). Thomas *et al.* (1979) found that almost 50% of patients had bilateral breast carcinoma by the time they reached autopsy. This included those tumours which had been detected in life and those that had been detected only after a detailed post mortem examination.

In the majority of cases the tumour on the opposite side is a second primary as judged by the presence of an *in situ* component. Although most bilateral tumours are of the infiltrative ductal type, there appears to be a disproportionately high number of lobular invasive carcinomas (Finney *et al.*, 1972; Lewis *et al.*, 1982).

CARCINOMAS TREATED BY RADIOTHERAPY AND CHEMOTHERAPY

The appearance of tumours treated with radiotherapy or cytotoxic drugs is essentially similar but varies significantly according to the response obtained. At one extreme no neoplastic cells may be found; in these cases there is usually an irregular zone of scarring that denotes the site of the pre-existing tumour. A variety of changes may be seen with partial responses. The tumour may be very poorly circumscribed, the malignant cells being widely dispersed in an unusually large amount of stroma (Fig. 11.38). The cells may exhibit no obvious cytological change (Fig. 11.39) or they may appear atypical with large bizarre nuclei with a dense hyperchromatic clumped chromatin pattern. The cytoplasm is often vacuolated. These cytological changes make grading inappropriate. The stroma may contain aggregates of coarse elastin fibres and collections of macrophages, which may have foamy cytoplasm or contain haemosiderin. Necrosis is not usually seen. There is often a poor correlation between response as judged by radiological and pathological examination. On the one hand residual tumour may not be visualized by mammography, and on the other the residual acellular scars may, quite reasonably, be interpreted as residual, viable tumour (Vinnicombe *et al.*, 1996).

CARCINOMAS DETECTED BY MAMMOGRAPHIC SCREENING

Carcinomas detected by screening are more likely to be of the ductal *in situ* type, which accounts for 15–20% of cancers detected in the UK national programme compared to about 5% of those occurring in symptomatic women (Moss *et al.*, 1995). In comparison with symptomatic carcinomas, invasive carcinomas detected by screening are, on average, smaller and of lower grade, have fewer mitoses and less necrosis and are less likely to exhibit aneuploidy and vascular or perineural invasion. Lymph node positivity is also less frequent and the number of involved nodes generally lower (Anderson *et al.*, 1991; Joensuu *et al.*, 1991). Tubular and invasive cribriform carcinomas are more frequent in screened women, although lobular, mucinous and medullary carcinomas are neither over- nor underrepresented (Rajakariar and Walker,

1995; Cowan *et al.*, 1997). The lower incidence of high-grade tumours and nodal metastases persists after correction for tumour size (Klemi *et al.*, 1992). Histological calcification is not found more frequently in the screen-detected invasive tumours.

Immunohistological studies using antibodies to cell products related to tumour biology or prognosis have produced conflicting findings. Thus Cowan *et al.* (1997) found that immunostaining for EGFR, c-erbB-2 protein, oestrogen and progesterone receptors, cathepsin D, p53 and retinoblastoma protein did not distinguish symptomatic and screen-detected cancers. This led them to conclude that these do not differ biologically but are essentially the same lesions detected at an earlier stage in their natural history. In contrast, Rajakariar and Walker (1995) found that screen-detected cancers were less likely to be positive for EGFR, c-erbB-2, retinoblastoma protein, p53 and cathepsin D, and more likely to be positive for oestrogen receptors and the oestrogen-regulated molecule PS2. The reasons for this discrepancy are not clear but to some extent reflect the general lack of agreement about the significance of many cell products detected by immunohistology in breast carcinomas, possibly resulting from differences in fixation and the choice of antibodies, staining methods and scoring systems employed.

Another probable reason for the discrepant findings is patient selection: Rajakariar and Walker's study was restricted to impalpable tumours detected in the prevalent round, whereas that of Cowan *et al.* included all screen-detected cancers, although most were detected in the prevalent round. Klemi *et al.* (1992) found that cancers detected by screening were more likely to have a higher oestrogen and progesterone receptor concentration than non-screen-detected tumours, their study also being restricted to the prevalent round.

Interval cancers are those that present between screening rounds. 'True' interval cancers are those for which no sign of tumour can be seen on the last screening mammogram and which are consequently likely to have arisen between screening rounds. In other cases cancers may have been detectable at screening but were missed through observer or technical error or because the mammographic changes were insufficiently well developed to justify a biopsy. An overrepresentation of unfavourable pathological prognostic features is seen in the 'true' interval cases (von Rosen, 1992). Cancers are more likely to be missed on screening mammography if they occur in radiologically dense breasts or if they are not associated with calcification (Bird *et al.*, 1992).

CARCINOMAS OCCURRING IN YOUNG WOMEN AND CHILDREN

There is very good evidence that breast carcinomas are more aggressive in young women. Kingsley Pillers (1992) found a higher proportion of high-grade carcinomas in younger women, but the effect was seen only in women under 35, where 76% of tumours were grade 3 compared to 53% for all ages. In a later study Kollias *et al.* (1997) divided patients into three age groups: under 35, 35–50 and 51–70 years. Compared to the other two groups, patients under 35 years of age had higher-grade cancers, a greater frequency of vascular invasion and reduced metastasis-free and actuarial survival. There were no differences in tumour size or lymph node stage.

Nixon *et al.* (1994) identified 107 women less than 35 years of age from a group of 1398 stage I or II breast cancer patients treated by breast-conserving therapy. These younger patients had a significantly higher overall recurrence rate as well as a greater risk of developing distant metastases. Their tumours were more likely to be grade 3, and exhibit vascular invasion, necrosis and oestrogen receptor negativity. The worse prognosis in women under 35 was, however, only partly explained by adverse histological factors.

Using multivariate analysis in a study of over 500 patients with T1, T2, N0 and N1a invasive carcinomas, Fourquet *et al.* (1989) found that young age was the most important risk factor for local recurrence after local excision and adjuvant radiotherapy. Peer *et al.*

(1996) found it more difficult to improve survival in younger women through earlier detection, the survival advantage associated with small tumour size being greater in women over 50. They concluded that this effect is probably related to the earlier metastatic potential of tumours in young women. This seems to be supported by the higher incidence of vascular invasion found in carcinomas in younger women by other workers. It should be remembered that a higher proportion of young women with breast cancer would have inherited gene mutations.

The most significant difference in histological type of carcinoma between children and adults is the greatly higher proportion of secretory carcinomas in the former.

CARCINOMAS OCCURRING IN PREGNANT WOMEN

The relationship between pregnancy and prognosis associated with breast cancer has attracted controversy. Statistically significant data are difficult to acquire as, fortunately, very few pregnant patients develop breast cancer. Furthermore, there may be a bias towards detecting higher-stage tumours as smaller lesions may not be discovered until some time after pregnancy and lactation have ceased.

The age at which pregnancy-associated cancer occurs may also be important. In a large study of women under 30 years old, Guinee et al. (1994) found that women whose cancers were diagnosed in pregnancy were significantly more likely to die from the disease than those who had never been pregnant. The relative risk was reduced only slightly when adjustment was made for tumour size and axillary node involvement. For each 1-year increment in time between the latest previous pregnancy and breast cancer diagnosis, the risk of dying decreased by 15%. Anderson et al. (1996) also found that women of 30 years of age or younger experienced decreased survival but as a consequence of having larger, more advanced cancers. Pregnancy appeared to have no prognostic effect on women with early-stage cancers.

In Bonnier et al.'s (1997) study, 5-year disease-free and overall survival were reduced in 154 patients with pregnancy-associated cancer compared to non-pregnancy-associated controls. Pregnancy was found to be an independent prognostic factor. Petrek et al. (1991), on the other hand, did not find any difference in the survival of patients with pregnancy-associated and non-pregnancy-associated cancer when corrected for stage. In the author's opinion the balance of evidence favours a worse prognosis in pregnancy, but it is not clear whether this is because of later presentation or of some effect of pregnancy on the biology of the tumour.

Although there is strong evidence that early age at first pregnancy has a strong protective effect against breast cancer, there is no evidence that breast cancers in parous women are associated with a prognosis any different from that of non-parous women (von Schoultz et al., 1995).

CARCINOMAS OCCURRING IN PATIENTS WITH INHERITED CANCER SYNDROMES

Mutations in the BRCA-1 and BRCA-2 genes account for most of the obviously inherited carcinomas, being responsible for about 85% of families with four or more cases of breast cancer diagnosed under the age of 60 years. Inherited mutations in BRCA-1 are associated with a risk of developing breast cancer of about 80% and a risk of ovarian cancer of about 40% by the age of 70. The BRCA-1 gene is located on chromosome 17q21 (Hall et al., 1990) and encodes a 220 kDa cell cycle-regulated nuclear phosphoprotein of 1863 amino acids that includes a zinc ring finger domain. Murine BRCA-1 is expressed during embryonic development and its mRNA level increases markedly in breast epithelial cells during pregnancy. Expression is inducible by oestrogens (Marquis et al., 1995). At the time of writing there are few data on immuno-staining, and there are doubts about the specificity of some of the antibodies. Some appear to react with EGFR (Thomas et al., 1996; Wilson et al., 1996).

The *BRCA-2* gene is located on chromosome 13q12–q13 (Wooster *et al.*, 1995) and encodes a protein of 3418 amino acids without extensive sequence homology with any other known proteins. Current estimates indicate that *BRCA-2* mutations are associated with a risk of developing breast cancer similar to that of *BRCA-1*, but the risk of ovarian cancer is lower and the risk of male breast cancer higher.

Inherited and acquired mutations of the *TP 53* gene may occur in breast cancer, the former in association with the Li–Fraumeni syndrome, a familial cancer syndrome characterized by diverse multiple neoplasms including soft tissue sarcomas, osteosarcomas, brain tumours, leukaemia and adrenocortical tumours, as well as breast and other carcinomas.

Other genes known to confer an elevated risk of breast cancer are *PTEN* on chromosome 10q23.3, responsible for Cowden's disease (Nelen *et al.*, 1996), and in men the androgen receptor (Wooster *et al.*, 1992). Breast cancer predisposition has also been reported in individuals with the constitutional *translocation 11q;22q* (Lindblom *et al.*, 1994).

In addition to a very high risk of developing breast cancer in those who inherit gene mutations, there is also a higher probability of contracting the disease at a young age and/or in both breasts.

There is evidence that familial carcinomas tend to be of higher grade than sporadic tumours. In two studies of a large number of patients with *BRCA-1* and *BRCA-2* mutations undertaken by the International Breast Cancer Linkage Consortium and Lakhani *et al.* (1997, 1998), cancers from both groups of patients had a higher average grade than those of age-matched controls. When the three components of the grade were considered separately, tumours in *BRCA-1* carriers were found to show more pleomorphism, less tubule formation and a higher mitotic rate than the controls. In addition these tumours were more likely to exhibit pushing margins and a heavier lymphocytic infiltrate. In contrast carcinomas arising in carriers of a *BRCA-2* mutation showed less tubule formation, and greater circumscription than control cancers. There was, however, no significant difference in mitotic count or pleomorphism. Tumours in the *BRCA-1* group are more likely to be negative for oestrogen and progesterone receptors and c-erbB-2 (Johannsson *et al.*, 1997) and to exhibit *p53* mutations (Crook *et al.*, 1997; Gretarsdottir *et al.*, 1998).

Despite these adverse histological features, hereditary breast cancer patients do not appear to have a higher incidence of lymph node metastases or a worse prognosis than age-matched patients with sporadic tumours (Marcus *et al.*, 1996; Eisinger *et al.*, 1998).

CARCINOMA IN ACCESSORY BREAST TISSUE

Accessory breast tissue may occur as supernumerary breasts along the milk lines or as aberrant breast tissue extending beyond the normal peripheral limits of the breast, usually in the axilla, infraclavicular region or epigastrium (see Chapter 5). Carcinomas arising in accessory breast tissue are very rare, but their histological appearance and behaviour are similar to those arising in the normally situated breast.

These tumours present as subcutaneous nodules and are often difficult to distinguish from primary sweat gland carcinomas or metastatic carcinomas (Petrek *et al.*, 1980). Residual non-neoplastic breast tissue around the periphery of the tumour should be sought and, ideally, an *in situ* component identified. It is important to remember that *in situ* carcinoma within sweat glands may sometimes resemble that seen in the breast (*see* Fig. 0.00). In the absence of an obvious *in situ* component, a search should be made for a primary carcinoma in the breast or elsewhere.

REFERENCES

Abati A.D., Kimmel M., Rosen, P.P. (1990) Apocrine mammary carcinoma. A clinico-pathologic study of 72 cases. *Am. J. Clin. Pathol.*, **94**, 371–7.

Aboumrad M.H., Horn R.C., Fine G. (1963) Lipid-secreting mammary carcinoma: report of a case associated with Paget's disease of the nipple. *Cancer*, **16**, 521–5.

Agnantis N.T., Rosen P.P. (1979) Mammary carcinoma with osteoclast-like giant cells. *Am. J. Clin. Pathol.*, **72**, 383–9.

Ahmed A. (1980) Ultrastructural aspects of human breast lesions. *Pathol. Ann.*, **15**, 411–43.

Anderson B.O., Petrek J.A., Byrd D.R., Senie R.T., Borgen P.I. (1996) Pregnancy influences breast cancer stage at diagnosis in women 30 years of age and younger. *Ann. Surg. Oncol.*, **3**, 204–11.

Anderson T.J., Lamb J., Donnan P. *et al.* (1991) Comparative pathology of breast cancer in a randomised trial of screening. *Br. J. Cancer*, **64**, 108–13.

Andreola S., Di Re E., Merson M., Maggiulli L., De Palma P. (1988) Immunohistochemical study of ten cases of argyrophilic carcinoma (carcinoid) of the breast. *Tumori*, **74**, 295–302.

Anthony P.P., James P.D. (1975) Adenoid cystic carcinoma of the breast: prevalence, diagnostic criteria, and histogenesis. *J. Clin. Pathol.*, **28**, 647–55.

Ashikari R., Huvos A.G., Urban J.A., Robbins G.F. (1973) Infiltrating lobular carcinoma of the breast. *Cancer*, **31**, 110–16.

Azzopardi J.G. (1979) *Problems in Breast Pathology*. London, W.B. Saunders.

Azzopardi J.G., Eusebi V. (1977) Melanocyte colonization and pigmentation of breast carcinoma. *Histopathology*, **1**, 21–30.

Azzopardi J.G., Laurini R.N. (1974) Elastosis in breast cancer. *Cancer*, **33**, 174–83.

Azzopardi J.G., Muretto P., Goddeeris P., Eusebi V., Lauweryns J.M. (1982a) 'Carcinoid' tumours of the breast: the morphological spectrum of argyrophil carcinomas. *Histopathology*, **6**, 549–69.

Barsky S.H., Grotendorst G.R., Liotta L.A. (1982) Increased content of type V collagen in desmoplasia of human breast carcinoma. *Am. J. Pathol.*, **108**, 276–83.

Battersby S., Dely C.J., Hopkinson H.E., Anderson T.J. (1992) The nature of breast dense core granules: chromogranin reactivity. *Histopathology*, **20**, 107–14.

Berx G., Cleton-Jansen A.-M., Nollet F. *et al.* (1995) E-cadherin is a tumour/invasion supressor gene mutated in human breast cancers. *EMBO J*, **14**, 6107–15.

Bird R.E., Wallace T.W., Yankaskas B.C. (1992) Analysis of cancers missed at screening mammography. *Radiology*, **184**, 613–17.

Bloom H.J.G., Richardson W.W. (1957) Histological grading and prognosis in breast cancer. *Br. J. Cancer*, **11**, 359–77.

Bonnier P., Romain S., Dilhuydy J.M. *et al.* (1997) Influence of pregnancy on the outcome of breast cancer: a case-control study. *Int. J. Cancer*, **72**, 720–7.

Boyages J., Recht A., Connolly J.L. *et al.* (1990) Early breast cancer: predictors of breast recurrence for patients treated with conservative surgery and radiation therapy. *Radiother. Oncol.*, **19**, 29–41.

Bulman A.S., Lindley R.P., Parsons P., Ellis H. (1988) Pathological features of invasive breast cancer associated with a high risk of local recurrence after tumour excision and radical radiotherapy. *Ann. Roy. Coll. Surg. Engl.*, **70**, 289–92.

Capella C., Eusebi V., Mann B., Azzopardi J.G. (1980) Endocrine differentiation in mucoid carcinoma of the breast. *Histopathology*, **4**, 613–30.

Carter D. (1986) Margins of 'lumpectomy' for breast cancer. *Hum. Pathol.*, **17**, 330–2.

Cooper D.J. (1974) Mucin histochemistry of mucous carcinomas of breast and colon and non-neoplastic breast epithelium. *J. Clin. Pathol.*, **27**, 311–14.

Cornford E.J., Wilson A.R.M., Athanassiou E. (1995) Mammographic features of invasive lobular and invasive ductal carcinoma of the breast: a comparative analysis. *Br. J. Radiol.*, **68**, 450–3.

Cornog J.L., Mobini J., Steiger E., Enterline H.T. (1971) Squamous carcinoma of the breast. *Am. J. Clin. Pathol.*, **55**, 410–17.

Cowan W.K., Kelly P., Sawan A. *et al.* (1997) The pathological and biological nature of screen-detected breast carcinomas: a morphological and immuno-histochemical study. *J. Pathol.*, **182**, 29–35.

Coyne J., Haboubi N.Y. (1992) Micro-invasive breast carcinoma with granulomatous stromal response. *Histopathology*, **20**, 184–5.

Crook T., Crossland S., Crompton M.R., Osinm P., Gusterson B.A. (1997) p53 mutation in BRCA1-associated familial breast cancer. *Lancet*, **350**, 638–9.

Cubilla A.L., Woodruff J.M. (1977) Primary carcinoid tumor of the breast. *Am. J. Surg. Pathol.*, **1**, 283–92.

Deos P.H., Norris H.J. (1982) Well-differentiated (tubular) carcinoma of the breast: a clinicopathologic study of 145 pure and mixed cases. *Am. J. Clin. Pathol.*, **78**, 1–7.

Diamiani S., Riccioni L., Pasquinelli G., Eusebi V. (1997) Poorly differentiated myoepithelial carcinoma of the breast. *Histopathology*, **30**, 542–8.

Di Constanzo D., Rosen P.P., Gareen I., Franklin S., Lesser M. (1990) Prognosis in infiltrating lobular carcinoma: an analysis of 'classical' and variant tumors. *Am. J. Surg. Pathol.*, **14** (1), 12–23.

Drudis T., Arroyo C., Van Hoeven K., Cordon-Cardo C., Rosen P.P. (1994) The pathology of low grade adenosquamous carcinoma of the breast. *Pathol. Ann.*, **29 (part 2)**, 181–97.

DuToit R.S., Locker A.P., Ellis I.O., Elston C.W., Nicholson R.I., Blamey R.W. (1989) Invasive lobular carcinomas of the breast – the prognosis of histopathological subtypes. *Br. J. Cancer.*, **60**, 605–9.

Egan R.L. (1982) Multicentric breast carcinomas: clinical-radiographic-pathologic whole organ studies and 10-year survival. *Cancer*, **49**, 1123–30.

Eggers J.W., Chesney T.M. (1984) Squamous cell carcinoma of the breast: a clinicopathologic analysis of eight cases and review of the literature. *Hum. Pathol.*, **15**, 526–31.

Eisinger F., Nogues C, Birnbaum D, Jacquemier J, Sobol H. (1998). Low frequency of lymph-node metastasis in BRCA1-associated breast cancer. *Lancet*, **351**, 1633–4.

Ekblom P., Miettinen M., Forsman L., Andersson L.C. (1984) Basement membrane and apocrine epithelial antigens in differential diagnosis between tubular carcinoma and sclerosing adenosis of the breast. *J. Clin. Pathol.*, **37**, 357–63.

Ellis I.O., Galea M., Broughton N., Locker A., Blamey R.W., Elston C.W. (1992) Pathological prognostic factors in breast cancer. II. Histological type. Relationship with survival in a large study with long-term follow-up. *Histopathology*, **20**, 479–89.

Elston C.W., Ellis I.O. (1991) Pathological prognostic factors in breast cancer. I. The value of histological grade in breast cancer: experience from a large study with long term follow up. *Histopathology*, **19**, 403–10.

European Commission (1996) *European Guidelines for Quality Assurance in Mammography Screening*, 2nd edn. Office for Official Publications of the European Communities.

Eusebi V., Pich A., Macchioriatti E., Bussolati G. (1977) Morphofunctional differentiation in lobular carcinoma of the breast. *Histopathology*, **1**, 301–14.

Eusebi V., Betts C.M., Bussolati G. (1979) Tubular carcinoma: a variant of secretory breast carcinoma. *Histopathology*, **3**, 407–19.

Eusebi V., Betts C., Haagensen D.E., Gugliotta P., Bussolati G., Azzopardi J.G. (1984) Apocrine differentiation in lobular carcinoma of the breast: a morphologic, immunologic and ultrastructural study. *Hum. Pathol.*, **15 (2)**, 134–40.

Eusebi V., Millis R.R., Cattini M.G., Bussolati G., Azzopardi J.G. (1986) Apocrine carcinoma of the breast. A morphological and immunocytological study. *Am. J. Pathol.*, **123**, 532–41.

Eusebi V., Casadei G.P., Bussolati G., Azzopardi J.G. (1987) Adenomyoepithelioma of the breast with a distinctive type of apocrine adenosis. *Histopathology*, **11**, 305–15.

Eusebi V., Magalhaes F., Azzopardi J.G. (1992) Pleomorphic lobular carcinoma of the breast: an aggressive tumor showing apocrine differentiation. *Hum. Pathol.*, **23 (6)**, 655–62.

Fechner R.E. (1975) Histologic variants of infiltrating lobular carcinoma of the breast. *Hum. Pathol.*, **6**, 373–8.

Finney G.G. Jr., Finney G.G., Montague A.C.W., Stonesifer G.L., Brown C.C. (1972) Bilateral breast cancer, clinical and pathological review. *Ann. Surg.*, **175**, 635–46.

Fisher E.R. (1976) Ultrastructure of the human breast and its disorders. *Am. J. Clin. Pathol.*, **66**, 291–375.

Fisher E.R., Gregorio R.M., Redmond C., Vellios F., Sommers S.C., Fisher B. (1975) Pathologic findings from the National Surgical Adjuvant Breast Project (Protocol No. 4). I. Observations concerning the multicentricity of mammary cancer. *Cancer*, **35**, 247–54.

Fisher E.R., Gregorio R.M., Redmond C., Fisher B. (1977) Tubulolobular invasive breast cancer: a variant of lobular invasive cancer. *Hum. Pathol.*, **8**, 679–83.

Fisher E.R., Kenny J.P., Sass R., Dimitrov N.V., Siderits R.H., Fisher B. (1990) Medullary cancer of the breast revisited. *Breast Cancer Res. Treat.*, **16**, 215–29.

Flotte T.J., Bell D.A., Greco M.A. (1980) Tubular carcinoma and sclerosing adenosis: the use of basal lamina as a differential feature. *Am. J. Surg. Pathol.*, **4**, 75–7.

Foschini M.P., Fulcheri E., Baracchini P., Ceccarelli C., Betts C.M., Eusebi V. (1990) Squamous cell carcinoma with prominent myxoid stroma. *Hum. Pathol.*, **21 (8)**, 859–65.

Fourquet A., Campana F., Zafrani B. *et al.* (1989) Prognostic factors of breast recurrence in the conservative management of early breast cancer: a 25 year follow up. *Int. J. Radiat. Biol. Phys.*, **17**, 719–25.

Gallager H.S., Martin J.E. (1969) Early phases in the development of breast cancer. *Cancer*, **24**, 1170–8.

Gamallo C., Palacios J., Suarez A. *et al.* (1993) Correlation of E-cadherin expression with differentiation grade and histological type in breast carcinoma. *Am. J. Pathol.*, **142**, 987–993.

Gatalica Z. (1997) Immunohistochemical analysis of apocrine breast lesions. Consistent over-expression of androgen receptor accompanied by the loss of estrogen and progesterone receptors in apocrine metaplasia and apocrine carcinoma *in situ*. *Pathol. Res. Pract.*, **193**, 753–8.

Gersell D.J., Katzenstein A.A. (1981) Spindle cell carcinoma of the breast: a clinicopathologic and ultrastructural study. *Hum. Pathol.*, **12**, 550–61.

Geschickter C.F. (1945) *Diseases of the Breast*. Philadelphia, J.B. Lippincott.

Gorski C.M., Niepolomska W., Nowak K. *et al.* (1968) Clinical evaluation and pathological grading in relation to other prognostic factors. In Forrest

A.P.M., Kunkler C.B. (eds), *Prognostic Factors in Breast Cancer*. Baltimore, Williams & Wilkins.

Gretarsdottir S., Thorlacius S., Valgardsgottier R. *et al.* (1998) BRCA2 and p53 mutations in primary breast cancer in relation to genetic instability. *Cancer Res.*, 58, 859–62.

Guarino M., Reale D., Micoli G. (1993) The extracellular matrix in sarcomatoid carcinomas of the breast. *Virchows Archiv A, Pathol. Anat.*, 423, 131–6.

Guinee V.F., Olsson H., Moller T. *et al.* (1994). Effect of pregnancy on prognosis for young women with breast cancer. *Lancet*, 343, 1587–9.

Gusterson B.A., Warburton M.J., Mitchell D., Ellison M., Neville A.M., Rudland P.S. (1982) Distribution of myoepithelial cells and basement membrane proteins in the normal breast and in benign and malignant breast diseases. *Cancer Res.*, 42, 4763–70.

Hall J.M., Lee M.K., Newman B. *et al.* (1990) Linkage of early onset familial breast cancer to chromosome 17q21 *Science.*, 250, 1684–9.

Hamperl H. (1970) The myoepithelia (myoepithelial cells) normal state; regressive changes; hyperplasia; tumors. *Curr. Top. Pathol.*, 53, 161–213.

Hashizume R., Koizumi H., Ihara A., Ohta T., Uchikoshi T. (1996) Expression of β catenin in normal breast tissue and breast carcinoma: a comparative study with epithelial cadherin and α-catenin. *Histopathology*, 29, 139–46.

Holland R., Veling S.H.J., Mravunac M., Hendriks J.H.C.L. (1985) Histologic multifocality of Tis, T1-2 breast carcinomas. *Cancer*, 56, 979–90.

Holland R., Connolly J.L., Gelman R. *et al.* (1990) The presence of an extensive intraductal component following a limited excision correlates with prominent residual disease in the remainder of the breast. *J. Clin. Oncol.*, 8 (1), 113–18.

Hood C.I., Font R.L., Zimmerman L.E. (1973) Metastatic mammary carcinoma in the eyelid with histiocytoid appearance. *Cancer*, 31, 793–800.

Hull M.T., Priest J.B., Broadie T.A., Ransburg R.C., McCarthy L.J. (1981) Glycogen-rich clear cell carcinoma of the breast: a light and electron microscopic study. *Cancer*, 48, 2003–9.

Huvos A., Lucas J., Foote F. (1973) Metaplastic breast carcinoma: rare form of mammary cancer. *N.Y. J. Med.*, 73, 1078–82.

International Breast Cancer Linkage Consortium (1997) The pathology of familial breast cancer: differences between breast cancers in carriers of BRCA-1 or BRCA-2 mutations and sporadic cases. *Lancet*, 349, 1505–10.

Jacquemier J., Kurtz J.M., Amalric R., Brandone H., Ayme Y., Spitalier J.M. (1990) An assessment of extensive intraductal component as a risk factor for local recurrence after breast-conserving therapy. *Br. J. Cancer*, 61, 873–76.

Jao W., Recant W., Swerdlow M.A. (1976) Comparative ultrastructure of tubular carcinoma and sclerosing adenosis of the breast. *Cancer*, 38, 180–6.

Jensen M.L., Kiaer H., Melsen F. (1996) Medullary breast carcinoma vs. poorly differentiated ductal carcinoma: an immunohistochemical study with keratin 19 and oestrogen receptor staining. *Histopathology*, 29, 241–5.

Jensen M.L., Kiaer H., Andersen J., Jensen V., Melsen F. (1997) Prognostic comparison of three classifications for medullary carcinomas of the breast. *Histopathology*, 30, 523–32.

Joensuu H., Toikkanen S., Klemi P.J. (1991) Histological features, DNA content and prognosis of breast carcinoma found incidentally or in screening. *Br. J. Cancer*, 64, 588–92.

Johanssonn O.T., Idvall I., Anderson C., *et al.* (1997) Tumour biological features of BRCA-induced breast and ovarian cancer. *Eur. J. Cancer*, 33, 362–71.

Kiaer H., Nielsen B., Paulsen S., Soresen I.M., Dyreborg V., Blichert-Toft M. (1984) Adenomyoepithelial adenosis and low grade malignant adenomyoepithelioma of the breast. *Virchows Archiv*, 405, 55–67.

Kingsley Pillers E.M. (1992) Histological grade of breast cancer in younger women. *Lancet*, 339, 1483.

Klemi P.J., Joensuu H., Toikkanen S. *et al.* (1992) Aggressiveness of breast cancers found with and without screening. *Br. Med. J.*, 304, 467–9.

Kollias J., Elston C.W., Ellis I.O., Robertson J.F., Blamey R.W. (1997) Early-onset breast cancer – histopathological and prognostic considerations. *Br. J. Cancer*, 75, 1318–23.

Kovi J., Duong H.D., Leffall L.D. (1981) High-grade mucoepidermoid carcinoma of the breast. *Arch. Pathol. Lab. Med.*, 105, 612–14.

Kraus F.T., Neubecker R.D. (1962) The differential diagnosis of papillary tumours of the breast. *Cancer*, 15, 444–55.

Krausz T., Jenkins D., Grontoft O., Pollock D.J., Azzopardi J.G. (1989) Secretory carcinoma of the breast in adults: emphasis on late recurrence and metastasis. *Histopathology*, 14, 25–36.

Krecke K.N., Gisvold J.J. (1993) Invasive lobular carcinoma of the breast: mammographic findings and extent of disease at diagnosis in 184 patients. *Am. J. Roentgenol.*, 161, 957–60.

Kurebayashi J., Izuo M., Ishida T., Kurosumi M., Kawai T. (1988) Two cases of lipid-secreting carcinoma of the breast: case reports with an electron microscopic study. *Jpn J. Clin. Oncol.*, 18 (3), 249–54.

Kuwubara H., Uda H. (1997) Clear cell mammary malignant myoepithelioma with abundant glycogens. *J. Clin. Pathol.*, 50, 700–2.

Lagios M.D., Rose M.R., Margolin F.R. (1980) Tubular carcinoma of the breast: association with multicentricity, bilaterality, and family history of mammary carcinoma. *Am. J. Clin. Pathol.*, 73, 25–30.

Lagios M.D., Westdahl P.R., Rose M.R. (1981) The concept and implications of multicentricity in breast carcinoma. *Pathol. Ann.*, **16**, 83–102.

Lakhani S.R., O'Hare M.J., Monaghan P., Winehouse J., Gazet J.C., Sloane J.P. (1995) Malignant myoepithelioma (myoepithelial carcinoma) of the breast: a detailed cytokeratin study. *J. Clin. Pathol.*, **48**, 164–7

Lakhani S.R., Easton D.F., Stratton M.R. *et al.* (1997) Pathology of familial breast cancer: differences between breast cancers in carriers of *BRCA1* or *BRCA2* mutations and sporadic cases. *Lancet*, **349**, 1505–10.

Lakhani S.R., Jacquemier J., Sloane J.P. *et al.* (1998) Multifactorial analysis of differences between sporadic breast cancer and cancers involving BRCA1 and BRCA2 mutations. *J. Natl Cancer Inst.*, **90**, 1138–45.

Lawrence J.B., Mazur M.T. (1982) Adenoid cystic carcinoma: a comparative pathologic study of tumors in salivary gland, breast, lung, and cervix. *Hum. Pathol.*, **13**, 916–24.

Levine P., Steinhorn S., Ries L. *et al.* (1985) Inflammatory breast cancer. The experience of the Surveillance, Epidemiology and End Results Program. *J. Natl Cancer Inst.*, **74**, 291–7.

Lewis T.R., Casey J., Buerk C.A., Cammack K.V. (1982) Incidence of lobular carcinoma in bilateral breast cancer. *Am. J. Surg.*, **144**, 635–8.

Lindblom A., Sandelin K., Iselius L. *et al.* (1994) Predisposition for breast cancer in carriers of constitutional translocation 11q;22q. *Am. J. Hum. Genet.*, **54**, 871–6.

Loose J.H., Patchefsky A.S., Hollander I.J., Lavin L.S., Cooper H.S,. Katz S.M. (1992) Adenomyoepithelioma of the breast: a spectrum of biologic behavior. *Am. J. Surg. Pathol.*, **16**, 868–76.

Lu Y.J., Xiao S., Yan Y.S. *et al.* (1993) Direct chromosome analysis of 50 breast carcinomas. *Cancer Genet. Cytogenet.*, **69**, 91–9.

Luna-More S., Gonzalez B., Acedo C., Rodrigo I., Luna C. (1994) Invasive micropapillary carcinoma of the breast: a new special type of invasive mammary carcinoma. *Pathol. Res. Pract.*, **190**, 668–74.

Lwin K.Y., Zuccarini 0., Sloane J.P., Beverley P.C.L. (1985) An immunohistological study of leucocyte localization in benign and malignant breast tissue. *Int. J. Cancer*, **36**, 433–8.

Maitra A., Tavassoli F.A., Albores-Saavedra J. *et al.* (1999) Molecular abnormalities associated with secretory carcinomas of the breast. *Hum. Pathol.*, **30**, 1435–40.

Maluf H.M., Zuckerberg L.R., Dickersin G.R., Koerner F.C. (1991) Spindle cell argyrophilic mucin-producing carcinoma of the breast: histological , ultrastructural and immunohistochemical studies of two cases. *Am. J. Surg. Pathol.*, **15**, 677–86.

Marcus J.N., Watson P., Page D.L. *et al.* (1996) Hereditary breast cancer : Pathology, Prognosis, and BRCA-1 and BRCA-2 gene linkage. *Cancer*, **77**, 697–709.

Marquis S.T., Rajan J.V., Wynshaw-Boris A., *et al.* (1995) The developmental pattern of Brca-1 expression implies a role in differentiation of the breast and other tissues. *Nature Genet.*, **11**, 17–26.

Martinez V., Azzopardi J.G. (1979) Invasive lobular carcinoma of the breast: incidence and variants. *Histopathology*, **3**, 467–88.

McDivitt R.W., Stewart F.W. (1966) Breast carcinoma in children. *J. Am. Med. Assoc.*, **195**, 144–6.

McDivitt R.W., Stewart F.W., Berg J.W. (1968) *Tumors of the Breast: Atlas of Tumor Pathology, Fascicle 2*, Washington, DC, Armed Forces Institute of Pathology.

McDivitt R.W., Boyce W., Gersell D. (1982) Tubular carcinoma of the breast: clinical and pathological observations concerning 135 cases. *Am. J. Surg. Pathol.*, **6**, 401–11.

McKay M.J., Mayo F.M., Bilous A.M. (1992) Massive carcinoidlike tumor of the breast. *Breast Disease*, **5**, 125–30.

Michal M., Baumruk L., Burger J., Manhalova M. (1994) Adenomyoepithelioma of the breast with undifferentiated carcinoma component. *Histopathology*, **24**, 274–6.

Mies C.M. (1993) Recurrent secretory carcinoma in residual mammary tissue after mastectomy. *Am. J. Surg. Pathol.*, **17**, 715–21.

Mitnick J.S., Vasquez M.F., Harris M.N., Schechter S., Roses D.F. (1990) Invasive papillary carcinoma of the breast: mammographic appearance. *Radiology*, **177**, 803–6.

Moll R., Mitze M., Frixen U.H., Birchmeier W. (1993) Differential loss of E-cadherin expression in infiltrating ductal and lobular breast carcinomas. *Am. J. Pathol.*, **143**, 1731–42.

Moss S.M., Michel M., Patnick J., Johns L., Blanks R., Chamberlain J. (1995) Results from the NHS Breast Screening Programme 1990–1993. *J. Med. Screening*, **2**, 186–90.

National Coordinating Group for Breast Screening Pathology (1995) *Pathology Reporting in Breast Cancer Screening*. NHSBSP Publication No.3.

Nelen M.R., Padberg G.W., Peeters E.A.J. *et al.* (1996) Localisation of the gene for Cowden's disease to chromosome 10q22–23. *Nature Genet.*, **13**, 114–16.

Nixon A.J., Neuberg D., Hayes D.F. *et al.* (1994) Relationship of patient age to pathologic features of the tumor and prognosis for patients with stage I or II breast cancer. *J. Clin. Oncol.*, **12** (5), 888–94.

Norris H.J., Taylor H.B. (1965) Prognosis of mucinous (gelatinous) carcinoma of the breast. *Cancer*, **18**, 879–85.

Oberman H.A. (1987) Invasive carcinoma of the breast with granulomatous response. *Am. J. Clin. Pathol.*, **88** (6), 718–21.

Ohtake T., Abe R., Kimijima I. *et al.* (1995) Intraductal extension of primary invasive breast carcinoma treated by breast-conservative surgery: computer graphic three-dimensional reconstruction of the mammary duct-lobular systems. *Cancer*, **76**, 32–45.

Oka H., Shiozaki H., Kobayashi K. *et al.* (1993) Expression of E-cadherin cell adhesion molecules in human breast cancer tissues and its relationship to metastasis. *Cancer Res.*, **53**, 1696–701.

Ozzello L. (1971) Ultrastructure of the human mammary gland. *Pathol. Ann.*, **6**, 1–59.

Page D.L., Dixon J.M., Anderson T.J., Lee D., Stewart H.J. (1983) Invasive cribriform carcinoma of the breast. *Histopathology*, **7**, 525–36.

Pandis N., Jin Y., Gorunova L. *et al.* (1995) Chromosomal analysis of 97 primary breast carcinomas: identification of eight karyotypic sub-groups. *Genes Chromosomes Cancer*, **12**, 173–85.

Papotti M., Macri L., Finzi G., Capella G., Eusebi V., Bussolati G. (1989) Neuroendocrine differentiation in carcinomas of the breast: a study of 51 cases. *Semin. Diagn. Pathol.*, **6**, 174–88.

Papotti M., Gherardi G., Eusebi V., Pagani A., Bussolati G. (1992) Primary oat cell (neuroendocrine) carcinoma of the breast. *Virchows Archiv A, Pathol. Anat.*, **420**, 103–8.

Patchefsky A.S., Frauenhoffer C.M., Krall R.A., Cooper H.S. (1979) Low-grade mucoepidermoid carcinoma of the breast. *Arch. Pathol. Lab. Med.*, **103**, 196–8.

Pedersen L., Holck S., Schiodt T., Zedeler K., Mouridsen H.T. (1989) Inter- and intra observer variability in the histopathological diagnosis of medullary carcinoma of the breast and its prognostic implications. *Breast Cancer Res. Treat.*, **14**, 91–9.

Pedersen L., Zedeler K., Holck S., Schiodt T., Mouridsen H.T. (1991) Medullary carcinoma of the breast, proposal for a new simplified histopathological definition. *Br. J. Cancer*, **63**, 591–5.

Peer P.G., Verbeek A.L., Mravunac M., Hendriks J.H., Holland R. (1996) Prognosis of younger and older patients with early breast cancer. *Br. J. Cancer*, **73**, 382–5.

Pereira H., Pinder S.E., Sibbering D.M. *et al.* (1995) Pathological prognostic factors in breast cancer. Should you be a typer or grader? A comparative study of two histological prognostic features in operable breast carcinoma. *Histopathology*, **27**, 219–26.

Peterse J.L. (1993) Breast carcinomas with an unexpected inside-out growth pattern. Rotation of polarisation associated with angioinvasion. *Path. Res. Pract.*, **189**, 780.

Petrek J., Rosen P.P., Robbins G.F. (1980) Carcinoma of aberrant breast tissue. *Clin. Bull.*, **10**, 13–15.

Petrek J.A., Dukoff R., Rogatko A. (1991) Prognosis of pregnancy-associated breast cancer. *Cancer*, **67**, 869–72.

Prescott R.J., Eyden B.P., Reeve N.L. (1992) Sebaceous differentiation in a breast carcinoma with ductal, myoepithelial and squamous elements. *Histopathology*, **21**, 181–4.

Rajakariar R., Walker R.A. (1995) Pathological and biological features of mammographically detected invasive breast carcinomas. *Br. J. Cancer*, **71**, 150–4.

Ramos C.V., Taylor H.B. (1974) Lipid-rich carcinoma of the breast: a clinicopathologic analysis of 13 examples. *Cancer*, **33**, 812–19.

Rapin V., Contesso G., Mouriesse H. *et al.* (1988) Medullary breast carcinoma: a reevaluation of 95 cases of breast cancer with inflammatory stroma. *Cancer*, **61**, 2503–10.

Ravichandran D., Al-Talib R.K., Carty N.J., Theaker J.M., Royle G.T. (1996) Giant cell carcinoma of the breast. *Breast*, **5**, 434–6.

Ridolfi R.L., Rosen P.P., Port A., Kinne D., Mike V. (1977) Medullary carcinoma of the breast: a clinicopathologic study with 10-year follow-up. *Cancer*, **40**, 1365–85.

Rigaud C., Theobald S., Noel P. *et al.* (1993) Medullary carcinoma of the breast: a multicenter study of its diagnostic consistency. *Arch. Pathol. Lab. Med.*, **117**, 1005–7.

Ro J.Y., Silva E.G., Gallagher H.S. (1987) Adenoid cystic carcinoma of the breast. *Hum. Pathol.*, **18 (12)**, 1276–81.

Robbins G.F., Berg J.W. (1964) Bilateral primary breast cancers: a prospective clinicopathological study. *Cancer*, **17**, 1501–27.

Roncaroli F., Lamovec J., Zidar A., Eusebi V. (1996) Acinic cell-like carcinoma of the breast. *Virchows Archiv*, **429**, 69–74.

Rosen P.P. (1979) Multinucleated mammary stromal giant cells: a benign lesion that simulates invasive carcinoma. *Cancer*, **44**, 1305–8

Rosen P.P., Cranor M.L. (1991) Secretory carcinoma of the breast. *Arch. Pathol. Lab. Med.*, **115**, 141–4.

Rosen P.P., Menendez-Botet C.J., Nisselbaum J.S. *et al.* (1975) Pathological review of breast lesions analyzed for estrogen receptor protein. *Cancer Res.*, **35**, 3187–94.

Santini D., Pasquinelli G., Alberghini M., Martinelli G.N., Taffurelli M. (1992) Invasive breast carcinoma with granulomatous response and deposition of unusual amyloid. *J. Clin. Pathol.*, **45**, 885–8.

Schnitt S.J., Connolly J.L., Harris J.R. *et al.* (1984) Pathological predictors of early local recurrence in stage I and II breast cancer treated by primary radiation therapy. *Cancer*, **53**, 1049–57.

Schnitt S.J., Connolly J.L., Khettry U. *et al.* (1987) Pathological findings on re-excision of the primary site in breast cancer patients considered for treatment by primary radiation therapy. *Cancer*, **59**, 675–81.

Schoorl R., de la Riviere A.B., von dem Borne A.E.G., Feltkamp-Vroom T.M. (1976) Identification of T and

B lymphocytes in human breast cancer with immuno-histochemical techniques. *Am. J. Pathol.*, **84**, 529–44.

Schurch W., Lagace R., Seemayer T.A. (1982) Myofibroblastic stromal reaction in retracted scirrhous carcinoma of the breast. *Surg. Gynecol. Obstet.*, **154**, 351–8.

Scopsi L., Andreola S., Pilotti S. *et al.* (1992) Argyrophilia and granin (chromogranin/ secre-togranin) expression in female breast carcinomas. *Am. J. Surg. Pathol.*, **16** (6), 561–76.

Silverberg S.G., Kay S., Chitale A.R., Levitt S.H. (1971) Colloid carcinoma of the breast. *Am. J. Clin. Pathol.*, **55**, 355–63.

Simkovich A.H., Sclafani L.M., Masri M., Kinne D.W. (1993) Role of contralateral breast biopsy in infil-trating lobular cancer. *Surgery*, **114** (3), 555–7.

Siriaunkgul S., Tavassoli F.A. (1993) Invasive micropap-illary carcinoma of the breast. *Mod. Pathol.*, **6**, 660–2.

Sloane J.P. Amendoeira I., Apostolikas N. *et al.* (1999) Consistency achieved by 23 European pathologists from 12 countries in diagnosing breast disease and reporting prognostic features of carcinomas. *Virchows Archiv*, **434**, 3–10.

Swann C.A., Kopans D.B., Koerner F.C., McCarthy K.A., White G., Hall D.A. (1987) The halo sign and malig-nant breast lesions. *Am. J. Roentgenol.*, **149**, 1145–7.

Tamai M. (1992) Intraductal growth of malignant mammary myoepithelioma. *Am. J. Surg. Pathol.*,16, 1116–25.

Tanaka H., Hori M., Ohki T. (1992) High endothelial venule and immunocompetent cells in typical medullary carcinoma of the breast. *Virchows Archiv A, Pathol. Anat.*, **420**, 253–61.

Tavassoli F.A. (1991) Myoepithelial lesions of the breast. Myoepitheliosis, adenomyepithelioma and myoep-ithelial carcinoma. *Am. J. Surg. Pathol.*, **15**, 554–68.

Tavassoli F.T., Norris H.J. (1980) Secretory carcinoma of the breast. *Cancer*, **45**, 2404–13.

Tavassoli F.T., Norris H.J. (1986) Breast carcinoma with osteoclastlike giant cells. *Arch. Pathol. Lab. Med.*, **110**, 636–9.

Thomas J.E., Smith M., Rubinfield B., Gutowski M., Beckmann R.P., Polakis P. (1996) Subcellular locali-sation and analysis of apparent 180-kDa and 220-kDa proteins of the breast cancer susceptibility gene, BRCA1. *J. Biol. Chem.*, **271**, 28630–5.

Thomas J.M., Redding W.H., Sloane J.P. (1979) The spread of breast cancer: importance of the intratho-racic lymphatic route and its relevance to treatment. *Br. J. Cancer*, **40**, 540–7.

Toikkanen S., Joensuu H. (1991) Glycogen-rich clear-cell carcinoma of the breast: a clinicopathologic and flow cytometric study. *Hum. Pathol.*, **22**, 81–3.

Toikkanen S., Kujari H. (1989) Pure and mixed mucinous carcinomas of the breast: a clinicopatho-logic analysis of 61 cases with long-term follow up. *Hum. Pathol.*, **20** (8), 759–64.

Urban J.A. (1970) Bilaterality of breast cancer: biopsy of the contralateral breast. *Cancro*, **23**, 315–18.

Venable J.G., Schwartz A.M., Silverberg S.G. (1990) Infiltrating cribriform carcinoma of the breast: a distinctive clinicopathologic entity. *Hum. Pathol.*, **21**, 333–8.

Vinnicombe S.J., MacVicar A.D., Guy R.L. *et al.* (1996) Primary breast cancer: mammographic changes after neoadjuvant chemotherapy, with pathologic correla-tion. *Radiology*, **198**, 333–40.

Von Rosen A, Frisell J, Nilsson R, Wiege M, Auer G. (1992). Histopathologic and cytochemical character-istics of interval breast carcinomas from the Stockholm mammography screening project. *Acta Oncol.*, **31**, 399–402.

Von Schoultz E., Johansson H., Wilking N., Rutqvist L.E. (1995) Influence of prior and subsequent pregnancy on breast cancer prognosis. *J. Clin. Oncol.*, **13**, 430–4.

Wade P.M., Mills S.E., Read M., Cloud W., Lambert M.J. , Smith R.E. (1983) Small cell neuroendocrine (oat cell) carcinoma of the breast. *Cancer*, **52**, 121–5.

Walford N., Ten Velden J.T. (1989) Histiocytoid breast carcinoma: an apocrine variant of lobular carcinoma. *Histopathology*, **14**, 515–22.

Wargotz E.S., Norris H.J. (1989a) Metaplastic carcino-mas of the breast. I. Matrix-producing carcinoma. *Hum. Pathol.*, **20**, 628–35.

Wargotz E.S., Norris H.J. (1989b) Metaplastic carcino-mas of the breast. III. Carcinosarcoma. *Cancer*, **64**, 1490–9.

Wargotz E.S., Norris H.J. (1990a) Metaplastic carcinomas of the breast. V. Metaplastic carcinoma with osteo-clastic giant cells. *Hum. Pathol.*, **21** (11), 1142–50.

Wargotz E.S., Norris H.J. (1990b) Metaplastic carcino-mas of the breast: IV. Squamous cell carcinoma of ductal origin. *Cancer*, **65**, 272–6.

Wargotz E.S., Silverberg S.G. (1988) Medullary carci-noma of the breast: A clinicopathologic study with appraisal of current diagnostic criteria. *Hum. Pathol.*, **19** (11), 1340–6.

Wargotz E.S., Deos P.H., Norris H.J. (1989) Metaplastic carcinomas of the breast. II. Spindle cell carcinoma. *Hum. Pathol.*, **20** (8), 732–40.

Wheeler J.E., Enterline H.T. (1976) Lobular carcinoma of the breast *in situ* and infiltrating. *Pathol. Ann.*, **11**, 161–88.

Wilson C.A., Payton M.N., Pekar S.K. *et al.* (1996) BRCA1 protein products: Antibody sprecificity. *Nature Genet.*, **13**, 264–5.

Wooster R., Mangion J., Eeles R., *et al.* (1992). A germline mutation in the androgen receptor gene in two brothers with breast cancer and Reifenstein syndrome. *Nature Genet.*, **2**, 132–4.

Wooster R., Bignell G., Lancaster J. *et al.* (1995) Identification of the breast cancer susceptibility gene BRAC-2. *Nature*, **378**, 789–92.

12 Infiltrating carcinoma – morphological and molecular features of prognostic significance

Assessing the prognosis of women suffering from invasive breast carcinoma has become important in recent years for several reasons. First, there has been an increase in the number of treatment options, both surgical and medical. The major change in the former has been the more frequent use of breast-conserving surgery. It is now recognized that radical surgery does not prolong survival, and the detection of tumours at an earlier stage, as a consequence of mammographic screening and greater public awareness, makes it unnecessary to achieve local control in many cases. In the case of medical therapy, the use of hormonally active drugs and cytotoxic therapy has increased. Pathological features may be useful in planning therapy by predicting the natural history of the disease in the absence of treatment or in determining the possible response to a particular form of treatment. Most morphological features belong to the former category. A good example of the latter is the immunohistological determination of oestrogen receptor status in predicting the probable response to hormonal therapy, particularly in premenopausal women.

A second major reason for reporting pathological prognostic features is to monitor mammographic screening programmes. The success of breast screening is ultimately measured by the reduction in mortality from breast cancer in the invited population, but statistically significant mortality data do not become available for many years after the initiation of screening so surrogate measures are needed. These include pathological prognostic features, as the success of a screening programme will be reflected by the more favourable characteristics of the tumours detected.

The pathological grading and staging of breast cancer are also important for stratifying patients in clinical trials of new forms of treatment, auditing cancer units and enabling cancer registries to monitor changing patterns of disease. Finally, patients themselves may wish to know their chances of survival in order to make appropriate plans.

The major problem with reporting pathological prognostic features is interobserver and, to a lesser extent, intraobserver variability. The main reasons for the lack of consistency are the structural and/or cytological heterogeneity of many breast carcinomas and the inherent subjectivity of histopathological examination, particularly of features that form a continuum such as nuclear pleomorphism. Some of the inconsistencies can be overcome by using elaborate morphometric techniques, but they are time-consuming and expensive and thus not generally applicable to routine diagnostic histopathology.

Not surprisingly, there is some disagreement in the literature about the prognostic significance of certain histological and molecular characteristics of invasive carcinomas. This is the result of different study designs (mainly with respect to endpoints and follow-up periods), the subjectivity of histopathological examination and the variation in methodology associated with the measurement of biological markers. There is, however, a general consensus about the significance of some histological features, which should form part of the assessment of invasive breast carcinomas.

MORPHOLOGICAL FEATURES

Subtype

The prognostic significance of the various histological subtypes of breast carcinoma is discussed in Chapter 11. Lobular, tubular and mucinous carcinomas are the most common variants that exhibit significantly different behaviour from the usual invasive ductal (nst) carcinoma. The importance of an extensive intraduct component in determining local recurrence is discussed on p. 173. The major subtypes can be reported with reasonable consistency. In a recent study by a group of over 20 European pathologists, κ statistics (*see* Chapter 2) of 0.76, 0.56, 0.61, 0.92 and 0.51 were obtained for lobular, medullary, tubular, mucinous and ductal (nst) carcinomas

respectively (Sloane *et al.*, 1999). The relatively low value for ductal (nst) carcinomas is not surprising as this subtype is generally the alternative choice for tumours placed in all the other groups and, by its very nature, tends to be a repository for lesions that are difficult to classify. Several other groups have reported relative inconsistency in classifying medullary carcinomas (Pedersen *et al.*, 1989).

Grade

Numerous studies, carefully conducted by experienced workers, have demonstrated a highly significant relationship between tumour grade and prognosis (e.g. Bloom and Richardson, 1957; Freedman *et al.*, 1979; Rosen *et al.*, 1981; Elston *et al.*, 1982; Elston and Ellis, 1991). It is an independent prognostic factor in multivariate analysis for overall and disease-free survival in both pre- and postmenopausal women (Davis *et al.*, 1986).

There are three major methods of grading breast carcinoma. One is exemplified by that used by Black and Speer (1957), in which only the degree of nuclear differentiation is taken into account. The lower grades apply to the more poorly differentiated tumours and higher grades to well-differentiated lesions. The second is the UICC system, in which tumours are divided into well, moderately and poorly differentiated and anaplastic. Both these systems are now only rarely used, having been superseded by the Bloom and Richardson system (1957), which takes into account the structural and cytological features of tumours. Scores from 1 to 3 are given for the degree of tubule formation, pleomorphism and mitotic activity, these then being added together to give the overall grade. A version of this system modified by workers in Nottingham, UK, has been adopted for European Breast Screening Programmes (Elston and Ellis, 1991) as well as by many other workers throughout the world. The grading criteria for this system are as shown below.

12.1 (Left) The whole of this tumour exhibits tubule formation and consequently scores 1 using the Nottingham system (H&E).

12.2 (Right) About half the cell nests in this carcinoma exhibit tubule formation. Consequently it scores 2 using the Nottingham system (H&E).

12.3 (Left) There are no obvious tubules in this tumour, although very occasional tiny lumina can just be discerned, particularly on the left. This scores 3 on the Nottingham system (H&E).

12.4 (Right) A tubule of an invasive carcinoma is seen on the right and a normal lobule on the left. The nuclei are almost identical in the two structures. This tumour scores 1 for pleomorphism (H&E).

12.5 (Left) A tubule of an invasive carcinoma is seen on the left and part of a normal lobule on the right. The nuclei of the tumour are about 1.5 times the normal size and very uniform. The score for pleomorphism is 1 (H&E).

12.6 (Right) Part of an invasive ductal (nst) carcinoma is seen on the right and three normal acini on the left. The nuclei of the tumour are larger than normal (about twice the size) and more vesicular, and contain small but discernible nucleoli. The score for pleomorphism is 2 (H&E).

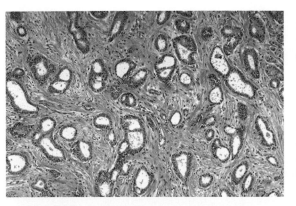

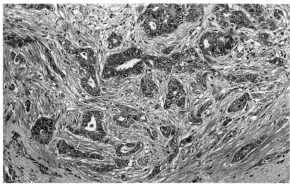

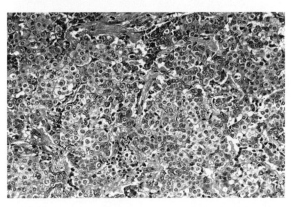

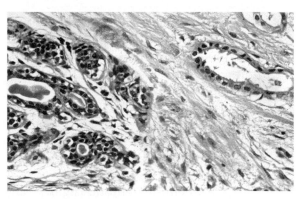

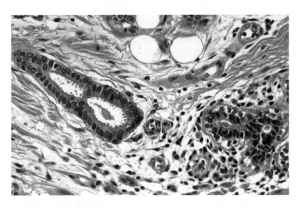

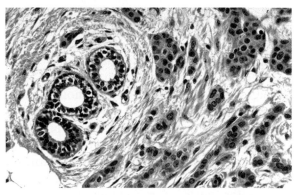

Tubule formation. Only structures with a clearly defined lumen, indicative of ductal or glandular differentiation, are included. Spaces formed as a consequence of other mechanisms, such as poor cellular cohesion or cellular necrosis, are excluded. The following percentages refer to the area of the carcinoma exhibiting tubule formation for each of the three scores:

- 1 = more than 75% (Fig. 12.1)
- 2 = between 10 and 75% (Fig. 12.2)
- 3 = less than 10% (Fig. 12.3).

Pleomorphism. The following criteria are used:

- 1 = The nuclei are small and exhibit little increase in size over that of normal breast epithelial cells. They have regular outlines and uniform nuclear chromatin, and show little variation in size (Figs 12.4 and 12.5).
- 2 = The cells are significantly larger than normal with open vesicular nuclei, discernible nucleoli and moderate variability in size and shape (Figs 12.6 and 12.7).

217

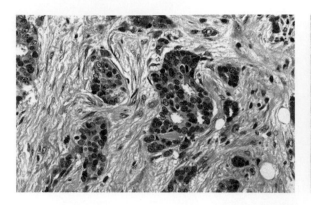

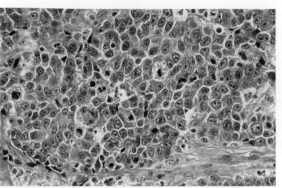

12.7 (Left) The nuclei of this tumour score 2 for pleomorphism. They are somewhat larger than normal, vesicular, and contain small nucleoli (H&E).

12.8 (Right) This tumour exhibits grossly pleomorphic nuclei that score 3 on the Nottingham system. They are much larger than normal and vesicular, containing very prominent nucleoli. There are also numerous mitotic figures (H&E).

12.9 Graph enabling mitotic counts to be corrected for field diameter. This graph was devised by Dr Clive Wells and colleagues at St Bartholomew's Hospital and has been adopted for use in European breast screening programmes. (Illustration reproduced with permission from the NHS Breast Screening Programme.)

- 3 = The nuclei are large and vesicular, often with prominent nucleoli, show a marked variation in size and shape and occasionally exhibit very large and bizarre forms (Fig. 12.8).

Pleomorphism is best assessed using the ×40 objective on the microscope and can thus be done at the same time as counting the mitoses.

Mitoses. Only definite mitotic figures are counted (Fig. 12.8); pyknotic nuclei resulting from apoptosis or any other cause are excluded. The score depends on the number of mitoses per 10 high-power fields, counted at the periphery of the tumour in areas deemed on lower power examination to be of average cellularity for the tumour under examination. It is best to scan the sections of several blocks to select the highest proliferative area as there may be a significant intra-tumour variation in mitotic activity (Jannink *et al.*, 1996).

A major cause of inaccuracy in counting mitoses is the field size, which varies from one microscope to another. For the purposes of the UK National Breast Screening Programme, a graph was devised that enables mitotic counts to be standardized (Fig. 12.9). Other European screening programmes have adopted this. The high-power field diameter is first measured with a graticule, and a vertical line is then drawn at this value on the graph. In Fig. 12.9, for a field diameter of 0.51 mm, a score of 1 is given for a count of 7 or fewer mitoses per 10 high-power fields, 2 for a count of 7–14 and 3 for more than 14. This calibra-

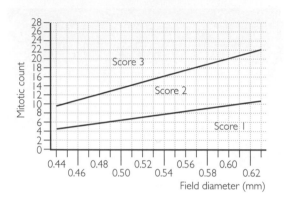

tion procedure needs to be undertaken only once for each microscope.

Overall grade. The scores for tubule formation, pleomorphism and mitoses are then added together:

- Grade 1 = score 3–5
- Grade 2 = score 6–7
- Grade 3 = score 8–9.

Grading breast carcinomas presents a number of difficulties. All tumours are to some extent heterogeneous, and sampling is thus important. Even if the blocks taken are representative of the whole tumour, there may still be a significant variation in differentiation and/or cellularity from field to field. Section quality is another important factor, particularly in assessing pleomorphism and mitotic activity, and a delay in fixation has been shown to affect the assessment of grade (Start *et al.*, 1991). One group (Robbins *et al.*, 1995) found that a higher level of grading consistency could be achieved using sections fixed in B5 rather than the more usual buffered formol saline.

Both inter- and intraobserver variability are important. Freedman *et al.* (1979), using the Bloom and Richardson system, found that the distribution of 1579 tumours over histological grades 1, 2 and 3 was approximately 3:5:6, whereas in Bloom and Richardson's original study of a similarly large number of patients, the proportions were nearer 1:2:1. Although one pathologist had graded all the tumours in Freedman's study, the proportion in each grade varied over the 8-year period of the study.

Other consistency studies of grading have been undertaken in recent years. Dalton *et al.* (1994) sent one slide from each of 10 invasive breast carcinomas to 25 pathologists working in 6 centres, ranging from small town community to large metropolitan hospitals. The slides were selected from 30 cases of invasive carcinomas of no special type to represent a spectrum of differentiation. Section quality was adequate in all cases. The slides were accompanied by a written description of the modified Bloom and Richardson (Nottingham) grading system. There was unanimity in three cases and more than 87% agreement in another six. The median weighted κ statistic was 0.7. In only one case did the participants' responses span all three grades. When the grades were broken down into their constituent scores, it was found that the participants' responses almost invariably clustered into adjacent scores and that disagreement concerning the overall grade of a particular tumour consequently occurred only when adjacent scores bridged grades, that is 5/6 and 7/8. As a consequence of this observation, the authors proposed a 5-grade system: low grade (3/4/5), 5/6, 6/7, 7/8 and high grade (8/9).

Perhaps the largest study of interobserver consistency in grading was undertaken by the UK National Co-ordinating Group for Breast Screening Pathology, who measured the consistency achieved by up to 250 pathologists in the UK National External Scheme using κ statistics (Sloane *et al.*, 1994). Kappa statistics of 0.36, 0.18 and 0.21 were obtained for grades 1, 2 and 3 respectively. The overall value for all grades was 0.26. The 20 or so members of the National Co-ordinating Group, not surprisingly, fared somewhat better but still achieved values of only 0.58, 0.40 and 0.38, for grades 1, 2 and 3, with an overall value of 0.46.

Guidance on how to apply the grading system had been circulated at the beginning of the scheme, but it was not clear whether the relatively poor consistency was caused by the inherent subjectivity of histological examination or a failure to follow the guidelines. More detailed guidance with illustrations was issued, and there is at the time of writing evidence of some improvement as evidenced by recent experience in the UK. Furthermore, a group of European pathologists following the same guidelines achieved an overall κ value of 0.53 (Sloane *et al.*, 1999). It thus seems likely that the maximum level of consistency that can be attained by large numbers of pathologists using the modified Bloom and Richardson (Nottingham) grading system lies in the moderate range as measured by the κ value.

Concerning the different components of the system, three studies (Dalton *et al.*, 1994; Frierson *et al.*, 1995; Sloane *et al.*, in preparation) have shown that nuclear pleomorphism is assessed least consistently, probably because it is the most subjective feature. Two of these studies (Dalton *et al.*, 1994, Sloane *et al.*, in preparation) found the mitotic rate to be the most consistent feature and one (Frierson *et al.*, 1995) the degree of tubule formation. Several workers have found mitotic count to be the most significant feature of the system in predicting clinical outcome (e.g. Clayton, 1991).

Grading is appropriate for histological subtypes for two main reasons. First, not all tumours are easy to type, and grading may provide useful prognostic information when typing is dubious. Second, there is evidence from studies on a large number of well-characterized patients that grading can add significantly to the prognostic assessment of patients with certain histological subtypes. In the study of Pereira *et al.* (1995) classic invasive lobular carcinomas of all three grades were encountered and were associated with different outcomes. Mucinous carcinomas were graded as 1 or 2, each being associated with a different prognosis. Conversely, tumours of the same grade but a different type were associated with different behaviour.

In conclusion there is widespread acceptance that the histological grading of invasive breast carcinomas provides powerful prognostic information, both cheaply and quickly. Interobserver inconsistency is not a surprising problem given the inherently subjective nature of grading, but there is now strong evidence that if grading protocols are strictly adhered to, at least a moderate level of consistency can be achieved. Observer variation can be overcome to some extent by the use of morphometric techniques that enable cytological and structural characteristics to be measured with some precision (Baak et al., 1982), but morphometry is very laborious and costly and, at its present stage of development, not applicable to routine diagnostic histopathology.

Tumour size

There is general agreement that tumour size has strong prognostic significance, smaller tumours being associated with longer survival. This applies not only to the common invasive ductal (nst) and lobular carcinomas, but also to the rarer special subtypes. Carter et al. (1989) examined data on 24 740 cases of invasive breast cancer recorded in the Surveillance, Epidemiology and End Results (SEER) Programme of the US National Cancer Institute and found tumour diameter to be a strong predictor of clinical outcome, independent of lymph node status. The relative 5-year survival was 91.3% for tumours less than 20 mm, 79.8% for tumours 20–50 mm and 62.7% for those over 50 mm in diameter. Size has been found to have more relevance to prognosis with tumours less than 30 mm in size than with larger lesions (Eggers et al, 1971; Elston et al., 1982).

The measurement of tumour size can be undertaken more simply and accurately than grading, but significant problems of consis-

tency can nevertheless be encountered. In the study undertaken by the UK National Breast Screening Programme (Sloane et al., 1994), a wide range was encountered in measuring all tumours on histological sections, although histograms generally showed tight groupings with a small number of outlying results, the reasons for which were not clear. Overall, for unicentric tumours, over 80% of measurements were within 3 mm of the median.

In some cases, however, there was a wide distribution of measurements, for which the main reasons appeared to be tumour asymmetry, poor circumscription (particularly where microscopic foci of tumour extended well beyond the macroscopic limits) and uncertainty about whether to include ductal carcinoma in situ extending beyond the invasive component.

All lesions should be measured macroscopically and histologically. If the two measurements are discrepant, the latter should be recorded if the tumour is small enough to be included in the section in its entirety. The problem of shrinkage of tissue in processing has been exaggerated, and there is generally little difference in size between fresh and processed specimens. Where lesions are too large to be sectioned in their entirety, the histological sections should be used to check the macroscopic measurement. This requires taking an adequate number of blocks from the tumour periphery. The largest dimension should be measured to the nearest millimetre. Where ductal carcinoma in situ extends for more than 1 mm beyond the edge of the invasive tumour, two measurements should be given: one for the invasive component alone and the other for the whole tumour including the in situ disease. This latter measurement allows the identification of carcinomas with extensive intraduct component (see p. 173). Foci of vascular invasion extending beyond the periphery of the lesion should not be included in the measurement. Despite these guidelines some tumours remain difficult to measure accurately, and in these circumstances the best estimate should be given, noting in the histological report that difficulty was experienced.

Regional lymph node involvement

There is universal agreement that the presence of breast carcinoma in the regional lymph nodes is the strongest pathological indicator of an unfavourable prognosis. In the SEER study of 24 740 patients referred to above, Carter *et al.* (1989) found that the 5-year survival rate for patients with tumours under 20 mm was 96.3% for those with negative nodes, 87.4% for those with 1–3 nodes involved and 66.0% for those with more than four nodes. The corresponding figures for tumours 20–50 mm were 89.4%, 79.9% and 58.7%, and for tumours over 50 mm 82.2%, 73% and 45.5%.

An interesting feature of this study was that, for each size group, there was a greater difference in 5-year survival between patients with up to three positive nodes involved and those with four or more than between those with negative nodes and those with 1–3 involved. This indicates that the size of the metastatic tumour burden as well as the mere presence of metastases is important. This finding may be of relevance to the studies on micrometastases discussed below. Other workers have also found that the number of involved nodes is important in predicting clinical outcome (Smith *et al.*, 1977; Fisher *et al.*, 1978).

Axillary lymph node spread is not an infallible guide, however, as some patients with metastases survive and some without evidence of secondaries eventually die of disseminated carcinoma. The reasons are not clearly understood, but the survival of node-positive patients may be due to the dormancy or regression of secondary deposits or the fact that the nodal metastases represent all the metastatic disease. The importance of tumour burden has been mentioned above.

Death from carcinoma of node-negative patients is also poorly understood, but plausible explanations are more forthcoming. The tumour may have spread to nodes other than those in the axilla (such as the internal mammary chain), or metastases may be exclusively blood-borne. An explanation that has attracted a great deal of attention is that secondaries may exist in the nodes in an occult form undetectable by conventional histopathological examination.

There have been many studies investigating the adequacy of histological sampling of lymph nodes. In 1948 Saphir and Amromin investigated 30 patients with breast carcinoma in whom the nodes had been reported as negative and examined an average of 332 serial sections from each block. Altogether a total of 149 axillary nodes was examined. Lymph node metastases were found in 10 (33%) of the 30 cases. Pickren (1961) later performed a similar study on a larger number of patients. Serial 12 μm sections were cut from the blocks of 51 radical axillary node resection specimens originally reported as negative, and metastases were found in 11 (22%). No difference in prognosis, however, was found between the 11 in which micrometastases were found and the remaining 40 in which the nodes remained negative after extensive sampling.

Wilkinson *et al.* (1982) studied 525 cases of invasive breast carcinoma in which the axillary nodes had been reported as negative. All the patients were followed up for at least 5 years. Serial sectioning revealed occult metastases in 89 (17%) of the 525 cases. In 18 of these cases, however, metastases were also found on reviewing the original sections, and in five metastases were present in the original sections but not in the serials. No significant difference in overall survival was found between those with and those without occult metastases. The 18 patients with overlooked metastases, however, exhibited a significantly increased death rate over those with true occult metastases or negative nodes. The presence of occult metastases could not be related to the site, size, grade or type of the primary tumour but did appear to occur more frequently in patients exhibiting evidence of vascular invasion.

A number of similar studies have been undertaken by other workers, and although there is general agreement that serial sectioning increases the detection rate of metastatic cancer, opinion is divided on whether the tumour detected by this method has prognostic significance. Fisher *et al.* (1978) also failed to demonstrate an effect on survival of micrometastatic tumour detected by serial sectioning. In contrast, however, the International Breast Cancer Study Group (1990) found that 83 patients in whom regional lymph node involvement was detected by this method suffered a worse clinical outcome than the 838 who remained node negative. This last study is clearly very large and statistically powerful.

Similar findings have been obtained using immunohistological staining with various antibodies to epithelial components, principally low molecular weight keratins and epithelial membrane antigen (Wells et al., 1984; Trojani et al., 1987; Springall et al., 1990; Galea et al., 1991; Cote et al.,1999). Virtually all studies have shown that the number of positive nodes and node-positive patients is increased by this method, particularly in cases of lobular carcinoma. Furthermore, more cases are identified using immunohistochemistry rather than serial sections stained with H&E (Cote et al., 1999). There is, however, disagreement about the clinical significance of the tumour so detected. In the studies referred to above, a survival effect was found in those of Wells et al., Springall et al. and Cote et al. but not in those of Trojani et al. or Galea et al. In Cote's study 10-year survival and disease-free survival were shorter but only in postmenopausal patients, in whom immunohistochemically detected tumour had independent prognostic significance.

The reasons for these discrepant findings are uncertain. That the number of involved nodes influences prognosis (see above) indicates that the burden of metastatic tumour is an important aspect of prognostication, and one would consequently expect to see a weaker association with prognosis with a smaller amount of tumour. Other possible explanations are that the prognostic significance of micrometastases only becomes clear after very long periods of follow-up or that it only applies to certain subgroups of patients, as in Cote et al.'s study. The methodology of some of the studies may also be significant. It is not acceptable to compare the detection rate using immunohistochemistry under research conditions with

that determined retrospectively on H&E-stained sections reported in routine diagnostic practice. Histological sections immunostained for the appropriate marker should be compared with adjacent H&E-stained sections cut specifically for the purpose of the study and examined under the same conditions.

There is some dispute about the relationship between the size of nodal tumour deposits detected conventionally and prognosis. Huvos et al. (1971) found that cases in which the nodal metastases were under 2 mm exhibited a prognosis similar to those in which metastases were not found. Fisher et al. (1978) found that metastases less than 1.3 mm were associated with survival and treatment failure rates similar to those associated with no nodal involvement, although their findings were based on a rather small sample size. Wilkinson et al. (1982) could find no effect on prognosis of nodal tumour size whether measured as diameter or as volume. Fisher et al. (1978) have also concluded that survival is more likely to be related to the number of nodes involved rather than the size of the deposits.

Extracapsular spread appears to have less significance in breast cancer than in cancers of other sites, for example squamous carcinomas of the head and neck. Pierce et al. (1995) found that an extracapsular spread of axillary nodal deposits was more likely to be found where a larger numbers of nodes were involved and where the primary tumour was of the invasive ductal (nst) type. There was a trend for extracapsular spread to be associated with reduced survival rather than recurrence specifically in the axilla, but the results did not achieve statistical significance.

In summary there is currently insufficient evidence to justify the serial sectioning or immunohistochemical examination of lymph nodes in routine diagnostic practice. Although these methods increase the number of positive samples, there is insufficient evidence that they are of practical prognostic value. Immunohistochemistry is, however, useful in clarifying the nature of suspicious cells in difficult cases, particularly of lobular carcinoma. Time should be spent cutting up axillary dissection specimens in order to identify as many nodes as possible. All should be examined thoroughly, but one H&E section per node is generally sufficient.

Nottingham Prognostic Index

Although lymph node status is the most important pathological factor in predicting prognosis, it is a time-dependent factor that takes no account of the innate aggressiveness of tumours. In a study of nine putative prognostic factors in nearly 400 patients with primary operable breast cancer, Haybittle *et al.* (1982) found that several showed a significant relationship to prognosis but only three – size, grade and lymph node status – remained significant on multivariate analysis The β values from the multivariate analysis were used to derive an index that became known as the Nottingham Prognostic Index (NPI) and is calculated as follows:

0.2 × size (in cm) + stage (lymph node, 1–3 by no. of nodes involved; 0 nodes = 1, 1–3 nodes = 2, > 3 nodes = 3) + grade (modified Bloom and Richardson [Nottingham], 1–3).

It can be seen that the higher the index, the worse the prognosis. A number of subsequent prospective studies have been undertaken to review the efficacy of the index in predicting the clinical outcome of an increasingly large number of patients with increasingly long follow-up times treated at the same unit (Todd

et al., 1987; Galea *et al.*, 1992). Figure 12.10 shows a recent update of the Nottingham series. An excellent prognostic group has also been recently defined to take account of patients whose tumours have been detected by screening. Galea *et al.* (1992) gave a simplified therapeutic guide based on the index. The efficacy of the index has been confirmed by workers in other centres (Baslev *et al.*, 1994). It is not necessary for pathologists to give the NPI in histological reports, and indeed it may not be possible if the lymph nodes have not been sampled. Otherwise it is essential to provide the data from which the NPI is calculated as they form part of the minimum dataset (see Chapter 2).

Lymphatic and blood vascular invasion

The assessment of blood and lymphatic vascular invasion by breast carcinoma is also subject to significant interobserver variation. Several studies have investigated the consistency with which vascular invasion is recognized. In that of Gilchrist *et al.* (1982), three pathologists examined several slides from each of 35 node-negative modified radical mastectomy specimens. All three concurred on the presence or absence of intralymphatic tumour in only 12 (34%) of the cases, which led the authors to conclude that the identification of intralymphatic disease is not a sufficiently reproducible finding on which to recommend systemic chemotherapy. In the later study of Orbo *et al.* (1990), however, two pathologists achieved a κ statistic of 0.6 in identifying lymphatic invasion in 95 invasive carcinomas. Two or more pathologists examined 400 cases in the study of Pinder *et al.* (1994), and there was overall agreement in 77%. The small number of pathologists involved in these studies is probably a major reason for their disparate findings.

The largest study to date is that of the European Commission Working Group on Breast Screening Pathology, in which 23 pathologists examined sections from 57 invasive carcinomas. Complete agreement on vascular invasion was obtained in 22 (39%) of the cases, and there was more than 80% agreement in over 70% of cases (Sloane *et al.*,

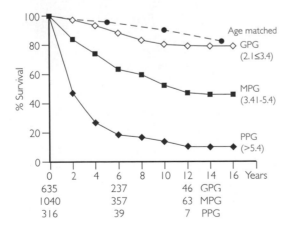

12.10 Survival according to the Nottingham Prognostic Index. (Illustration provided by Professor Christopher Elston and reproduced with permission from the NHS Breast Screening Programme.)

GPG = Good prognostic group
MPG = Moderate prognostic group
PPG = Poor prognostic group

1999). The overall κ statistic was, however, low at 0.38. The major problems lie in overlooking small tumour emboli in capillary vessels and distinguishing them from masses of tumour exhibiting retraction from the surrounding stroma as a result of processing artefact (Fig. 12.11). Larger blood vessels are more easily identifiable by the structure of their walls.

A clear rim of endothelium should be identified around the tumour before vascular invasion is diagnosed, but this is not always easy. The following points may therefore be helpful:

1. Clumps of carcinoma in spaces are more likely to indicate vascular invasion in the tissue around the periphery of the tumour than within the tumour itself.
2. Nests of tumour separated from the stroma by shrinkage artefact usually conform very well to the shape of the space in which they lie (Fig. 12.11), whereas an intravascular tumour usually exhibits noticeable differences in contour.
3. The proximity of larger lymphatics to blood vessels is of help in diagnosing lymphatic invasion as vessels generally run together (Fig. 12.12).
4. Blood vessel invasion is facilitated by the identification of erythrocytes and/or thrombus.
5. Immunohistological stains for factor VIII rag (Fig. 12.13), CD31 or CD34 are very useful in identifying blood vascular invasion in cases where there is doubt on the H&E sections.

At the time of writing, there are no satisfactory morphological or immunohistological methods for distinguishing lymphatic from blood vessels, so vascular invasion should be reported without further qualification.

It is often reported that infiltrative lobular carcinomas exhibit less frequent infiltration of the lymphatics than do invasive ductal (nst) carcinomas, but this may simply be the result of the lesser vascular distension produced by single cells and small clumps.

Despite these problems most researchers have found a significant relationship between

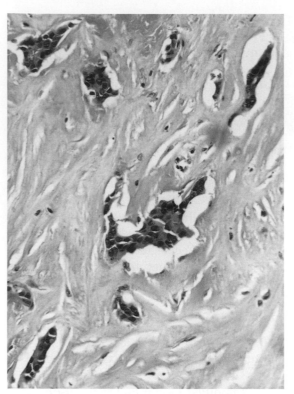

12.11 Infiltrative ductal carcinoma showing retraction from the surrounding stroma caused by a processing artefact. Note the lack of an endothelial lining (H&E).

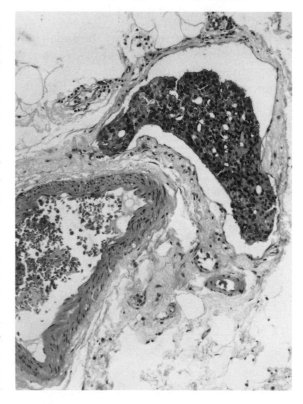

12.12 Metastatic carcinoma within a lymphatic vessel. An endothelial lining is visible, and the structure lies in close proximity to a large vein and a small artery (H&E).

the presence of vascular invasion and prognosis as judged by local recurrence, disease-free

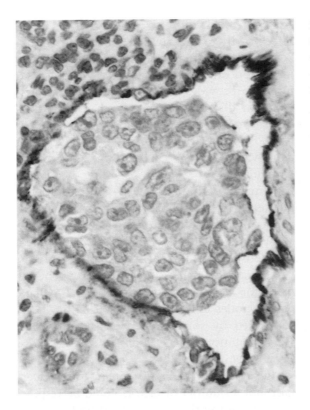

12.13 Metastatic carcinoma in a small blood vessel, which has been stained immunohistochemically for factor VIII rag.

survival or overall survival (Bettelheim and Neville, 1981; Rosen *et al.*, 1981; Roses *et al.*, 1982; Davis *et al.*, 1985; Pinder *et al.*, 1994). Vascular invasion has also been shown to be a predictor of lymph node status, tumour grade and size but not of oestrogen receptor (ER) or menopausal status (Orbo *et al.*, 1990; Pinder *et al.*, 1994). The incidence of vascular invasion in invasive carcinomas varies from study to study. Pinder *et al.* (1994) studied at least three H&E-stained sections from 1704 primary operable breast carcinomas without immunohistological stains and found vascular invasion to be definitely present in 23% of cases, absent in 60% and probably present in 17%.

Excision margins
Microscopic examination of the excision margins is usually undertaken to assess the adequacy of surgical excision and hence the probability of recurrence. Pathological assessment of the excision margins is, however, problematic. Residual tumour may not be present when the margins appear to be involved as the tumour may have reached but

not actually extended beyond the edge of the specimen. Alternatively, it may have extended beyond the margin but been destroyed by the surgical procedure. A false impression of complete excision may be given when the relevant part of the tumour is not included in the sections examined. Most breast carcinomas have an irregular, ill-defined outline, and determining the one nearest the excision margin on macroscopic examination can be very difficult. This is particularly true of poorly circumscribed or multicentric tumours. Re-excision specimens sometimes appear not to contain residual tumour owing to sampling error, giving an erroneous impression that the lesion was originally completely excised. In some cases more than one piece of tissue is excised, making it impossible to determine where the true excision margins are unless clear surgical marking makes it possible to reconstruct the whole specimen. The excision margins are usually marked with ink or dyes, which may track along the interstices of the specimen through defects in the surface. A major problem in comparing the results from different centres is the use of different definitions of margin clearance. Despite these problems it has, nevertheless, been found in most studies that when tumour reaches the excision margins, there is a significantly increased risk of local and distant recurrence.

There are two main groups of investigations in which pathological assessment of excision margins has been evaluated. In the first the distance between the tumour and the nearest margin of a local excision specimen is related to the presence or absence of tumour in a subsequent wider excision or mastectomy specimen. In the second it is related to local recurrence. The disadvantage of the former type of study is that it is not known whether the residual tumour is clinically relevant. The disadvantages of the second are that a long period of follow-up is required and that the picture is often complicated by adjuvant treatment.

Frazier *et al.* (1989) studied 87 patients who underwent more extensive surgery after local excision. The subsequent resection specimens contained tumour in 53% of those deemed to have involved margins, 32% of those with close margins and 26% of those in which the margins were clear. Thus 47% of patients with involved margins had no residual tumour, and 30% of those with close or clear margins had residual disease.

In their study of 181 patients with invasive ductal (nst) carcinoma treated by local excision and radiotherapy, Schnitt et al. (1994) defined three categories of adequacy of excision: positive, in which tumour was present at the inked margin; close, in which the tumour was within 1 mm; and negative, in which the tumour was more than 1 mm clear. The 5-year recurrence rate for those with negative, close, focally positive and more than focally positive margins was 0%, 4%, 6% and 21% respectively. Patients with positive margins were also more likely to have involved lymph nodes at presentation and to have distant metastases at 5 years, suggesting that margin involvement may be a manifestation of more aggressive disease. Patients with an extensive intraduct component were three times more likely to have recurrence, but even in these cases recurrence was infrequent when the excision margins were clear.

In contrast Solin et al. (1991) found no significant difference in 5-year overall or disease-free survival among patients with stage I or II invasive breast cancer with involved, close (2 mm or less) or negative (over 2 mm) margins after local excision. Patients with grossly positive margins were not included, however, as they were converted to mastectomy, leaving only those with focally involved margins. Furthermore, all patients received postoperative radiotherapy. These authors therefore concluded that patients with focally positive or close margins on histological examination could be adequately treated with definitive breast irradiation. Gross margin involvement has, however, been found to be a major risk factor for local recurrence after local excision in multivariate analysis even when adjuvant radiotherapy is given (Fourquet et al., 1989).

Angiogenesis

The growth of an invasive breast carcinoma beyond a very small size is dependent on the formation of new blood vessels. This vasculature also provides the tumour with a mechanism for distant metastatic spread. It is thus not surprising that there has been interest in the possible relationship between microvessel density in breast cancers and prognosis, particularly as immunostaining can be performed with a variety of endothelial markers to render small vessels easily visible and consequently relatively easy to enumerate. Weidner et al. (1991) found that microvessel density in the area of most intense vascularization may be an independent predictor of metastatic disease in axillary lymph nodes and distant sites. This has been confirmed by some groups (Gasparini et al., 1994) but not others (Axelsson et al., 1995; Costello et al., 1995).

The reasons for this discrepancy are uncertain, but a number of factors could be responsible, including the choice of antibody used to stain the vessels, the staining technique, including the method of antigen retrieval, the method of quantification and the uneven distribution of vessels throughout the tumour. Assessing microvessel density may be associated with significant interobserver inconsistency (Axelsson et al., 1995). Even if these factors can be controlled, there remain the complex molecular variables of metastasis associated with the tumour's ability to invade, penetrate vessel walls, extravasate and grow at a distant site. At present, therefore, there is insufficient evidence to recommend that the determination of microvessel density should form part of the routine histopathological assessment of breast carcinomas.

Other morphological features

There have been reports that the prognosis of breast carcinoma may be related to the intensity of stromal infiltration by leucocytes. Hamlin (1968) found that intense stromal mononuclear cell infiltration was associated with a better prognosis, but she included medullary carcinomas in her study. There is evidence that medullary carcinoma is associated with a prognosis better than that of other high-grade carcinomas, but this is a special histological subtype exhibiting other differences from ordinary carcinomas, and there is no evidence that the lymphoid infiltrate is responsible for the improved prognosis.

Later workers (Rosen *et al.*, 1981; Elston *et al.*, 1982) did not find that leucocyte infiltration was associated with improved behaviour in ordinary breast carcinomas. On the contrary, intense infiltration was associated with tumours of higher histological grade. Although there is still considerable interest in the possibility of a beneficial immune response to human tumours, there is no conclusive evidence that assessing mononuclear cell infiltration has any prognostic value in infiltrative breast carcinomas. Indeed, it is often forgotten that lymphocytes and macrophages are constituents of the normal breast epithelium and stroma. Lwin *et al.*(1985) found that the density of intraepithelial leucocytes was actually reduced in breast carcinomas, although it was increased in the stroma. Abnormal leucocyte localization is thus an equally plausible mechanism for the increase in stromal mononuclear cells in many carcinomas. The degree of lymphocytic infiltration of carcinomas does not therefore form part of the minimum dataset described in Chapter 2.

The relationship between prognosis and various reactive changes in the regional lymph nodes is discussed on p. 283.

Similar arguments apply to the question of tumour circumscription and the degree of stromal fibrosis or elastosis. A lower incidence of local recurrence is likely to be found in circumscribed tumours because they are easier to excise completely. Improved survival is likely to be associated with circumscribed tumours with little stromal fibrosis if medullary and colloid carcinomas are included, but there is no convincing evidence that either of these factors is a significant prognostic indicator in ordinary infiltrative ductal (nst) carcinomas. Furthermore, the proportion of infiltrative ductal and lobular carcinomas that are well circumscribed is low.

There has also been disagreement about the prognostic significance of stromal elastosis. In one study (Robertson *et al.*, 1981), a marginally better survival was found for patients with massive elastosis over those with none, but the difference was so small as to have little or no bearing on the overall duration of survival. It is probable, however, that the prognostic significance of elastosis is not independent of other variables such as tumour type and grade.

In conclusion, the most important histological features influencing the natural history of breast carcinoma, which can be reported with reasonable consistency by the histopathologist, are histological type, grade, tumour size, regional lymph node involvement and vascular invasion. The last of these is, however, subject to a greater inconsistency of reporting than the others.

MOLECULAR MARKERS OF PROGNOSIS

A very large number of studies attempting to correlate various molecular aspects of breast carcinomas with prognosis have been undertaken in the past decade, with two main objectives. The first is to improve the understanding of the mechanisms by which breast cancers exert their lethal effects, and the second is to search for methods that are more objective and reproducible in predicting the natural history and the response to treatment than are the traditional histological features described above. Moreover, whereas histological features may give information about the natural history of tumours, biological markers may also be able to predict the response to certain forms of treatment. In the case of ERs, this has proved to be true, but an accurate and reproducible prediction of response to other forms of therapy (e.g. cytotoxic drugs) is not possible at the time of writing. A recently updated version of the American Society of Clinical Oncology guidelines (1997) on the use of tissue tumour markers in the management of patients with breast cancer recommended that only oestrogen and progesterone receptors be measured.

Molecular studies have, however, suffered from a lack of reproducibility as great as or even greater than that associated with morphological assessment, for several reasons. First, the molecules under investigation have been studied from different points of view. In some cases changes in the genes themselves, for example point mutations, deletions and amplifications, have been identified. In others gene expression has been studied either at the mRNA level or by determining the amount of the protein product. Furthermore, different methods have been used to study these different aspects; some have been biochemical, involving the extraction of DNA, RNA or protein from the tissue, and others histochemical, demonstrating changes by techniques such as *in situ* hybridization and immunohistochemistry. The former have the advantage of quantitation and the latter that of being able to relate molecular changes to morphology and thus overcome some (but not all) of the problems associated with tumour heterogeneity and sampling. Immunohistochemistry has, for obvious reasons, been popular with histopathologists working in this field, but inconsistencies have occurred as a result of using different antibodies, processing schedules and staining methods. With the current exception of the ER, external quality assessment schemes have not been introduced to minimize interlaboratory variation.

Another major factor is that the prognosis of breast carcinoma is not always defined in the same way. Some studies have related molecular changes to the risk of recurrence, either local and/or distant, and others to overall survival, which may itself be crude or actuarial. The length of follow-up may vary considerably from study to study, and knowing this will be vital if the molecular change is associated with survival in the longer term. In some reports the changes are related not to clinical outcome but to the stage of the disease at presentation, usually to the presence or absence of regional lymph node metastases or to the morphological features of established prognostic significance described above. Finally, different conclusions from different centres about the prognostic significance of molecular variables may even reflect geographical variations.

The molecular changes that have been investigated are numerous, and it is beyond the scope of this book to deal with all of them. A brief account is given below of those that have been most extensively studied.

Steroid receptors

ER status is increasingly being determined in histopathology laboratories using immunohistochemistry on formalin-fixed, paraffin-embedded sections (for methods of assessment, *see* p. 31). It has been found that this method is superior to the ligand-binding assay and that the degree of positivity, as measured by the proportion of positive cells and their staining intensity, correlates well with the probability of response to endocrine therapy (Harvey *et al.*, 1999).

In recent years the introduction of the anti-oestrogenic drug tamoxifen has made the determination of ER status less critical, as it is relatively non-toxic and a trial of treatment can be given regardless of the knowledge of receptor status. Indeed, evidence of significant benefit from endocrine treatment has been observed in patients whose tumours contain as few as 1% positive cells (Clark *et al.*, 1997). There is clearly, however, a significant economic advantage in not prescribing the drug for patients who will not benefit from it. Elledge and Osborne (1997) have argued that when the cut-off point is stringently low and the assay of high quality, patients with ER-negative tumours will experience little or no benefit from tamoxifen, especially when it is used as adjuvant treatment. Significant financial savings can thus be made by not using the drug indiscriminately. In many centres ER determination is performed as a requirement for the entry of patients into clinical trials.

The expression of the *progesterone receptor* (PR) is also a predictor of response to endocrine therapy and can improve prediction when combined with that of ERs. ER+/PR+ tumours thus respond more frequently than those that are ER+/PR–, which in turn respond more frequently than the small number that are ER–/PR+ (NIH Consensus Development Conference, 1980). The determination of PR status is not usually carried out in routine clinical practice as clinicians are generally prepared to decide treatment on the knowledge of ER status alone, and as there are limited external quality assessment schemes for PR at the time of writing. PR immunostaining can be restricted to ER-negative tumours to reduce costs. Despite the value of ER and PR status in predicting response to endocrine therapy, these are relatively weak prognostic indicators of long-term relapse and mortality, and it is not recommended that they are used *alone* to assign patients to prognostic groupings (American Society of Clinical Oncology, 1996).

Oestrogen-inducible molecules

Studies on the relationship between *cathepsin D* and prognosis have been conflicting and confusing, some finding that its expression is associated with a worse (e.g. Thorpe *et al.*, 1989) and some a better (e.g. Henry *et al.*, 1990) outcome. Some of the confusion has arisen because cathepsin D is found in stromal macrophages as well as tumour cells, and the distinction between these two sources cannot be made in immunoassays of tumour extracts. Even immunohistochemical studies, however, have failed to demonstrate a consistent relationship to prognosis, mainly as a consequence of the use of different antibodies, staining methods and interpretations. The problem is compounded by there being at least three molecular forms, which may be present in different concentrations and have varying affinities for the different antibodies. The American Society of Clinical Oncology (1996) has concluded that present data are insufficient to recommend use of cathepsin D measurements in the management of patients with breast cancer.

Expression of pS2 by breast cancers is usually only encountered in the presence of ERs (Henry *et al.*, 1989) and has been found to be associated with the response to endocrine therapy (Henry *et al.*, 1991), but not all investigators have confirmed its prognostic significance. Thor *et al.* (1992) found that pS2 expression correlated with

tumour grade and oestrogen receptor positivity but not with lymph node metastases, tumour type or patient age. A univariate analysis of lymph node-negative patients showed that pS2 expression was associated with a better outcome, but this did not have independent significance in multivariate analysis or in univariate analysis when all the patients were considered. It is therefore not recommended that immunostaining for pS2 be performed in routine practice.

Type 1 growth factor receptors and their ligands

An increased level of *epidermal growth factor receptor* (EGFR, c-erbB-1) has been found in breast carcinomas in 35–40% of cases (Sainsbury *et al.*, 1987), having an inverse correlation with ER and PR but, perhaps surprisingly, no correlation with c-erbB-2 status (see below). The increased expression is generally not caused by gene amplification, as is the case with c-erbB-2, but by a higher level of mRNA, which generally correlates well with the level of protein. Most groups have not found a relationship with tumour size or subtype, although positivity seems somewhat lower in mucinous and tubular carcinomas. Reports on the relationship between EGFR expression, tumour grade, proliferation rate and lymph node status are contradictory, but most groups have found a positive relationship with aneuploidy. There is little agreement on the prognostic value of EGFR, although most studies indicate a weak association between EGFR and reduced disease-free or overall survival, with a tendency for any prognostic effect to decrease with longer follow-up (Klijn *et al.*, 1992). There is also no agreement on the subgroups of patients in which EGFR status may have a discriminative prognostic effect. Consequently, it is not recommended that EGFR immunostaining be performed on a routine basis.

Some workers have found an association between c-erbB-2 overexpression and poor survival (Paik *et al.*, 1990; Winstanley *et al.*, 1991) but not necessarily disease-free survival (Paik *et al.*, 1990). Gusterson *et al.* (1992) studied 1506 breast cancers immunohistochemically with the monoclonal antibody ICR 12. Approximately half were node negative. Sixteen per cent of the node-negative and 19% of the node-positive cases expressed detectable c-erbB-2, and in both groups there was a negative correlation with ER and PR status and a positive one with high tumour grade.

The last of these findings has been confirmed in many other studies. Lobular carcinomas were all negative. Immunopositivity was significantly associated with poor prognosis in node-positive cases only. Positive tumours were less responsive to chemotherapy with cyclophosphamide, methotrexate and fluorouracil. O'Reilly et al. (1991) also found that the relationship between c-erbB-2 and prognosis applied only to node-positive patients, whereas others have found that patients with immunoreactive tumours are at increased risk of relapse and death irrespective of nodal status (Gullick et al., 1991). Paterson et al. (1991) found that a gene amplification of more than 6 copies was associated with poor prognosis in node-negative patients. In the study of Wolman et al., (1991), however, c-erbB-2 positivity was found with equal frequency in tumours from patients in both good and poor prognostic groups. An association between c-erbB-2 immunoreactivity and a high thymidine labelling index (Barnes et al., 1991a), a high S-phase fraction (O'Reilly et al., 1991) and DNA aneuploidy (Anbazhagan et al., 1991) has also been reported.

The American Society of Clinical Oncology (1996) concluded that data available at the time were insufficient to recommend the use of c-erbB-2 gene amplification or overexpression for management of patients with breast cancer. One exception is now the necessity to demonstrate the overexpression of c-erbB-2 by immunohistochemistry or gene amplification by in situ hybridization in order to select patients with advanced breast cancer for treatment with the humanized anti-c-erbB-2 antibody Herceptin. Standardized immunohistochemistry is needed as sensitivity varies with different antibodies and staining methods.

Quinn et al. (1994) found an increased expression of c-erbB-3 in approximately one third of invasive carcinomas, a normal level in one third and negativity in the remaining third. Immunostaining was restricted to the cytoplasm. There was no significant relationship between c-erbB-3 positivity and ER or c-erbB-2 status, histological grade, lymph node positivity or survival. Later Travis et al. (1996) reported heterogeneous cytoplasmic staining in both primary operable and advanced carcinomas. There was some association with tumour size, type and the probability of local recurrence in the former group but otherwise no association with other prognostic factors or measures of clinical outcome. The immunohistological demonstration of c-erbB-3 thus appears to have no value in the clinical investigation of patients with breast disease.

Other growth factors and their receptors

Transforming growth factor-α, amphiregulin and cripto-1 have been studied immunohistochemically in invasive carcinomas and found to be positive in about 80% of cases. In the study of Qi et al. (1994), no relationship was found with ER or lymph node status, grade, size, proliferation index, loss of heterozygosity at chromosome 17p or survival. Gobbi et al. (2000) found a significant inverse correlation between transforming growth factor-β type II receptor expression and tumour grade, mitotic count and clinical stage, but not ER expression or lymph node status. At the time of writing there is no justification for determining the expression of these growth factors in routine clinical practice.

Products of genes concerned with apoptosis or growth arrest

About 40% of invasive breast carcinomas show positive immunostaining for the p53 protein, which is associated with high tumour grade, ER negativity, the overexpression of c-erbB-2 and EGFR expression (Poller et al., 1992). Barnes et al. (1993) found that patients whose carcinomas expressed p53 in the majority of cells (19% of cases) had a considerably worse prognosis than those who did not. The effect was seen on disease-free survival, overall survival and survival after relapse in node-positive and node-negative patients. Immunostaining for p53 should be interpreted with caution, however, as the overexpression of the protein is not invariably associated with an underlying gene mutation. Van Slooten *et al.* (1999) found that p53 immunopositivity was more likely to be found in tumours with missense mutations or microdeletions than in those with frameshift or nonsense mutations, where immunostaining was generally negative.

Kovach *et al.* (1996), using methodology that detects virtually all mutations of the *TP53* gene, found that mutation was a very strong predictive indicator of disease-free and overall survival and had a much greater prognostic value than immunostaining. Recent evidence indicates that prognosis may be related to the actual site of the mutation: Borresen *et al.* (1995) found a particularly poor survival rate in cases with mutations in the zinc-binding domains. Berg *et al.* (1995) sequenced the complete coding region in breast cancers from 316 patients. Mutations in the evolutionary conserved coding regions II and V were associated with a significantly worse prognosis. Furthermore, adjuvant systemic therapy, especially with tamoxifen, along with radiotherapy seemed to be of less value in tumours with *TP53* mutations, possibly because of the reduced ability of these treatments to induce apoptosis.

Van Slooten *et al.* (1999) found that invasive carcinomas with *TP53* mutations were more likely to have high mitotic *and* apoptotic activity, suggesting that the gene is unimportant in inducing cell death in breast cancers. Furthermore, they showed that mutations in the zinc-binding functional domains or in the residues that directly bind DNA were not associated with an adverse histological appearance. Detecting and localizing mutations are very time-consuming processes, and the American Society of Clinical Oncology (1996) concluded that there were insufficient data to recommend the use of p53 measurements for management of patients with breast cancer.

The p21 protein is an essential part of the p53 growth arrest pathway and has been detected in at least some of the nuclei of over 80% of invasive breast carcinomas by immunohistochemistry. It does not relate to ER status or endocrine response but has been found to correlate with prognosis, particularly if taken into account with p53. Thus p21+/p53– patients have been found to have good survival characteristics, whereas p21–/p53+ patients do poorly (McClelland *et al.*, 1999). Further work is needed before any recommendations about immunostaining in routine diagnostic practice can be made.

In the study of Nathan *et al.* (1994) bcl-2 was overexpressed in 70% of invasive breast carcinomas but without the translocation of chromosomes 14 and 18 that occurs in follicular lymphomas. A highly significant inverse correlation was seen with c-erbB-2 expression and a positive correlation with ER and PR status. Sylvestrini *et al.* (1994) also found an association with ER positivity as well as small tumour size, low proliferation rate and negative immunostaining for p53. bcl-2 immunopositivity was associated with improved relapse-free and overall survival in univariate analysis but not in multivariate analysis, where its predictive role was found to be dependent on p53 expression. It is not recommended that bcl-2 immunostaining is undertaken in routine clinical practice.

Genes involved in metastasis

Several studies have been undertaken to investigate the relationship between the expression of the *nm23* gene and prognosis using either *in situ* hybridization for nm23 mRNA or immunohistochemistry for the NDP-K protein. The results have been conflicting. Bevilaqua *et al.* (1989) found that the level of RNA was in general lower in node-positive tumours, although some exhibited a high level. Hennessy *et al.* (1991) found a relationship between low RNA level and poor survival. In two studies using immunohistochemistry (Barnes *et al.*, 1991b; Hirayama *et al.*, 1991), nm23 positivity was associated with a good prognosis, whereas in another two no relationship with prognosis was found (Sastre-Garau *et al.*, 1992; Sawan *et al.*, 1994). Three different antibodies were used in these four studies, the same being employed in the last two. The present evidence is thus inconclusive.

Cell cycle proteins

Amplification of the *cyclin D1* gene has been found in about 20% of human breast cancers (Buckley *et al.* 1993) and is overexpressed at the protein level in about 40–80%. There have been conflicting reports about the relationship between cyclin D1 expression and prognosis. McIntosh *et al.* (1995) found no correlation with prognosis or established prognostic factors. Michalides *et al.* (1996) also found no relationship with clinical outcome but noted a positive correlation with ER expression. On the other hand, Gillett *et al.* (1996) found that cyclin D1 overexpression correlated positively with not only ER expression, but also low histological grade and a favourable prognosis. A major reason for these discrepant findings is likely to be the use of a different antibody in each study. There is no justification for determining cyclin D1 expression in routine histological practice.

The monoclonal antibodies Ki67 and MIB-1 have been used to stain sections of breast and bind to a protein expressed throughout the cell cycle except in early G1. The proliferative activity of breast carcinomas provides important prognostic information, and the MIB-1 labelling index correlates with histological features and clinical outcome. Perhaps surprisingly, assessing proliferative index by counting Ki67-positive cells has been shown to be associated with low interobserver consistency. This, and the additional cost of immunohistology in time and money, means that counting mitotic figures still remains the method of assessing proliferation in routine diagnostic practice, particularly in grading invasive tumours by the Nottingham method (for a review, see Pinder *et al.*, 1996).

Matrix metalloproteinases

Using immunohistochemistry Jones *et al.* (1999) investigated the expression and distribution of type IV collagenases, their inhibitors and the activator MTI–MMP in a series of invasive breast carcinomas. Matrix metalloproteinase-2 (MMP-2) and MTI–MMP were expressed in more than 90% of all cases with predominantly stromal

and tumour cell cytoplasmic staining. Reactivity localized to tumour cell membranes was, however, recorded for MMP-2 in only 34% of cases with a monoclonal antibody and 55% with a polyclonal antibody, and for MTI-MMP in 68%. In each case this pattern of staining was strongly associated with the presence of lymph node metastases. Tumour cell and stromal staining was seen with TIMP-2 but exhibited no correlation with metastatic status. Expression of the 92 kDa gelatinase MMP-9 was more frequent and homogeneous in the cytoplasm of the tumour cells in invasive lobular carcinomas.

The authors pointed out that previous immunohistochemical studies had been inconsistent in demonstrating an association between MMP expression and clinical outcome. Probable explanations for the inconsistency were the failure to distinguish membrane and cytoplasmic positivity and the inability of immunohistochemistry to distinguish between the active and latent forms of the enzymes. More work is clearly needed before any recommendation can be made about investigating matrix metalloproteinases in the assessment of patients with breast cancer.

GENETIC CHANGES

A number of *conventional cytogenetic analyses* have been undertaken on invasive breast carcinomas. Although no specific abnormality has been linked to prognosis, survival appears to be more favourable in patients with less complex karyotypes (Cervantes and Glassman, 1996). Similarly, Isola *et al.* (1995) found that the total number of genetic aberrations per tumour detected by *comparative genomic hybridization* was significantly greater in node-negative patients who relapsed or died.

Molecular genetic studies have revealed the presence of *allelic imbalance* at a large number of loci, with a highly variable incidence. In some cases the imbalance occurs at loci where there are known tumour suppressor genes, such as *BRCA-1, BRCA-2, RB1* and *TP53* (Chen *et al.*, 1995; Cleton-Jansen, 1995; Beckmann *et al.*, 1996; Hamann *et al.*, 1996). In most cases, however, its significance is not understood except as a non-specific manifestation of genomic instability, and it has no known prognostic significance. Allelic imbalance involving the *BRCA-1* locus may be seen in ductal (nst) and lobular carcinomas and has been found to be associated with larger tumour size and higher grade. Allelic imbalance at the *BRCA-2* locus has been found to correlate with higher grade and aneuploidy (Beckmann *et al.*, 1996; Hamann *et al.*, 1996).

There have been many studies of *microsatellite instability* in invasive breast carcinoma, but the findings have been very variable. At the extremes Patel *et al.* (1994) found microsatellite instability in all 13 cases studied, in contrast to Peltomaki *et al.* (1993), who found no evidence of it in any of their 84 cases. Not surprisingly, the clinical significance is unclear.

REFERENCES

American Society of Clinical Oncology (1996) Clinical practice guidelines for the use of tumor markers in breast and colorectal cancer. *J. Clin. Oncol.*, **14**, 2843–77. 1997 update (1998) *J. Clin. Oncol.*, **16**, 793–5.

Anbazhagan R., Gelber R.D., Bettelheim R., Goldhirsch A., Gusterson B.A. (1991) Association of c-erbB-2 expression and S-phase fraction in the prognosis of node positive breast cancer. *Ann. Oncol.*, **2**, 47–53.

Axelsson K., Ljung B.M.E., Dan H. *et al.* (1995) Tumor angiogenesis as a prognostic assay for invasive ductal breast carcinoma. *J. Natl Cancer Inst.*, **87 (13)**, 997–1008.

Baak J.P.A., Kurver P.H.J., De Snoo-Niewlaat A.J.E., De Graef S., Makkink B., Boon M.E. (1982) Prognostic indicators in breast cancer – morphometric methods. *Histopathology*, **6**, 327–39.

Barnes D.M., Meyer J.S., Gonzalez J.G., Gullick W.J., Millis, R.R. (1991a) Relationship between c-erbB-2 immunoreactivity and thymidine labelling index in breast carcinoma in situ. *Breast Cancer Res. Treat.*, **18**, 11–17.

Barnes R., Shahla M., Barker E. *et al.* (1991b) Low nm23 protein expression in infiltrating ductal breast carcinomas correlates with reduced patient survival. *Am. J. Pathol.*, **139**, 245–50.

Barnes D.M., Dublin E.A., Fisher C.J., Levison D.A., Millis R.R. (1993) Immunohistochemical detection of p53 protein in mammary carcinoma: an important new independent indicator of prognosis? *Hum. Pathol.*, **24 (5)**, 469–76.

Baslev I., Axelsson C.K., Zedeler K., Rasmussen B.B., Carstensen B., Mouridsen H.T. (1994) The Nottingham Prognostic Index applied to 9,149 patients from the studies of the Danish Breast Cancer Cooperative Group (DBCG). *Breast Cancer Res. Treat.*, **32**, 281–90.

Beckmann M.W., Picard F., An H.X. *et al.* (1996) Clinical impact of detection of loss of heterozygosity of BRCA1 and BRCA2 markers in sporadic breast cancer. *Br. J. Cancer*, **73**, 1220–6.

Berg J., Norberg T., Sjogren S., Lindgren A., Holmberg L. (1995) Complete sequencing of the p53 gene provides prognostic information in breast cancer patients, particularly in relation to adjuvant systemic therapy and radiotherapy. *Nature Med.*, **1**, 1029–34.

Bettelheim R., Neville A.M. (1981) Lymphatic and vascular channel involvement within infiltrative breast carcinomas as a guide to prognosis at the time of primary surgical treatment. *Lancet*, **ii**, 631.

Bevilacqua G., Sobel M.E., Lance A., Liotta L.A., Sreeg P.S. (1989) Association of low nm23 RNA levels in human primary ductal breast carcinoma with lymph node involvement and other histopathological indicators of high metastatic potential. *Cancer Res.*, **49**, 5185–90.

Black M.M., Speer F.D. (1957) Nuclear structure in cancer tissues. *Surg. Gynecol., Obstet.*, **105**, 97–102.

Bloom H.J.G., Richardson W.W. (1957) Histological grading and prognosis in breast cancer. *Br. J. Cancer*, **11**, 359–77.

Borresen A.L., Andersen T.I., Eyfjord J.E. *et al* (1995) Tp53 mutations and breast cancer prognosis: particularly poor survival rates for cases with mutations in the zinc-binding domains. *Genes, Chromosomes Cancer*, **14**, 71–5.

Buckley M.F., Sweeney K.J., Hamilton J.A. *et al.* (1993) Expression and amplification of cyclin genes in human breast cancer. *Oncogene*, **8**, 2127–33.

Carter C.L., Allen C., Henson D.E. (1989) Relation of tumor size, lymph node status, and survival in 24,740 breast cancer cases. *Cancer*, **63**, 181–7.

Cervantes M., Glassman A.B. (1996) Breast cancer cytogenetics: a review and proposal for clinical application. *Ann. Clin. Lab. Sci.*, **26**, 208–14.

Chen Y.H., Li C-D., Yap E.P.H., McGee J.O'D. (1995) Detection of loss of heterozygosity of p53 gene in paraffin embedded breast cancers by non-isotopic PCR-SSCP. *J. Pathol.*, **177**, 129–34.

Clark G.M., Harvey J.M., Osborne C.K., Allred D.C. (1997) Estrogen receptor status determined by immunohistochemistry is superior to biological ligand-binding assay for evaluating breast cancer patients. *Proc. Am. Soc. Clin. Oncol.*, **16**, 129.

Clayton F. (1991) Pathologic correlates of survival in 378 lymph node-negative infiltrating ductal breast carcinomas. Mitotic count is the best single predictor. *Cancer*, **68**, 1309–17.

Cleton-Jansen A.-M., Collins N., Lakhani S.R. *et al.* (1995) Loss of heterozygosity in sporadic breast tumours at the BRCA2 locus on chromosome 13q12-q13. *Br. J. Cancer*, **72**, 1241–4.

Costello P., McCann A., Carney D.N., Dervan P.A. (1995) Prognostic significance of microvessel density in lymph node negative breast carcinoma. *Hum. Pathol.*, **26**, 1181–4.

Cote R.J., Peterson H.F., Chaiwun B. *et al.* (1999) Role of immunohistochemical detection of lymph-node metastases in management of breast cancer. *Lancet*, **354**, 896–900.

Dalton L.W., Page D.L., Dupont W.D. (1994) Histologic grading of breast carcinoma. *Cancer*, **73**, 2765–70.

Davis B.W. (1985) Prognostic significance of peritumoral vessel invasion in clinical trials of adjuvant therapy for breast cancer with axillary lymph node metastasis. *Hum. Pathol.*, **16**, 1212–18.

Davis B.W., Gelber R.D., Goldhirsch A. *et al.* (1986) Prognostic significance of tumour grade in clinical trials of adjuvant therapy for breast cancer with axillary lymph node metastasis. *Cancer*, **58**, 2662–70.

Eggers C., de Cholnoky T., Jessup D.S. (1971) Cancer of the breast. *Ann. Surg.*, **113**, 321–40.

Elledge R.M., Osborne C.K. (1997) Oestrogen receptors and breast cancer. *BMJ*, **28**, 1843–4.

Elston C.W., Ellis I.O. (1991) Pathological prognostic factors in breast cancer. I. The value of histological grade in breast cancer: experience from a large study with long term follow up. *Histopathology*, **19**, 403–10.

Elston C.W., Gresham G.A., Rao G.S. *et al.* (1982) The Cancer Research Campaign (Kings/Cambridge) trial for early breast cancer: clinico-pathological aspects. *Br. J. Cancer*, **45**, 655–69.

Fisher E.R., Palekar A., Rockette H., Redmond C., Fisher B. (1978) Pathologic findings from the National Surgical Adjuvant Breast Project (Protocol No. 4). V. Significance of nodal micro and macrometastastes. *Cancer*, **42**, 2032–8.

Fourquet A., Campana F., Zafrani B. *et al.* (1989) Prognostic factors of breast recurrence in the conservative management of early breast cancer: a 25 year follow up. *Int. J. Radiat. Biol. Phys.*, **17**, 719–25.

Frazier T.G., Wong R.W.Y., Rose D. (1989) Implications of accurate pathologic margins in the treatment of primary breast cancer. *Arch. Surg.*, **124**, 37–8.

Freedman L.S., Edwards D.N., McConnell E.M., Downham D.Y. (1979) Histological grade and other prognostic factors in relation to survival of patients with breast cancer. *Br. J. Cancer*, **40**, 44–55.

Frierson H.F., Wolber R.A., Berean K.W. *et al.* (1995) Interobserver reproducibility of the Nottingham modification of the Bloom and Richardson histologic grading scheme for infiltrating ductal carcinoma. *Am. J. Clin. Pathol.*, **103**, 195–8.

Galea M., Athananassiou E., Bell J. *et al.* (1991) Occult regional lymph node metastases from breast carcinoma: immunohistological detection with antibodies CAM 5.2 and NCRC 11. *J. Pathol.*, **165**, 221–7.

Galea M.H., Blamey R.W., Elston C.E., Ellis I.O. (1992) The Nottingham Prognostic Index in primary breast cancer. *Breast Cancer Res. Treat.*, **22**, 207–19.

Gasparini G., Weidner N., Bevilacqua P. *et al.* (1994) Tumor microvessel density, p53 expression, tumor size and peritumoral lymphatic vessel invasion are relevant prognostic markers in node-negative breast carcinoma. *J. Clin. Oncol.*, **12 (3)**, 454–66.

Gilchrist K.W., Gould V.E., Hirschl S. *et al.* (1982) Interobserver variation in the identification of breast carcinoma in intramammary lymphatics. *Hum. Pathol.*, **13**, 170–2.

Gillett C.E., Smith P., Gregory W. *et al.* (1996) Cyclin D1 and prognosis in human breast cancer. *Int. J. Cancer (Pred. Oncol.).*, **69**, 92–9.

Gobbi H., Arteaga CL, Jensen RA et al. (2000) Loss of expression of transforming growth factor beta type II receptor correlates with high tumour grade in human breast in-situ and invasive carcinomas. *Histopathology*, **36**, 168–77.

Gullick W.J., Love S.B., Wright C., Barnes D.M., Gusterson B., Harris A.L. (1991) c-erbB-2 protein overexpression in breast cancer is a risk factor in patients with involved and uninvolved lymph nodes. *Br. J. Cancer*, **63**, 434–8.

Gusterson B.A., Gelber R.D., Golhirsch A. *et al.* (1992) Prognostic importance of c-erbB-2 expression in breast cancer. *J. Clin. Oncol.*, **10**, 1049–56.

Hamann U., Herbold C., Costa S. *et al.* (1996) Allelic imbalance on chromosome 13: evidence for involvement of BRCA2 and RB1 in sporadic breast cancer. *Cancer Res.*, **56**, 1988–90.

Hamlin I.M.E. (1968) Possible host resistance in carcinoma of the breast, a histological study. *Br. J. Cancer*, **22**, 383–401.

Harvey J.M., Clark G.M., Osborne C.K., Allred D.C. (1999) Estrogen receptor status by immunohistochemistry is superior to the ligand binding assay for predicting response to adjuvant endocrine therapy in breast cancer. *J. Clin. Oncol.*, **17**, 1474–81.

Haybittle J.L., Blamey R.W., Elston C.W. *et al.* (1982) A prognostic index in primary breast cancer. *Br. J. Cancer*, **45**, 361–6.

Hennessy C., Henry J.A., May F.E.B., Westley B.R., Angus B., Lennard T.W.J. (1991) Expression of the antimetastic gene nm23 in human breast cancer: an association with good prognosis. *J. Natl Cancer Inst.*, **83**, 281–5.

Henry J.A., Nicholson. S. Hennessy C. *et al* (1989) Expression of the estrogen-regulated pNR-2 mRNA in human breast cancer: relation to oestrogen receptor mRNA levels and response to tamoxifen therapy. *Br. J. Cancer*, **61**, 32–8.

Henry J.A., McCarthy A.L., Angus B. *et al.* (1990) Prognostic significance of the estrogen-regulated protein, cathepsin D, in breast cancer. *Cancer*, **65**, 265–71.

Henry J.A., Piggott. N.H., Mallick. UK *et al* (1991) pNR-2/pS2 immunohistochemical staining in breast cancer. Correlation with prognostic factors and endocrine response. *Br. J. Cancer.*, **62**, 615–22.

Hirayama R., Sawai S., Takagi Y. *et al.* (1991) Positive relationship between expression of anti-metastatic factor (nm23 gene product or nucleoside diphosphate kinase) and good prognosis in human breast cancer. *J. Natl. Cancer Inst.*, **83**, 1249–50.

Huvos A.H., Hutter R.V.P., Berg J.W. (1971) Significance of axillary macrometastases and micrometastases in mammary cancer. *Ann. Surg.*, **173**, 44–6.

International Breast Cancer Study Group (1990) Prognostic importance of occult axillary lymph node micrometastases from breast cancers. *Lancet*, **335**, 1565–8.

Isola J.J., Kallioniemi O.-P., Chu L.W *et al.* (1995). Genetic aberrations detected by comparative genomic hybridisation predict outcome in node-negative breast cancer. *Am. J. Pathol.*, **147**, 905–11.

Jannink I., Risberg B., Van Diest P.J., Baak J.P.A. (1996) Heterogeneity of mitotic activity in breast cancer. *Histopathology*, **29**, 421–8.

Jones J.L., Glynn P., Walker R.A. (1999). Expression of MMP-2 and MMP-9, their inhibitors, and the activator MT1-MMP in primary breast carcinomas. *J. Pathol.*, **189**, 161–8.

Klijn J.G.M., Berns P.M.J.J., Schmitz P.I.M., Foekens J.A. (1992) The clinical significance of Epidermal Growth Factor Receptor EGF-R in human breast cancer: a review on 5232 patients. *Endocrine Rev.*, **13**, 3–17.

Kovach J.S., Hartmann A., Blaszyk H., Cunningham J., Schaid D., Sommer S.S. (1996) Mutation detection by highly sensitive methods indicates that p53 gene mutations in breast cancer can have important prognostic value. *Proc. Natl Acad. Sci. USA*, **93**, 1093–6.

Lwin K.Y., Zuccarini O., Sloane J.P., Beverley P.C.L. (1985) An immunohistological study of leucocyte localization in benign and malignant breast tissue. *Int. J. Cancer*, **36**, 433–8.

McClelland R.A., Gee J.M.W., O'Sullivan L. *et al.* (1999) p21[WAF1] expression and endocrine response in breast cancer. *J. Pathol.*, **188**, 126–32.

McIntosh G.G., Anderson J.J., Milton I. *et al.* (1995) Determination of the prognostic value of cyclin D1 overexpression in breast cancer. *Oncogene*, **11**, 885–91.

Michalides R., Hageman P., van Tintern H. *et al.* (1996) A clinicopathological study on overexpression of cyclin D1 and of p53 in a series of 248 patients with operable breast cancer. *Br. J. Cancer*, **73**, 728–34.

Nathan B., Gusterson B.A., Jadayel D. *et al.* (1994) Expression of BCL-2 in primary breast carcinoma and its correlation with tumour phenotype. *Ann. Oncol.*, **5**, 409–14.

NIH Consensus Development Conference (1980). Steroid Receptors in Breast Cancer. *Cancer*, **46**, 2759–963.

Orbo A., Stalsberg H., Kunde D. (1990) Topographic criteria in the diagnosis of tumor emboli in intramammary lymphatics. *Cancer*, **66**, 972–7.

O'Reilly S.M., Barnes D.M., Camplejohn R.S., Bartkova J., Gregory W.M., Richards M.A. (1991) The relationship between c-erbB-2 expression, S-phase fraction and prognosis in breast cancer. *Br. J. Cancer*, **63**, 444–6.

Paik S., Hazan R., Fisher E.R. *et al.* (1990) Pathologic findings from the National Surgical Adjuvant Breast and Bowel Project: prognostic significance of c-erbB-2 protein overexpression in primary breast cancer. *J. Clin. Oncol.*, **8**, 103–12.

Patel U., Grundfest-Broniatowski S., Gupta M., Banerjee S. (1994) Microsatellite instabilities at five chromosomes in primary breast tumours. *Oncogene*, **9**, 3695–700.

Paterson M.C., Dietrich K.D., Danyluk J. *et al.* (1991) Correlation between c-erbB-2 amplification and risk of recurrent disease in node negative breast cancer. *Cancer Res.*, **51**, 556–7.

Pedersen L., Holck S., Schiodt T., Zedeler K., Mouridsen H.T. (1989) Inter- and intra observer variability in the histopathological diagnosis of medullary carcinoma of the breast and its prognostic implications. *Breast Cancer Res. Treat.*, **14**, 91–9.

Peltomaki P., Lothe R.A., Aaltonen L.A. *et al.* (1993) Microsatellite instability is associated with tumours that characterise the hereditary non-polyposis colorectal carcinoma syndrome. *Cancer Res.*, **53**, 5853–5.

Pereira H., Pinder S.E., Sibbering D.M. *et al.* (1995) Pathological prognostic factors in breast cancer. Should you be a typer or grader? A comparative study of two histological prognostic features in operable breast carcinoma. *Histopathology*, **27**, 219–26.

Pickren J.W. (1961) Significance of occult metastases: a study of breast cancer. *Cancer*, **14**, 1266–1271.

Pierce L.J., Oberman H.A., Strawderman M.H., Lichter A.S. (1995) Microscopic extracapsular extension in the axilla: is this an indication for axillary radiotherapy? *Int. J. Radiat. Oncol. Biol. Phys.*, **33**, 253–9.

Pinder S.E., Ellis I.O., Galea M., O'Rouke S., Blamey R.W., Elston. C.W. (1994) Pathological prognostic factors in the breast cancer. III. Vascular invasion: relationship with recurrence and survival in a large study with long -term follow up. *Histopathology*, **24**, 41–7.

Pinder S.E., Elston C.W., Ellis I.O. (1996) Proliferative activity in invasive breast carcinoma. *J. Clin. Pathol.*, **49**, 868–9

Poller D.N., Hutchings C.E., Galea M. *et al.* (1992) p53 protein expression in human breast carcinoma: relationship to expression of epidermal growth factor receptor, c-erbB-2 protein overexpression, and oestrogen receptor. *Br. J. Cancer*, **66**, 583–8.

Qi C.-F., Liscia D.S., Normanno N., *et al.* (1994) Expression of transforming growth factor α, amphiregulin, and cripto-1 in human breast carcinomas. *Br. J. Cancer*, **69**, 903–10.

Quinn C.M., Ostrowski J.L., Lane S.A. *et al.* (1994) c-erbB-3 protein expression in human breast cancer: comparison with other tumour variables and survival. *Histopathology*, **25**, 247–52.

Robbins P., Pinder S., deKlerk N. *et al.* (1995) Histological grading of breast carcinomas: a study of interobserver agreement. *Hum. Pathol.*, **26**, 873–9.

Robertson A.J., Brown R.A., Cree I.A., MacGillivray J.B., Slidders W., Swanson-Beck J. (1981) Prognostic value of measurement of elastosis in breast carcinoma. *J. Clin. Pathol.*, **34**, 738–43.

Rosen P.P., Saigo P.E., Braun D.W., Weathers E., DePalo A. (1981) Predictors of recurrence in Stage I (T1N0M0) breast carcinoma. *Ann. Surg.*, **193**, 15–25.

Roses D.F., Bell D.A., Flotte T.J., Taylor R., Ratech H., Dubin N. (1982) Pathological predictors of recurrence in stage I (T1N0M0) breast cancer. *Am. J. Clin. Pathol.*, **78**, 817–20.

Sainsbury J.R.C., Needham G.K., Malcolm A., Farndon J.R., Harris A.L. (1987) Epidermal growth factor receptor status as predictor of early recurrence of and death from breast cancer. *Lancet*, **i**, 1398–402.

Saphir O., Amromin G.D. (1948) Obscure axillary lymph node metastases: a study of breast cancer. *Cancer*, **1**, 238–41.

Sastre-Garau X., Lacombe M., Louve M., (1992) Nucleoside diphosphate kinase/nm 23 expression in breast cancer: lack of correlation with lymph node metastasis. *Int. J. Cancer*, **50**, 533–8.

Sawan A., Lascu. I., Veron M. *et al.* (1994) NDP-K/nm23 expression in human breast cancer in relation to relapse, survival, and other prognostic factors: an immunohistochemical study. *J. Pathol.*, **172**, 27–34.

Schnitt S.J., Abner A., Gelman R. *et al.* (1994) The relationship between microscopic margins and the risk of local recurrence in patients with breast cancer treated with breast-conserving surgery and radiation therapy. *Cancer*, **74**, 1746–51.

Sloane J.P. and members of the National Coordinating Group for Breast Screening Pathology (1994) Consistency of histopathological reporting of breast lesions detected by screening: findings of the UK National EQA Scheme. *Eur. J. Cancer*, **30A**, 1414–19.

Sloane J.P. Amendoeira I., Apostolikas N. *et al.* (1999) Consistency achieved by 23 European pathologists from 12 countries in diagnosing breast disease and reporting prognostic features of carcinomas. *Virchows Archiv*, **434**, 3–10.

Smith J.A. III, Gamez-Araujo J.J., Gallager H.S., White E.C., McBride C.M. (1977) Carcinoma of the breast: analysis of total lymph node involvement versus level of metastasis. *Cancer*, **39**, 527–32

Solin L.J., Fowble B.L., Schultz D.J., Goodman R.L. (1991) The significance of the pathology margins of the tumor excision on the outcome of patients treated with definitive irradiation for early stage breast cancer. *Int. J. Radiat. Oncol. Biol. Phys.*, **21**, 279–87.

Springall R.J., Ryina E.R.C., Millis R.R. (1990) Incidence and significance of micrometastases in axillary lymph nodes detected by immunohistological techniques. *J. Pathol.*, **160**, 174A.

Start R.D., Flynn. M.G, Cross S.S., Rogers K., Smith J.H.F. (1991) Is the grading of breast carcinomas affected by a delay in fixation? *Virchows Archiv. Pathol. Anat.*, **419**, 475–7.

Sylvestrini R., Veneroni S., Daidone M.G. *et al.* (1994). The Bcl-2 protein; a prognostic indicator strongly related to p53 protein in lymph node-negative breast cancer patients. *J. Natl Cancer Inst.*, **86**, 499–504.

Thor A.D., Koerner F.C., Edgerton S.M., Wood W.C., Stracher M.A., Schwartz L.H. (1992) pS2 expression in primary breast carcinomas: relationship to clinical and histological features and survival. *Breast Cancer Res. Treat.*, **21**, 111–19.

Thorpe S.M., Rochefort H., Garcia M. *et al* (1989) Association between high concentrations of 52K cathepsin-D and poor prognosis in primary breast cancer. *Cancer Res.*, **49**, 6008–14.

Todd J.H., Dowle M.R., Williams M.R. *et al.* (1987). Confirmation of a prognostic index on primary breast cancer. *Br. J. Cancer*, **56**, 489–92.

Travis A., Pinder S.E., Robertson J.F.R. *et al.* (1996) C-erbB-3 in human breast carcinoma: expression and relation to prognosis and established prognostic indicators. *Br. J. Cancer*, **74**, 229–33.

Trojani M., Mascarel I.D., Coindre J.M., Bonichon F. (1987) Micrometastases to axillary lymph nodes from carcinoma of the breast: detection by immuno-histochemistry and prognostic significance. *Br. J. Cancer*, **55**, 303–6.

Van Slooten H.-J., van De Vijver M., Borresen A.-L. *et al.* (1999) Mutations in the p53 gene, independent of type and location, are associated with increased apoptosis and mitosis in invasive breast carcinoma. *J. Pathol.*, **189**, 504–13.

Weidner N., Simple J.P., Welch W.R., Folkman J. (1991) Tumor angiogenesis and metastasis – correlation in invasive breast carcinoma. *N. Engl. J. Med.*, **324**, 1–8.

Wells C.A., Heyret A., Brochier J., Gatter K.C., Mason D.Y. (1984) The immunocytochemical detection of axillary micrometasases in breast cancer. *Br. J. Cancer*, **50**, 193–7.

Wilkinson E.J., Hause L.L., Hoffman R.G., *et al.* (1982) Occult lymph node metastases in invasive breast carcinoma: characteristics of the primary tumor and significance of the metastases. *Pathol. Ann.*, **17**, 67–91.

Winstanley J., Cooke T., Murray G.D. *et al.* (1991) The long term significance of c-erbB-2 in primary breast cancer. *Br. J. Cancer*, **63**, 447–50.

Wolman S.R., Feiner H.D., Schinella R.A. *et al.* (1991) A retrospective analysis of breast cancer based on outcome differences. *Hum. Pathol.*, **22**, 475–80.

13 Fibroadenoma, adenoma and phyllodes tumour

FIBROADENOMA

Fibroadenomas are benign, circumscribed tumours composed of varying amounts of stromal and epithelial tissue. Although usually no more than 30 mm in size, they occasionally reach large proportions; large size is not, however, indicative of malignancy (see below).

Fibroadenomas usually arise in young women and are the most common primary tumours in younger age groups. They are usually solitary, but a few patients may develop more than one. There may very rarely be multiple bilateral lesions that are difficult to eradicate. Occasionally, they are found incidentally in otherwise normal breasts. Frantz *et al.* (1951) found fibroadenomas in

13.1 Pericanalicular fibroadenoma. The epithelial component consists of normal-appearing lobular and ductal epithelium separated by cellular stroma (H&E).

9% of breasts of women with no history of breast disease at autopsy, but Cheatle (1923) and Bartow *et al.* (1987) found them in about 25%. In the last study the incidence rose with age up to the 35-44 age group and declined thereafter.

There are two types of growth pattern – pericanalicular and intracanalicular. In the former the epithelial component consists of rounded duct-like structures around which the stromal component often has a concentric arrangement (Fig. 13.1). In the latter type there is considerable elongation, thinning and distortion of the epithelial elements, with a consequent reduction in the size of the lumina (Fig. 13.2). Although fibroadenomas have been classified according to growth pattern, it is now generally agreed that this is not worthwhile as there is no difference in behaviour and both patterns may occur in the same tumour.

The epithelial structures, although usually resembling interlobular ducts, are largely of lobular origin and undergo secretory changes in pregnancy and lactation, with the production of α-lactalbumin (Bailey *et al.*, 1982) (Fig. 13.3). The degree of similarity between the epithelium of the fibroadenoma and that in the lobules of the surrounding lactating breast varies from tumour to tumour but is usually

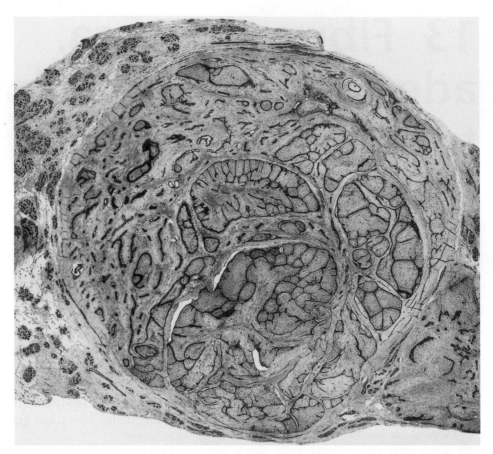

13.2 Intracanalicular fibroadenoma showing elongation, distortion and thinning of the epithelial elements (H&E).

close. These changes may result in a very rapid growth of the tumour, particularly in the first half of pregnancy, and lead to a clinical suspicion of carcinoma. Geschickter and Lewis (1938) found foci of non-encapsulation, an extension of epithelial tissue into the surrounding fat and marked mitotic activity in pregnancy, all of which could also lead to a suspicion of malignancy.

Apart from pregnancy changes the epithelial component may undergo other changes found in breast lobules. Thus fibroadenomas may contain cysts or exhibit foci of apocrine metaplasia, sclerosing adenosis, atypical and non-atypical hyperplasia and even carcinoma. Fibroadenomas containing carcinoma are rare and tend to occur in older women. Buzanowski-Konakry *et al.* (1975) found only five examples out of 4000 cases of fibroadenoma. Most are *in situ* carcinomas; in some series there is a disproportionately high number of lobular carcinomas *in situ*

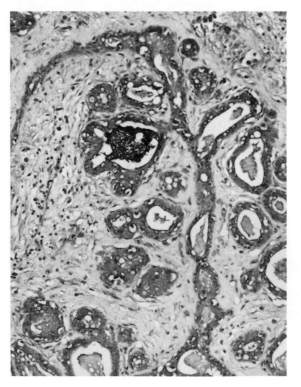

13.3 Formalin-fixed, paraffin-embedded section of a fibroadenoma removed from a patient in mid-pregnancy stained for α-lactalbumin by the indirect immunoperoxidase technique. The epithelium shows secretory changes consistent with the stage of pregnancy, and lactalbumin staining is present in the lumina and epithelial cells, especially in the upper centre of the picture. (Illustration reproduced with permission from the *Journal of Pathology*.)

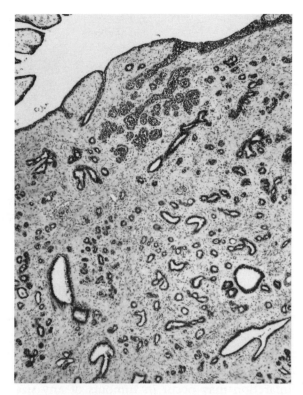

13.4 Fibroadenoma containing a focus of lobular carcinoma *in situ* (top) (H&E).

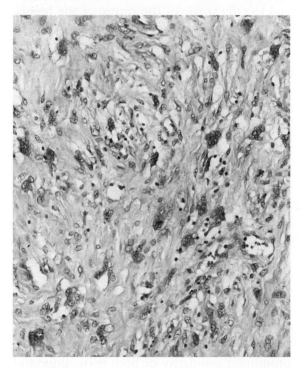

13.5 Benign multinucleate giant cells in a fibroadenoma. The nuclei do not show the gross pleomorphism or hyperchromatism of malignant giant cells, and the intervening tissue lacks the cytological features of malignancy (H&E).

(McDivitt *et al.*, 1967) (Fig. 13.4), although in others there is an equal mixture of ductal and lobular types (Diaz *et al.*, 1991). The extent of the malignant change may vary from a few small microscopic foci to an almost complete replacement of the epithelial component.

Of the 26 cases reviewed by Buzanowski-Konakry *et al.* (1975), 11 were also found to have carcinoma in the breast outside the fibroadenoma, and in three there was also carcinoma in the contralateral breast. In a later paper Ozzello and Gump (1985) reported 38 patients with unsuspected lobular neoplasia, ductal carcinoma *in situ* or invasive carcinoma in fibroadenomas and reviewed 56 other cases in the literature. They concluded that the biological and clinical behaviour of these malignancies was the same as those unassociated with fibroadenoma and that patient management should therefore be the same as if they had arisen in the usual setting.

Fibroadenomas have long been thought not to be associated with the subsequent development of carcinoma, but in the studies of Carter *et al.* (1988) and McDivitt *et al.* (1992) they were associated with an increased relative risk of developing breast cancer of 1.7. In a retrospective cohort study of 1835 patients, Dupont *et al.* (1994) found that the risk of developing invasive cancer was 2.17 times higher among patients with a fibroadenoma than among controls. The relative risk increased to 3.10 in patients with complex fibroadenomas (those containing cysts, sclerosing adenosis, epithelial calcifications or papillary apocrine changes) and to 3.88 in those in whom benign proliferative disease was identified in the breast adjacent to the fibroadenoma. Patients with complex fibroadenomas and a family history of breast cancer had a relative risk of 3.72 compared to controls with such a family history. The majority of patients, however, had non-complex fibroadenomas and no family history, and they were not at increased risk.

Eusebi and Azzopardi (1980) described the *in situ* proliferation of neurosecretory granule-containing, endocrine-type cells within fibroadenomas in young patients, taking the form of nests, clumps, tubules or endophytic buds. This appears to be a very rare phenomenon. The significance of the change is obscure but appears to be yet another manifestation of the ability of breast epithelial cells to exhibit neuroendocrine characteristics.

The stromal component of fibroadenomas may exhibit considerable variation in cellularity. The less cellular tumours tend to occur in older subjects and may occasionally be completely hyalinized. Care should be taken to distinguish lesions with densely cellular stroma from phyllodes tumours (see below), especially in older patients. Myxoid change may occur in the stroma of a fibroadenoma and often tends to be more pronounced around the epithelium. Pseudoangiomatous hyperplasia is not uncommon. Very occasionally, multinucleated stromal giant cells may be seen and may be very numerous (Fig. 13.5). These cells are similar to those occasionally seen in the non-lesional interlobular stroma of benign and malignant breasts. Despite their bizarre appearance they are benign and should not lead to a diagnosis of phyllodes tumour or any other malignancy. Immunohistochemical and ultrastructural studies have confirmed their mesenchymal and specifically fibroblastic nature (Berean et al., 1986).

The stroma usually appears entirely fibroblastic. Immunostaining reveals the presence of CD34+ fibroblasts showing varying myxoid, collagenous and myofibroblastic differentiation, accompanied by a number of factor XIIIa-positive dendritic histiocytes (Silverman and Tamsen, 1996). Elastin is not demonstrable by conventional methods, a finding consistent with the lobular origin of the lesion. Other mesenchymal elements such as adipose tissue or smooth muscle (Fig. 13.6) may, however, be seen on rare occasions. The frequent location of smooth muscle-containing lesions near the nipple has led to the suggestion that the myoid component may sometimes be derived from the erector muscles (Goodman and Taxy, 1981). Foci of cartilage or bone are very rare (Willis, 1967).

Ultrastructurally, the epithelial cells resemble those of the normal or hyperplastic breast. The luminal microvilli are often numerous and irregular, but the intercellular junctions comprise the usual terminal bars and desmosomes (Fisher, 1976; Jao et al., 1978).

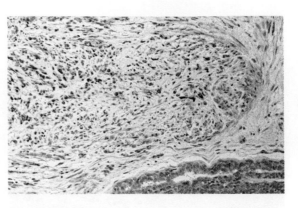

13.6 Stroma of a fibroadenoma stained immunohistochemically for desmin, revealing the presence of smooth muscle fibres.

Intracytoplasmic lumina are rarely encountered. The basal lamina is intact, but the myoepithelial layer is often attenuated or incomplete. The fibroblasts may show an increase in organelles.

Fibroadenomas may undergo infarction, but this is an uncommon complication: Majmudar and Rosales-Quintana (1975) found only two cases out of 404 fibroadenomas. Infarction may occur in tumours of any size and usually involves the centre of the lesion. The resulting necrosis may lead to confusion with carcinoma, especially on frozen sections. The cause of the infarction is not usually demonstrable; there is generally no evidence of vascular disease of either a thrombo-occlusive or an inflammatory nature. Most cases occur in pregnancy, which has led to the suggestion that the necrosis may be caused by relative vascular insufficiency resulting from increased metabolic demands.

Few molecular genetic studies have been undertaken. Reid et al. (1995) studied 13 formalin-fixed, paraffin-embedded fibroadenomas using comparative genomic hybridization. None revealed any genomic imbalance.

The term juvenile fibroadenoma is sometimes used to describe highly cellular, rapidly growing tumours that usually occur in juveniles and young women but may also be seen in older patients. These lesions exhibit a prominent cellularity of both epithelium and stroma and are occasionally multiple (Pike and Oberman, 1985). In some cases the epithelial hyperplasia is severely atypical and may even be suggestive of in situ carcinoma (Mies and Rosen, 1987). It may assume a

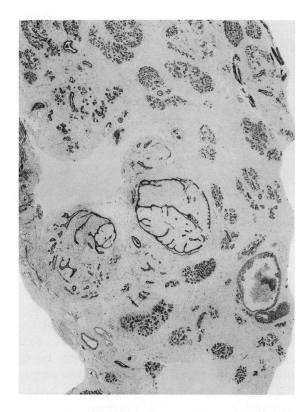

13.7 Fibroadenomatoid hyperplasia. Two loosely coalescent lobules exhibit fibroadenoma-like changes (H&E).

carcinomas were *in situ*: one an intraduct papillary carcinoma in the contralateral breast and the other an *in situ* lobular carcinoma in the same breast. There thus appears to be no increased risk of developing carcinoma, particularly in young patients. Patients with juvenile fibroadenomas, including those with atypical hyperplasia, have no increased incidence of exogenous hormone usage, menstrual irregularity or family history of breast cancer (Mies and Rosen, 1987).

FIBROADENOMATOID HYPERPLASIA

Fibroadenoma-like changes may occasionally occur in individual breast lobules, which may be discrete or loosely coalescent, forming an irregular ill-defined mass (Fig. 13.7). These lesions may or may not be clinically detectable, depending on their size. The term fibroadenoma seems inappropriate to describe such ill-defined lesions, so fibroadenomatoid hyperplasia is both descriptively accurate and convenient. Such lesions are, however, usually recorded as fibroadenomas in breast-screening databases. The strong resemblance of these lobular lesions to fibroadenomas is further evidence that the latter are of lobular origin.

Bittesini *et al.* (1994) described a fibroepithelial tumour of the breast with digital fibroma-like inclusions in the stromal component in a 34-year-old woman. The lesion was nodular but ill delimited from the surrounding breast. Focally, it exhibited the structural features of fibroadenomatoid hyperplasia or phyllodes tumour. The epithelial component displayed apocrine cysts and prominent epithelial hyperplasia. The stroma was composed of plump spindle cells intermingled with bundles of collagen fibres. Up to two stromal mitoses were seen per 10 high-power fields, with no atypical forms. The most striking feature of the stromal cells was the presence of intracytoplasmic round inclusion bodies evenly distributed within about 30% of the tumour cells. The morphological, immunohistochemical and ultrastructural findings indicated that the inclusions represented packed actin filaments. Apart from infantile digital fibromas, such inclusions

cribriform or solid growth pattern and involve duct and lobule-like structures, some of which may exhibit cystic dilatation. The cribriform zones may display well-delineated secondary lumina. The proliferating cells usually have small uniform hyperchromatic nuclei, reminiscent of those of low nuclear grade ductal carcinoma *in situ*. Mitoses may be observed, but necrosis is usually absent. The epithelial proliferation does not extend outside the fibroadenoma into the surrounding breast. The stroma is generally fibroblastic and may exhibit variable cellularity from case to case and within individual lesions. Atypia of the stromal cells is lacking, and mitoses are not usually seen. An infiltrate of lymphocytes and plasma cells is common; eosinophils and mast cells are rare.

Recurrences do not usually occur after local excision except in multiple cases (Pike and Oberman, 1985). In the series reported by Mies and Rosen, 2 of 28 patients followed up for 1–19 years (average 7 years) developed carcinoma. These patients were, however, 47 and 59 years old when their fibroadenomas were diagnosed, and both the subsequent have also been described in leiomyomas and intranodal myofibroblastomas. The morphology of the lesion suggested that it was benign, but the patient had been followed up for only 1 year at the time of the report.

ADENOMAS OF THE BREAST

There has been much confusion about the precise definition of adenoma of the breast, many recorded cases being merely fibroadenomas exhibiting a predominant epithelial component. A breast adenoma is a benign epithelial tumour in which the stroma shows no evidence of neoplasia and is present in no greater amount than would be expected merely to provide a supportive function. As thus defined, breast adenomas are rare.

Tubular adenoma

These are sharply demarcated but non-encapsulated lesions that are composed of numerous closely packed, small (30–50 μm), uniform, tubular structures lined by an inner epithelial and an outer, attenuated myoepithelial layer (Fig. 13.8). Occasional large ductal structures are seen. The cells are cytologically benign and virtually indistinguishable from those of normal lobules at both the light and electron microscope levels (Hertel *et al.*, 1976). The lesion often gives the impression of numerous enlarged but otherwise normal lobules that have coalesced to form a circumscribed mass. Hyperplasia of the lobules may be seen in the surrounding breast. LeGal (1961) found that a small number of tubular adenomas are composed of columnar or cuboidal apocrine cells arranged in tubules and solid trabeculae. Tubular adenomas may occur in childhood and old age, the average being in the early 20s. The size is usually between 10 and 40 mm.

Adenoma of the nipple (subareolar duct papillomatosis)

This condition also goes under the names of florid papillomatosis and florid adenomatosis of the nipple ducts. Grossly, it has the appearance of a nodule or mass, usually less than 15 mm in size, with ill-defined borders in the

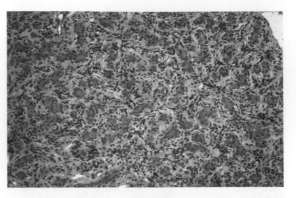

13.8 Tubular adenoma. There are numerous small tubules, mostly with poorly defined or indiscernible lumina separated by loosely textured stroma. The appearance is strongly suggestive of a greatly enlarged lobule (H&E).

region of the nipple. It is often associated with erosion of the skin, and there may be a serous or blood-stained discharge. Pain, tenderness and pruritus are not uncommon, and there may be a clinical impression of Paget's disease. It is seen in women of any age and occasionally in men (Taylor and Robertson, 1965).

Histologically, the lesion is usually well circumscribed but not encapsulated, being situated in the superficial stroma of the nipple (Fig. 13.9). There may be many small, irregularly distributed duct-like structures producing an adenomatous appearance that may reach the nipple surface. There is usually prominent intraductal hyperplasia (Fig. 13.10), especially within the larger ducts, often exhibiting a micropapillary growth pattern. Sometimes, however, the growth pattern is solid and

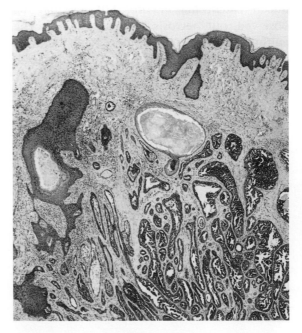

13.9 Adenoma of the nipple. There are many large and small duct-like structures exhibiting prominent hyperplasia at the bottom right of the picture. Note the two squamous-lined cysts in the centre left. At the top is the epidermis of the nipple (H&E).

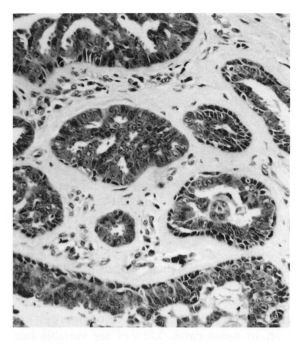

13.10 Detail of Fig. 13.9. The ducts show a varying degree of hyperplasia of usual type; in most of them the myoepithelial layer is well defined (H&E).

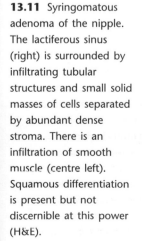

13.11 Syringomatous adenoma of the nipple. The lactiferous sinus (right) is surrounded by infiltrating tubular structures and small solid masses of cells separated by abundant dense stroma. There is an infiltration of smooth muscle (centre left). Squamous differentiation is present but not discernible at this power (H&E).

results in total luminal occlusion. The involved ducts may be greatly distended and convoluted. There is often focal necrosis of the hyperplastic epithelium, and mitoses may be found, although they are rarely numerous. The ducts without hyperplasia have a two-layered structure with columnar epithelial cells, often with apical snouts and cuboidal or flattened myoepithelial cells. Apocrine metaplasia may be present. Squamous-lined cysts are often seen in the subepidermal portion of the lesion and appear to be derived from the collecting ducts (*see* Fig. 13.9 above). Rarely the hyperplastic epithelium extends onto the surface of the nipple. The overlying squamous epithelium may be hyperplastic and is occasionally ulcerated.

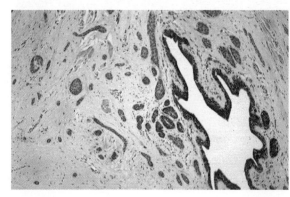

Rosen and Caicco (1986) divided their cases into three types depending on the predominant growth pattern: sclerosing papillomatosis, papillomatosis and adenosis. A mixed type was also recognized. No prognostic significance, however, could be attached to these different patterns. Follow-up data were available on 22 of the 51 cases treated by local excision. None recurred over an average period of 8.3 years. A further five cases were treated by biopsy alone, one recurring locally. Some cases are associated with carcinoma. Rosen and Caicco found 173 cases in the literature in addition to the 51 they reported themselves. Of the 224 cases there was concurrent carcinoma in 31 (14%), being within the nipple lesion in 8 (4%), in the ipsilateral breast but separate from the nipple lesion in 17 (8%) and in the contralateral breast in 6 (3%). Carcinoma subsequently developed in only 2 (1%). Paget's disease may be seen in cases in which carcinoma is present within the lesion itself. Patients with adenoma of the nipple should therefore be investigated carefully to exclude the presence of co-existent carcinoma, but there appears to be little value in long-term follow-up.

In a separate paper Rosen (1984) described five cases of a syringomatous type of nipple adenoma similar to the syringoma of skin adnexal origin. Four occurred in women aged 28–41 and one in a man aged 76. The lesions were all solitary and unilateral, being characterized on gross examination by minute cystic areas. Histologically, the tumour infiltrated among but did not replace the lactiferous ducts and lobules, although an invasion of smooth muscle bundles occurred (Fig. 13.11). Epithelial proliferation of the ducts and lobules was not seen. The tumour cells formed ductal structures, epithelial strands and foci of squamous differentiation with or without cyst formation. The intervening stroma was dense and generally plentiful. Focal calcification was noted in areas of keratinization. Follow-up data were available on four patients, one of whom experienced a gradual enlargement of the lesion over a period of 22 years after incomplete excision. The other patients remained disease-free.

Four similar syringomatous tumours arising deep in the breast were described by Suster *et al.* (1991) and are described in more detail below.

Ductal adenoma

Azzopardi and Salm (1984) first described this variety of breast adenoma, reporting 24 examples. All were from females, their age range being 26–73 years with a mean of 51. The tumours presented clinically as unilateral palpable lumps without nipple discharge, although the latter symptom has been rarely noted in other series. In over half the cases the mass consisted of multiple nodules that were three-dimensionally discontinuous and sometimes involved adjacent duct systems. The remaining lesions were solitary. The whole mass did not usually exceed 30 mm, individual nodules in the multiple cases rarely being larger than 20 mm.

Histologically, the lesions generally arise in interlobular ducts, either near the nipple or in the periphery. The ducts undergo marked distension, and the wall may in some cases be extensively destroyed by the expansile growth of the lesion. The epithelial elements comprise round or ovoid tubular structures lined by a double layer of epithelial and myoepithelial cells, with no evidence of a papillary growth pattern. Foci of solid epithelial hyperplasia may also be present.

The myoepithelial cells may be cuboidal with pale cytoplasm or flattened, and in some areas may overgrow the epithelium to produce spindle cell masses. The epithelial cells may exhibit apical snouts, and apocrine metaplasia is common although not usually prominent. In some cases the epithelial nuclei focally exhibit significant pleomorphism and hyperchromatism with inclusion-like nuclei, the significance of which is not clear (Gusterson *et al.*, 1987). Intraluminal calcospherites are seen in some cases. Mitoses are variable but usually few in number.

The fibrous stroma is usually loose but may be dense in places and usually contains elastin fibres. Myxoid change in the stroma is

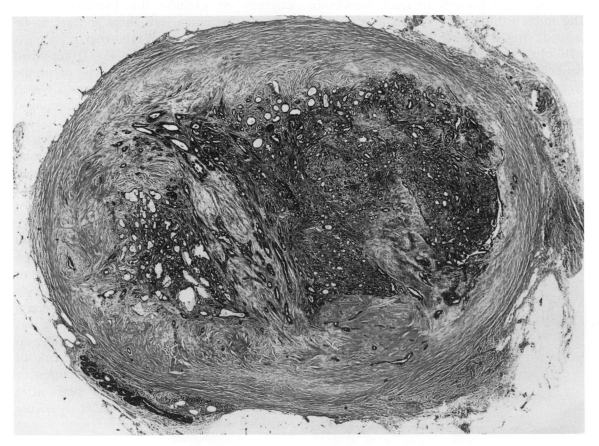

13.12 Ductal adenoma surrounded by a densely fibrous ductal wall. The fibrosis imparts an infiltrative appearance to the epithelium in many places (H&E). (Illustration reproduced with permission from the *Journal of Pathology*.)

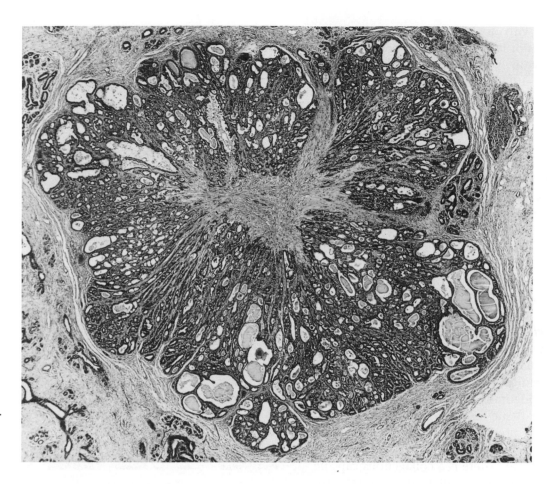

13.13 Ductal adenoma with a central scar (H&E). (Illustration reproduced with permission from the *Journal of Pathology*.)

uncommon and cartilaginous metaplasia rare (Lammie and Millis, 1989)

Two types of tumour were recognized by Azzopardi and Salm (1984). One was clearly within a duct, the wall of which was fibrosed and sometimes calcified (Fig. 13.12). There was often considerable peripheral fibrosis, sometimes entrapping epithelium to produce an infiltrative appearance like that seen in some intraduct papillomas. Sometimes there was a stellate central scar, giving a floral appearance (Fig. 13.13). The second type was not obviously confined to a ductal lumen, although the tumour margins were well delineated and smooth-contoured. The occurrence of irregular fibrosis in the presence of the cytological atypia mentioned above may give rise to a false impression of malignancy.

Azzopardi and Salm (1984) recommended the separation of the solitary and multiple types, at least provisionally, in view of the marked difference in behaviour exhibited by the solitary and multiple forms of intraduct papilloma. Ductal adenomas, however, appear to arise from ducts rather than terminal duct–lobular units and are not bilateral. Furthermore, although 2 of 24 cases exhibited co-existent *in situ* carcinoma (one ductal and one lobular in patients aged 56 and 60 years respectively), there was no evidence of any merging of the benign and malignant tissue. To the author's knowledge there have been no subsequent reports suggesting that solitary or multiple ductal adenomas are associated with an increased risk of malignancy.

Ductal adenomas are distinguished from carcinoma by their benign cytological appearances, the presence of two cell types in the tubules and often the presence of apocrine metaplasia. The distinction from intraduct papilloma is by the lack of a papillary growth pattern.

Patients with ductal adenoma usually have no previous or family history of breast disease, and follow-up is usually uneventful (Lammie and Millis, 1989).

Pleomorphic salivary type adenoma

These tumours are rare in the breast but are important as they produce hard, gritty masses easily mistaken for carcinoma on clinical, mammographic and even macroscopic pathological examination. Mastectomy has been unnecessarily performed in some cases. The lesions are well circumscribed (Fig. 13.14) and usually measure between 10 and 40 mm, although they may attain a very large dimension if untreated. Some tumours are multifocal (Moran et al., 1990). They occur in women and men, the median age being around 53 (Sheth et al., 1978; Makek and von Hochstetter, 1980). They are detected as a palpable mass, either by the patient or on routine medical examination, by mammography or incidentally in the process of examining breast tissue excised for other reasons. There is no predilection for any part of the breast (Moran et al., 1990).

Histologically, there is a collagenous capsule into which extensions of tumour epithelium may project. Satellite nodules are occasionally encountered. The epithelial cells are cytologically benign and are arranged in acini, solid islands or trabeculae (Fig. 13. 15). Glandular and ductal structures usually have a double layer of epithelial and myoepithelial cells, the latter staining for smooth muscle actin, S100 and vimentin (Moran et al., 1990). Solid masses of myoepithelial cells may be seen. The stroma is myxomatous and contains a large amount of hyaluronidase-resistant acid mucin in which there may be zones of cartilage, osteoid and bone (Fig. 13.16). Stromal elastin may be present. Oestrogen receptor positivity has been reported (Segen et al., 1986).

Difficulties may be encountered on frozen section examination. Distinction from carcinoma may be difficult, especially in the more densely cellular zones. Furthermore, the clinical and mammographic data as well as the hard, gritty macroscopic appearance may heavily influence the pathologist. The

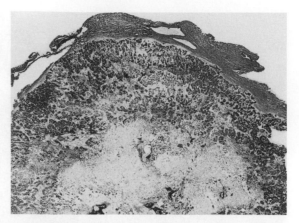

13.14 Pleomorphic adenoma. The tumour is well circumscribed and has a fibrous capsule. The periphery is cellular, but the central zone shows extensive cartilage and bone formation (H&E).

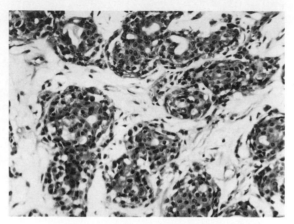

13.15 Pleomorphic adenoma. There are nests of benign epithelial and myoepithelial cells separated by myxoid stroma. Lumen formation is seen in many places (H&E).

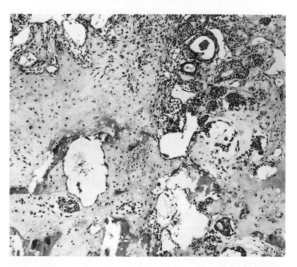

13.16 Pleomorphic adenoma. Epithelial elements are seen at the top right of the picture and contain some well-differentiated, two-layered tubules. There is extensive cartilage and bone formation in the lower part of the illustration (H&E).

tumours are sometimes so heavily calcified that frozen section examination cannot be performed.

Ultrastructural examination shows that the epithelial cells contain few organelles and exhibit normal surface microvilli and intercellular contacts. The outer myoepithelial cells contain myofilaments and are attached by hemidesmosomes to an outer basal lamina in the usual way (McClure *et al.*, 1982).

Pleomorphic adenomas may be confused with breast carcinomas containing metaplastic bone and cartilage (*see* p. 198) but can be distinguished from them by their cytologically benign features. Distinction from phyllodes tumour is by the lack of the characteristic fibroadenomatous growth pattern.

Pleomorphic adenomas behave in a benign fashion but may recur locally if excision is incomplete (Soreide *et al.*, 1988).

Lactating adenoma

This term is used to describe adenomas that are composed of dilated tubules lined by vacuolated cells identical to those seen in the pregnant or lactating breast. They usually present in pregnancy. Copious secretion may be present in the lumina, and immunostaining for the milk proteins lactoferrin and α-lactalbumin is positive. Mitoses may be frequent, and foci of necrosis are sometimes encountered that may lead to an erroneous diagnosis of malignancy. The precise appearance of the lesion will depend upon the stage of gestation. Although lactating adenomas conform to the definition of adenoma given above, it is possible that some of them are derived from pre-existing fibroadenomas, tubular adenomas or hamartomas (Slavin *et al.*, 1993) in which the epithelial proliferation obliterates the stroma as it does in the normal pregnant and lactating breast. It should be noted, however, that not all fibroadenomas show a secretory change in pregnancy (James *et al.*, 1988).

Other adenomas

Adenomas strongly resembling tumours of sweat gland origin have been reported. Hertel *et al.* (1976) reported two such lesions, one like an eccrine spiradenoma and the other a clear cell hidradenoma. An apocrine adenoma with papillary architecture was reported by Tesluk *et al.* (1986), who identified one previous case in the literature.

Suster *et al.* (1991) described four syringomatous squamous tumours occurring as a palpable mass in women 37–70 years of age. They resembled those occurring in the nipple (see above), but all the lesions were located deep in the breast, and there was no connection with the overlying skin. They formed clearly defined but non-encapsulated nodules with ill-defined, pseudo-infiltrative borders that were composed of teardrop- or comma-shaped islands of squamous epithelium separated by densely cellular stroma. The cellular islands often exhibited central lumina and were in many cases lined by eosinophilic cuticles. Cytological atypia, significant mitotic activity and necrosis were not seen. All lesions were treated by local excision, none recurring over a follow-up period of 1–6 years.

Tumours exhibiting a mixed appearance of adenoma and fibroadenoma have also been described.

PHYLLODES TUMOUR

A phyllodes tumour has the same architecture as a fibroadenoma, usually the intracanalicular type, but has the potential for local recurrence and metastasis. The essential point of distinction from fibroadenoma is the more densely cellular stroma that may or may not be cytologically malignant. Phyllodes tumour has also been called giant fibroadenoma, an unsuitable name as the two tumours are histologically different. Furthermore, although phyllodes tumours tend to be larger than fibroadenomas, they are by no means invariably so. Phyllodes tumours may occur at any age, a few cases having been reported in juveniles. The median age, however, is about 45 (Norris and Taylor, 1967), which is significantly higher than that for fibroadenoma.

Macroscopically, the tumours appear circumscribed and usually exhibit soft fleshy and hard gritty zones. Gelatinous foci may be seen. There is a large range in size: in Norris and Taylor's study of 94 cases, the size varied from 10 to 450 mm with a median of about 60 mm. Bilateral tumours are very rare.

Histologically, the degree of circumscription is variable. The edge of the tumour is usually

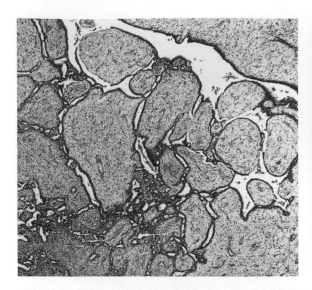

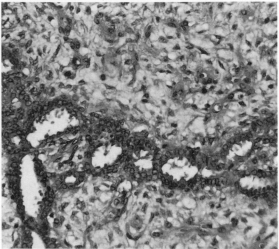

13.17 (Left) Phyllodes tumour. The growth pattern is essentially that of an intracanalicular fibroadenoma, but there are many club-like projections covered by epithelium, extending into cyst-like spaces (H&E).

13.18 (Right) Detail of Fig. 13.17. The stroma does not exhibit cytological features of malignancy but is more densely cellular than that of a fibroadenoma (H&E).

well defined, but there are often irregular, rounded surface projections that may be cut through during surgical removal; some tumours exhibit infiltrative margins. Although the growth pattern is essentially similar to that of an intracanalicular fibroadenoma, large leaf- and club-like, epithelial-lined papillary projections pushing into cystic spaces are more prominent (Fig. 13.17). Unlike fibroadenomas, phyllodes tumours are more likely to undergo haemorrhage and necrosis, and exhibit large zones of stroma devoid of epithelium.

The stroma shows a greater degree of cellularity than is seen in fibroadenomas (Fig. 13.18) and may exhibit considerable variation in appearance even within the same tumour. The distinction of fibroadenomas and phyllodes tumours thus requires extensive sampling in some cases. The cells may have the appearance of uniform, spindle-celled fibroblasts or may exhibit marked pleomorphism, nuclear hyperchromatism and mitotic activity. The stroma may thus appear benign (Fig. 13.18), borderline (Fig. 13.19) or malignant (Fig. 13.20), the corresponding tumours being classified as low, intermediate and high grade. Myxoid change is common, and some tumours exhibit hyalinized areas.

Although the stroma usually has a non-specific, spindle-celled appearance, fat, smooth muscle and even cartilage and bone associated with osteoclast-like giant cells have

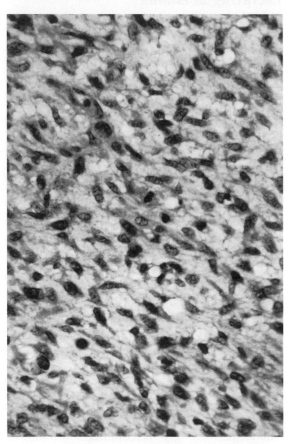

13.19 First recurrence of the tumour illustrated in Figs 13.17 and 13.18. Many areas of the tumour are devoid of epithelium, and the stroma now has the appearance of a low-grade fibrosarcoma. Mitoses and nuclear hyperchromasia are present, and the stroma is more cellular (H&E).

been reported (Norris and Taylor, 1967; Smith and Taylor, 1969). Tumours with liposarcomatous (Fig. 13.21) and malignant fibrous histiocytoma-like areas have also been described (Jimenez et al., 1986; Mentzel et al., 1991). Graadt van Roggen et al. (1998)

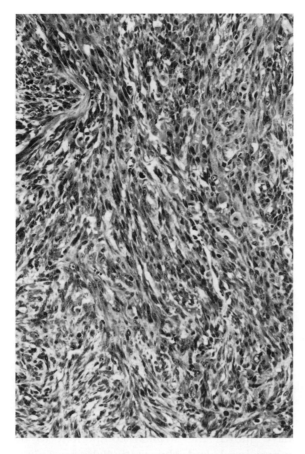

13.20 Second recurrence of the tumour illustrated in Figs 13.17–13.19. Hardly any epithelium was identified, and the stroma now has the appearance of a high-grade spindle-cell sarcoma (H&E).

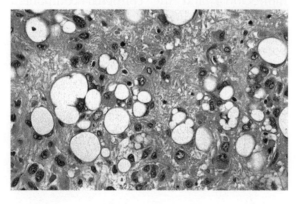

13.21 Phyllodes tumour with liposarcomatous stroma. A very large lipoblast is seen at the left/centre of the illustration (H&E).

reported a case with widespread differentiation towards telangiectatic osteosarcoma.

The epithelium is usually similar to that seen in the normal breast, although there may be zones of hyperplasia, which is sometimes atypical. Benign changes, such as cysts, apocrine metaplasia and sclerosing adenosis, seen not infrequently in fibroadenomas, are rare in phyllodes tumours. Squamous metaplasia, on the other hand, is more common.

There are occasional cases on record of co-existent carcinoma that may be confined to the phyllodes tumour itself. Norris and Taylor found infiltrating carcinoma in 2 of 94 cases. As with fibroadenomas there appears to be a disproportionately high incidence of lobular carcinomas (Rosen and Urban, 1975). Carcinomatous change in a phyllodes tumour is one possible mode of origin of a carcinosarcoma of the breast.

Norris and Taylor (1967) studied 94 patients with phyllodes tumour in an attempt to identify any pathological features related to clinical behaviour. Recurrence occurred in 28 patients, 15 of whom died of metastatic disease. Most recurrences occurred within 2 years and most deaths within 6. These authors found that a small size (less than 40 mm), a low mitotic rate (fewer than three mitotic figures per 10 high-power fields), pushing rather than infiltrative margins and minimal cytologic atypia were associated with a low risk of recurrence. No feature was wholly reliable, and a clear-cut separation of benign from malignant tumours could not be made.

Other workers have found necrosis (Cohn-Cedermark et al., 1991), stromal overgrowth (Kario et al., 1990; Hawkins et al., 1992; Moffat et al., 1995), mitotic activity (Kario et al., 1990; Hawkins et al., 1992), nuclear pleomorphism (Kario et al., 1990; Hawkins et al., 1992) and infiltrative margins (Hawkins et al., 1992) to be related to the probability of recurrence or death. In contrast, Keelan et al. (1992) found that histological evaluation provided no reliable clue to the natural history of an individual tumour.

There are several possible reasons for this lack of agreement. First, histological recognition of many of the putative prognostic features is especially subjective and consequently subject to lack of consistency; Oberman (1965), for example, found considerable variation in the relative proportion of histologically benign and malignant tumours in various published series, which reflected difficulties of classification. Second, the relatively small number and diverse nature of the clinical events (local recurrence, development of metastases and death) in different studies makes them difficult to compare and usually gives rise to a lack of statistical significance in any one series. Finally, the lesions may not be treated in a uniform way; in particular, those with more aggressive histological features may be more widely excised.

Moffat *et al.* (1995) reported 32 cases of phyllodes tumour and concluded that the presence of tumour at the margins of the excised specimen is the most important determinant of local recurrence and that the histological features are of secondary importance. They also reviewed data from 1612 previously reported cases. They drew several major conclusions:

1. Most phyllodes are histologically benign.
2. Benign and borderline cases recur locally in a high proportion of cases if initial surgical excision is incomplete.
3. Benign tumours rarely metastasize, and recurrence can usually be controlled by further surgery.
4. Histologically malignant phyllodes tumours may give rise to haematogenous metastases in up to 22% of cases.
5. More extensive initial surgery may reduce the risk of local recurrence in these cases but has not been shown to be effective in preventing metastatic spread.
6. Complete excision of the lesion with a minimum margin of 10 mm of surrounding breast appears to be the key to effective treatment.

If there is difficulty in deciding whether a lesion is a phyllodes tumour or a cellular fibroadenoma, it is best to err on the side of safety and ensure that it is excised with an adequate margin.

Phyllodes tumours metastasize largely by the haematogenous route, mostly to the lungs, pleurae and bone; axillary lymph nodes are rarely involved. Locally recurrent lesions may resemble the original tumour or exhibit a reduced epithelial component or a cytologically more malignant stroma (*see* Figs. 13.18–13.20 above). Distant metastases contain only the stromal component.

Increased immunoreactivity for p53 has been found in most high-grade phyllodes tumours but not in low-grade variants or fibroadenomas (Millar *et al.*, 1999). Feakins *et al.* (1999) found that p53 immunopositivity was associated high tumour grade, stromal overgrowth, nuclear pleomorphism, mitotic rate and infiltrative tumour margin but, rather surprisingly, did not predict tumour recurrence or patient survival.

X chromosome inactivation studies on DNA amplified by the polymerase chain reaction from small fragments of phyllodes tumours have shown the stromal component to be monoclonal and the epithelial component polyclonal. This is in contrast to fibroadenomas, in which both components are polyclonal (Noguchi *et al.*, 1993). The monoclonal nature of the phyllodes tumours has also been shown by cytogenetic analysis in which chromosomal changes, including t(6;12)–(q23;q13) and t(10;16)–(q22;p11), have been described (Birdsall *et al.*, 1992).

REFERENCES

Azzopardi J.G., Salm R. (1984) Ductal adenoma of the breast: a lesion which can mimic carcinoma. *J. Pathol.*, **144**, 15–23.

Bailey A.J., Sloane J.P., Trickey B.S., Ormerod M.G. (1982) An immunocytochemical study of a-lactalbumin in human breast tissue. *J. Pathol.*, **137**, 13–23.

Bartow S.A., Pathak D.R., Black W.C., Key C.R., Teaf S.R. (1987) Prevalence of benign, atypical, and malignant lesions in populations at different risk for breast cancer. *Cancer*, **60**, 2751–60.

Berean K., Tron V.A., Churg A., Clement P.B. (1986) Mammary fibroadenoma with multinucleated stromal giant cells. *Am. J. Surg. Oncol.*, **10**, 823–37.

Birdsall S.H., MacLennan K.A., Gusterson B.A. (1992) t(6;12)(q23;q13) and t(10;16)(q22;p11) in a phyllodes tumour of the breast. *Cancer Genet. Cytogenet.*, **60**, 74–7.

Bittesini L., Dei Tos A.P., Doglioni C., Della Libera D., Laurino L., Fletcher C.D.M. (1994) Fibroepithelial tumour of the breast with digital fibroma-like inclusions in the stromal component. *Am. J. Surg. Pathol.*, **18**, 296–301.

Buzanowski-Konakry K., Harrison E.G., Payne W.S. (1975) Lobular carcinoma arising in fibroadenoma of the breast. *Cancer*, **35**, 450–6.

Carter C.L., Corle D.K., Micozzi M.S., Schatzkin A., Taylor P.R. (1988) A prospective study of the development of breast cancer in 16,692 women with benign breast disease. *Am. J. Epidemiol.*, **128**, 467–77.

Cheatle G.L. (1923) Hyperplasia of epithelial and connective tissues in the breast: its relation to fibro-adenoma and other pathological conditions. *Br. Surg.*, **10**, 436–55.

Cohn-Cedermark G., Rutqvist L.E., Rosendahl I, Silfversward C. (1991) Prognostic factors in cytosar-coma phyllodes: a clinicopathologic study of 77 patients. *Cancer*, **68**, 2017–22.

Diaz N.M., Palmer J.O., McDivitt R.W. (1991) Carcinoma arising within fibroadenomas of the breast. A clinicopathologic study of 105 patients. *Am. J. Clin. Pathol.*, **95** (5), 614-22.

Dupont W.D., Page D.L., Parl F.F. *et al.* (1994) Long-term risk of breast cancer in women with fibroade-noma. *N. Engl. J. Med.*, **331**, 10–15.

Eusebi V., Azzopardi J.G. (1980) Lobular endocrine neoplasia in fibroadenoma of the breast. *Histopathology*, **4**, 413–28.

Feakins R.M., Mulcahy H.E., Nickols C.D., Wells C.A. (1999) p53 expression in phyllodes tumours is associated with histological features of malignancy but does not predict outcome. *Histopathology*, **35**, 162–9.

Fisher E.R. (1976) Ultrastructure of the human breast and its disorders. *Am. J. Clin. Pathol.*, **66**, 291–375.

Frantz V.K., Pickren J.W., Melcher G.W., Auchincloss H. (1951) Incidence of chronic disease in so-called 'normal breasts'; a study based on 225 post mortem examinations. *Cancer*, **4**, 762–83.

Geschickter C.F., Lewis D. (1938) Pregnancy and lacta-tion changes in fibro-adenoma of the breast. *Br. Med. J.*, **1**, 499–504.

Goodman Z.D., Taxy J.B. (1981) Fibroadenomas of the breast with prominent smooth muscle. *Am. J. Surg. Pathol.*, **5**, 99–100.

Graadt van Roggen J.F., Zonderland H.M., Welvaart K., Peterse J.L., Hogendoorn P.C.W. (1998) Local recur-rence of a phyllodes tumour of the breast presenting with widespread differentiation to a telagiectatic osteosarcoma. *J. Clin. Pathol.*, **51**, 706–8.

Gusterson B.A., Sloane J.P., Middwood C., *et al.* (1987) Ductal adenoma of the breast – a lesion exhibiting a myoepithelial/epithelial phenotype. *Histopathology*, **11**, 103–10.

Hawkins R.E., Schofield J.B., Fisher C., Wiltshaw E, McKinna A.J. (1992) The clinical and histologic crite-ria that predict metastases from cytosarcoma phyllodes. *Cancer*, **69** (1), 141–7.

Hertel B.F., Zaloudek C., Kempson R.L. (1976) Breast adenomas. *Cancer*, **37**, 2891–905.

James K., Bridger J., Anthony P. (1988) Breast tumour of pregnancy (lactating adenoma). *J. Pathol.*, **156**, 37–44.

Jao W., Vazquez L.T., Keh P.C., Gould V.E. (1978) Myoepithelial differentiation and basal lamina deposition in fibroadenoma and adenosis of the breast. *J. Pathol.*, **126**, 107–12.

Jimenez J.F., Gloster E.S., Perrot L.J., Mollitt D.L., Gollady E.S. (1986) Liposarcoma arising within a cystosarcoma phyllodes. *J. Surg. Oncol.*, **31**, 294–8.

Kario K., Maeda S., Mizuno Y., Makino Y., Tankawa H., Kitazawa S. (1990) Phyllodes tumor of the breast: a clinicopathologic study of 34 cases. *J. Surg. Oncol.*, **45**, 46–51.

Keelan P.A., Myers J.L., Wold L.E., Katzmann J.A., Gibney D.J. (1992) Phyllodes tumor: clinicopatho-logic review of 60 patients and flow cytometric analysis in 30 patients. *Hum. Pathol.*, **23**, 1048–54.

Lammie G.A., Millis R.R. (1989) Ductal adenoma of the breast – a review of fifteen cases. *Hum. Pathol.*, **20**, 903–8.

LeGal Y. (1961) Adenomas of the breast: relationship of adenofibroma to pregnancy and lactation. *Am. J. Surg.*, **27**, 14–22.

Majmudar B., Rosales-Quintana S. (1975) Infarction of breast fibroadenomas during pregnancy. *J. Am. Med. Assoc.*, **231**, 963–4.

Makek M., von Hochstetter A.R. (1980) Pleomorphic adenoma of the human breast. *J. Surg. Oncol.*, **4**, 281–6.

McClure J., Smith P.S., Jamieson G.G. (1982) 'Mixed' salivary type adenoma of the human female breast. *Arch. Pathol. Lab. Med.*, **106**, 615–19.

McDivitt R.W., Hutter R.V.P., Foote F.W., Stewart F.W. (1967) *In situ* lobular carcinoma: a prospective follow-up study indicating cumulative patient risks. *J. Am. Med. Assoc.*, **201**, 82–6.

McDivitt R.W., Stevens J.A., Lee N.C., Wingo P.A., Rubin G.L., Gersell D. (1992) Histologic types of benign breast disease and the risk for breast cancer. *Cancer*, **69**, 1408–14.

Mentzel T., Kosmehl H, Katenkamp D. (1991) Metastasising phyllodes tumour with malignant fibrous histiocytoma-like areas. *Histopathology*, **19**; 557–60.

Mies C., Rosen P.P. (1987) Juvenile fibroadenoma with atypical epithelial hyperplasia. *Am. J. Surg. Pathol.*, **11** (3), 184–90.

Millar E.K.A., Beretov J., Marr P. *et al.* (1999) Malignant phyllodes tumours of the breast display increased stromal p53 expression. *Histopathology*, **34**, 491–6.

Moffat C.J.C., Pinder S.E., Dixon A.R., Elston C.W., Blamey R.W., Ellis I.O. (1995) Phyllodes tumours of the breast: a clinicopathological review of thirty-two cases. *Histopathology*, **27**, 205–18.

Moran C.A., Suster S., Carter D. (1990) Benign mixed tumors (pleomorphic adenomas) of the breast. *Am. J. Surg. Pathol.*, **14** (10), 913–21.

Noguchi S., Motomura K., Inaji H., Imaoka S., Koyama H. (1993) Clonal analysis of fibroadenoma and phyllodes tumor of the breast. *Cancer Res.*, **53**; 4071–4.

Norris H.J., Taylor H.B. (1967) Relationship of histologic features to behavior of cystosarcoma phyllodes: analysis of ninety-four cases. *Cancer*, **20**, 2090–9.

Oberman H.A. (1965) Sarcomas of the breast. *Cancer*, **18**, 1233–43.

Ozzello L., Gump F.E. (1985) The management of patients with carcinomas in fibroadenomatous tumors of the breast. *Surg. Gynecol. Obstet.*, **160**, 99–104.

Pike A.M., Oberman H.A. (1985) Juvenile (cellular) adenofibromas – a clinicopathologic study. *Am. J. Surg. Pathol.*, **9 (10)**, 730–6.

Reid T., Just K.E., Holtgreve-Grez H. *et al.* (1995) Comparative genomic hybridisation of formalin-fixed, paraffin-embedded breast tumors reveals different patterns of chromosomal gains and losses in fibroadenomas and diploid and aneuploid carcinomas. *Cancer Res.*, **55**, 5415–23.

Rosen P.P., Caicco J.A. (1986) Florid papillomatosis of the nipple – a study of 51 patients, including nine with mammary carcinoma. *Am. J. Surg. Pathol.*, **10 (2)**, 87–101.

Rosen P.P., Urban J.A. (1975) Coexistent mammary carcinoma and cystosarcoma phyllodes. *Breast*, **1**, 9–15.

Rosen P.P. (1984) Syringomatous adenoma of the nipple. *Am. J. Surg. Pathol.*, **7**, 739–45.

Segen J.C., Foo M., Richer S. (1986) Pleomorphic adenoma of the breast with positive estrogen receptors. *N.Y. State J. Med.*, **86**; 265–6.

Sheth M.T., Hathway D., Petrelli M. (1978) Pleomorphic adenoma ('mixed' tumor) of human female breast mimicking carcinoma clinico-radiologically. *Cancer*, **41**, 659–65.

Silverman J.S, Tamsen A. (1996) Mammary fibroadenoma and some phyllodes tumour stroma are composed of CD34+ fibroblasts and factor XIIIa+ dendrophages. *Histopathology*, **29**, 411–19.

Slavin J.L., Billson V.R., Ostor A.G. (1993) Nodular breast lesions during pregnancy and lactation. *Histopathology*, **22**, 481–5.

Smith B.H., Taylor H.B. (1969) The occurrence of bone and cartilage in mammary tumours. *Am. J. Clin. Pathol.*, **51**, 610–18.

Soreide J.A., Oddvar A., Eriksen L., Holter J., Kjellevold K.H. (1988) Pleomorphic adenoma of the human breast with local recurrence. *Cancer*, **61**; 997–1001.

Suster S., Moran C.A., Hurt M.A. (1991) Syringomatous squamous tumors of the breast. *Cancer*, **67**; 2350–5.

Taylor H.B., Robertson A.G. (1965) Adenomas of the nipple. *Cancer*, **18**, 995–1002.

Tesluk H., Amott T., Goodnight J.E. (1986) Apocrine adenoma of the breast. *Arch. Pathol. Lab. Med.*, **110**, 351–2.

Willis R.A. (1967) *The Pathology of Tumours*, 4th edn. London, Butterworths.

14 Miscellaneous tumours

BENIGN MESENCHYMAL TUMOURS

Vascular tumours

Perilobular haemangiomas

These are small lesions usually discovered as an incidental finding in mastectomy specimens or benign breast biopsies; they are occasionally multiple. They are usually not detected on macroscopic inspection. Histologically, they consist of a meshwork of delicate, small, thin-walled, dilated blood-containing vascular channels with no significant muscle coat. The connective tissue is similar to that of the surrounding breast. Perilobular haemangioma is not an entirely satisfactory term as only some of the lesions are mingled with lobules, the remainder occuring in the extralobular stroma. The size usually varies between about 10 and 35 mm (Rosen and Ridolfi, 1977).

There is no known association between perilobular haemangioma and angiosarcoma, but care should be taken on histological examination as angiosarcomas of microscopic size have been reported (Donnell *et al.*, 1981; see below). A freely anastomosing growth pattern, nuclear hyperchromatism, tufting of the endothelial cells and solid zones of spindle cells are features that should arouse suspicion.

Cavernous haemangiomas

These may occur in the breast and resemble those seen in other parts of the body. Unlike perilobular haemangiomas, they usually present as a palpable mass. Occasional angiomatous lesions composed of dilated channels surrounded by prominent smooth muscle have also been reported (Donnell *et al.*, 1981). As with all other angiomas, care should be taken to exclude malignancy, as angiosarcomas may appear deceptively benign.

Juvenile haemangioendothelioma

This has been reported in the breast and may present diagnostic problems, as it does elsewhere (Donnell *et al.*, 1981). The lesion may exhibit dense cellularity with solid areas and even a moderate number of mitotic figures. The freely anastomosing growth pattern is lacking, however, and the endothelial cells do not exhibit nuclear hyperchromatism or tufting. The age of the patient is an important consideration.

Atypical haemangioma

Hoda *et al.* (1992) reported a series of 18 haemangiomas with atypical features. All patients were females between 18 and 82 years old (mean 60). Seven lesions presented as a mass, the rest being impalpable and detected by mammography. All were 20 mm or less in

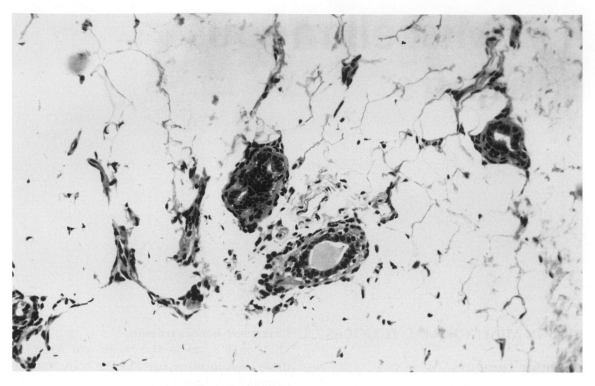

14.1 Adenolipoma. Clusters of normal-appearing epithelial structures occur in what is otherwise a straightforward lipoma (H&E).

size and unilateral. Fibrous septa often divided the lesions into segments or lobules, and a patchy infiltrate of mast cells was invariably found in the stroma. The lesions were regarded as atypical as all exhibited microscopic fields that, if viewed alone, would be suggestive of angiosarcoma.

There were four growth patterns: cavernous, compact capillary, capillary budding and combined cavernous and compact capillary.

1. *Cavernous* lesions were regarded as atypical if they exhibited focal endothelial hyperplasia, anastomosing vascular channels or invasive margins.
2. *Compact capillary* lesions comprised ill-defined lobules and invariably exhibited anastomosing channels.
3. The *capillary budding* lesions were all poorly circumscribed, exhibiting peripheral capillary offshoots bearing a superficial resemblance to Kaposi's sarcoma as a result of pronounced spindle cell proliferation. The centres of the lesions exhibited papillary endothelial hyperplasia with atypia. All were 10 mm or less and detected by mammography.
4. *Combined* tumours were the least frequent, the two patterns being separate but adjacent to each other.

None of the tumours showed solid neoplastic areas, blood lakes or haemorrhage, destructive invasion, necrosis (except in cases which had been needled) or microcalcification. Furthermore, the small size argued against angiosarcoma. Nine patients had no treatment after the initial biopsy, seven had a local re-excision and two underwent mastectomy. None had radio- or chemotherapy, and none developed a recurrence after a follow-up period averaging 44 months.

Lipoma and variants

Given the large amount of fat in the normal female breast, it is not surprising that lipomas are relatively common. They exhibit the same appearances and behaviour as in other parts of the body. *Angiolipomas* may also be encountered but are much less common. They are encapsulated and composed of a mixture of mature, adult-type adipose tissue and a fine meshwork of capillary vessels that may or may not contain erythrocytes. Small, ovoid

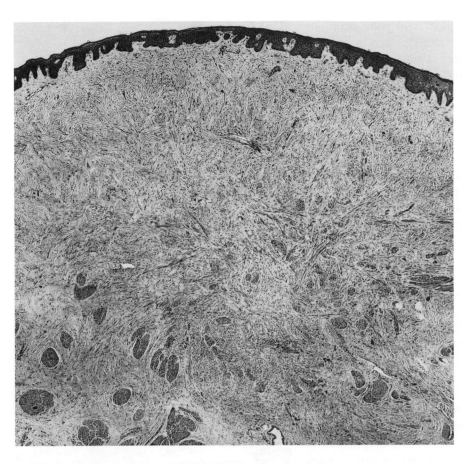

14.2 Leiomyoma arising from the smooth muscle bundles of the areola (H&E).

endothelial cells line the vascular channels. These tumours are distinguished from well-differentiated angiosarcomas invading fat by the absence of mitotic activity, nuclear atypia and tufting of the endothelial cells.

Lipomas containing epithelial structures have been termed *adenolipomas* (Haagensen, 1971) (Fig. 14.1). However, the epithelial elements resemble normal lobules, and it is unlikely that they are neoplastic, representing instead normal epithelium incorporated into the tumour. Marsh *et al*. (1989) reported a case of *chondrolipoma* composed of benign adipose tissue and lobules of mature cartilage. The tumour was well circumscribed and detected by mammography.

Leiomyoma

Leiomyomas of the breast are uncommon. They usually arise from the smooth muscle of the nipple and areola (Fig. 14.2), where they are generally small, non-encapsulated and quite often painful. They may recur if not completely excised, sometimes after a long interval (Nascimento *et al*., 1979). They are occasionally found deep in the breast or in the skin away from the nipple, where they tend to form well-circumscribed masses of very variable size.

Smooth muscle may also occur in breast hamartomas (see below), fibroadenomas and phyllodes tumours.

Neurilemmoma

There are in the literature occasional cases of neurilemmoma of the breast. These may be confused with carcinoma clinically in view of their hard consistency and tendency to cause skin retraction. The lesions may be solitary or associated with von Recklinghausen's disease (Krishnan and Krishnan, 1982).

Granular cell tumour

About 6% of granular cell tumours occur in the breast or overlying skin (Umansky and Bullock, 1968). The tumour appears to be more common in Negroes and may occur in males or females. The average age is around 35–40 years (Mulcare, 1968). The size is variable, most reported cases being between 10 and 60 mm. Macroscopically, they are well circumscribed or infiltrative and may exhibit a firm, gritty cut surface. There may thus be a strong resemblance to carcinoma on gross examination.

Histologically, the appearance is identical to those seen in other parts of the body, with clusters of cells surrounded by stroma that is usually fairly scanty and cellular but may be more abundant and fibrous. Nerve fibres may be present within the tumour, giving the impression of perineural infiltration. The low-power appearance may thus resemble that of an infiltrative ductal carcinoma (Fig. 14.3). At higher power, the cells exhibit the characteristic cytological appearance, with small hyperchromatic nuclei and abundant granular eosinophilic cytoplasm (Fig. 14.4).

Although the diagnosis is usually clear at this stage, confusion may still arise with some of the rare forms of breast carcinoma, such as the histiocytoid variant. Misdiagnosis is obviously most likely to occur on frozen sections, especially if they are not of good quality. The literature contains several cases of granular cell myoblastoma that have been mistaken for carcinoma and for which unnecessary mastectomy has been performed. Pseudoepitheliomatous hyperplasia may be seen where tumours extend close to the overlying skin, and this may be a useful diagnostic feature. As in other sites a few granular cell tumours exhibit malignant behaviour.

Myofibroblastoma

As this tumour occurs more frequently in the male breast, it is discussed on p. 292.

Hamartoma

The occasional presence of mixed mesenchymal tissues has already been described in a number of breast lesions, for example fibroadenoma, phyllodes tumours, intraduct papilloma, pleomorphic adenoma of salivary type, infiltrating carcinoma and malignant

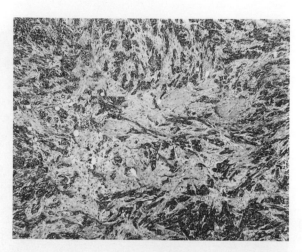

14.3 Granular cell tumour. There are irregular nests of cells surrounded by fibrous stroma, which is dense in the centre of the field (H&E).

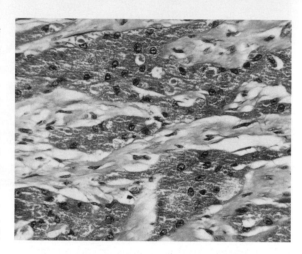

14.4 Higher-power view of Fig. 14.3. Note the small, uniform, darkly staining nuclei and the copious granular cytoplasm (H&E).

mixed mesenchymoma. There are in addition a few benign breast tumours that contain epithelium and a mixture of mesenchymal tissues but lack the growth pattern of a fibroadenoma or an intraduct papilloma.

Hamartomas are strictly malformations in which the normal components of an organ are present in an abnormal proportion or exhibit a disorderly arrangement or imperfect differentiation. Most breast hamartomas are thus composed of benign epithelium, fibrous tissue and fat and may resemble normal breast tissue so closely that they may be impossible to recognize by histological examination alone (Fig. 14.5a).

They are, however, readily identifiable macroscopically, forming well circumscribed

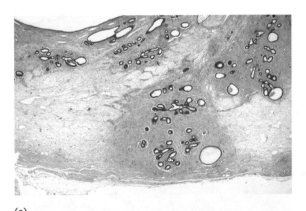

(a)

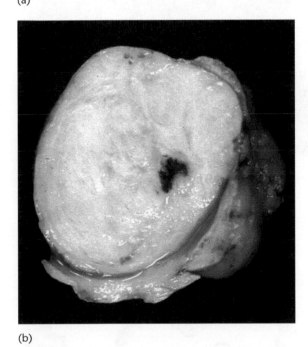

(b)

14.5 (a) Hamartoma. The epithelial and stromal elements are present in normal proportions, and the cytological and architectural features are normal apart from a minor degree of cystic change. The edge of the lesion is at the bottom of the illustration and is sharply delineated. Otherwise there are no histological clues to suggest that this section was taken from a tumour (H&E). (b) Macroscopic appearance of the same lesion, showing a well-circumscribed tumour that measured 50 mm in diameter.

but non-encapsulated, solitary rounded tumours (Fig. 14.5b). Most are palpable and visible on radiological examination provided the radiological density of the breast is not too great. The age at which they are discovered varies from adolescence to old age, the size range generally being 10–100 mm, although they may occasionally achieve a huge proportion: Linnell *et al.* (1979) reported one tumour weighing 1400 g.

Histologically, the relative proportion of epithelium, fat and fibrous tissues varies. The epithelium is generally normal but may show cystic change (*see* Fig. 14.5a), apocrine metaplasia and, rarely, ductal hyperplasia (Fisher *et al.*, 1992). Some tumours may

exhibit a gynaecomastia-like appearance with imperfect lobule formation (Oberman, 1989). The fibrous stroma may be slight but is always present around epithelial structures, in contrast to adenolipomas, in which the epithelial elements come into direct contact with the adipose tissue. In other cases the stroma may be dense and extensive, obliterating the normal intralobular stroma and forming concentric bands around the acini. Stromal proliferation does not, however, result in a distortion of epithelial structures as in fibroadenomas. Some cases have exhibited pseudoangiomatous hyperplasia of the stroma (Fisher *et al.*, 1992).

In addition to fibroadipose tissue the stroma may occasionally contain a variable amount of smooth muscle, in the form of either bundles or irregularly distributed fibres (Davies and Riddell, 1973; Oberman, 1989; Fisher *et al.*, 1992). Foci of mature cartilage have rarely been reported (Oberman, 1989). Strictly speaking, such tumours should not be regarded as hamartomas as cartilage is not a normal component of the breast, but they are identical to hamartomas in all other respects, and it is likely that the cartilage is metaplastic as in occasional fibroadenomas and papillomas.

The expression of steroid receptors was studied by Fisher *et al.* Using an immunohistological technique, they found staining for oestrogen and progesterone receptors in a variable number of epithelial cells, the latter giving the greater intensity and cell number.

Dworak *et al.* (1994) reported a case of hamartoma arising in an ectopic breast in the inguinal region.

MALIGNANT MESENCHYMAL TUMOURS

Angiosarcoma

Although the breast is a relatively favoured site for angiosarcoma, it is nevertheless a rare tumour, accounting for fewer than 10% of breast sarcomas. All but one of the 87 cases in the literature reviewed by Chen *et al.* (1980) occurred in females. Although there is a very wide age range from adolescence to old age, more than half the cases occur in the third

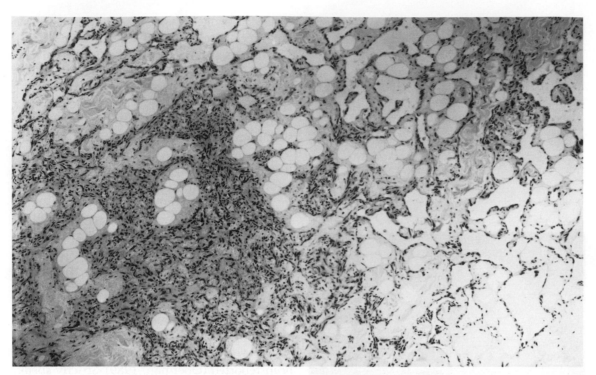

14.6 Angiosarcoma infiltrating breast adipose tissue. On the right the tumour consists of dilated vascular channels lined by hyperchromatic endothelial cells exhibiting intraluminal tufting. On the left there is a more solid zone of spindle cells (H&E).

and fourth decades, the mean age being about 35 years. This, together with a relatively frequent onset in pregnancy, has led to a suggestion of hormone dependency. Most cases arise spontaneously, but their origin in irradiated breasts and mastectomy scars has also been reported (Hamels *et al.* 1981; Givens *et al.*, 1989; Badwe *et al.*, 1991). Angiosarcomas may also occur in the lymphoedematous arm following treatment for breast carcinoma (Stewart–Treves syndrome).

The tumour may give rise to a discrete lump or produce a more diffuse enlargement of the breast. About one third of patients exhibit discoloration of the skin. The lesions are rarely painful or pulsatile. There is considerable variation in size: in the 40 cases reported by Donnell *et al.* (1981), the size varied from 20 to 110 mm, with a mean of 53 mm. Macroscopically, the tumours may appear as blood-filled spaces or simply as diffuse, ill-defined zones of induration. There is usually an extension beyond the macroscopic limits of the neoplasm.

The histological appearances are similar to those of angiosarcomas elsewhere in the body. Donnell *et al.* and later Rosen *et al.* (1988)

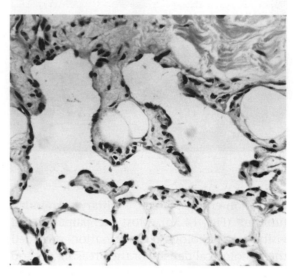

14.7 Detail of Fig. 14.6 showing hyperchromasia of endothelial cell nuclei and intraluminal papillary tufting. Note the infiltration of adipose tissue (bottom) (H&E).

divided breast angiosarcomas into three histological groups, each with a different prognostic significance. Features common to all groups were infiltration of the breast parenchyma by freely anastomosing vascular channels lined by endothelial cells exhibiting hyperchromatic nuclei and intraluminal tufting (Figs 14.6 and 14.7).

Type I tumours were composed entirely of well-formed anastomosing vascular channels invading the mammary fat and glandular parenchyma. The nuclei of the endothelial cells were hyperchromatic but tended to be flat with little or no papillary endothelial proliferation. Type II lesions largely resembled those of type I but also exhibited scattered microscopic foci of more solid neoplastic growth with papillary and/or solid components. The type III lesions exhibited prominent overtly malignant areas consisting of spindle cell sarcoma or papillary and solid endothelial patterns. Focal necrosis, haemorrhage and infarction were also present. Mitoses were rare or absent in group I, present only in the papillary areas of group II and numerous in group III. The estimated probability of 5-year disease-free survival was 76% for type I, 70% for type II and 15% for type III. The median length of disease-free survival was 15 years, 12 years and 15 months respectively.

Donnell et al. (1981) also reported four vascular tumours of microscopic size that had been discovered incidentally in breast biopsies exhibiting benign changes. These tumours showed a compact arrangement of vessels lined by endothelial cells exhibiting nuclear hyperchromasia. Although they fulfilled the histological criteria for angiosarcoma, the authors were reluctant to include them in their main series in view of their microscopic size. Three patients had mastectomies and one a local excision; all survived, but more information on this well-differentiated microscopic variant is needed. Small size is a favourable prognostic sign in the ordinary macroscopic lesions: none of Donnell et al.'s patients with a tumour less than 30 mm died.

The cells of angiosarcomas may exhibit both tight junctions and desmosomes on electron microscopy, and the cytoplasm usually contains pinocytotic vesicles. Foci of haemopoiesis have occasionally been reported (Stout, 1943).

Angiosarcomas should be completely excised, mastectomy usually being necessary. Radiotherapy appears to have little effect. Metastases may develop in the lungs, skin and subcutis, bone, liver, brain and ovary but only very rarely in the regional lymph nodes.

The histological diagnosis of angiosarcoma may prove difficult. Many tumours exhibit a deceptively benign appearance and may be mistaken for benign vascular lesions (see above). Of the cases reviewed by Chen et al. (1980), 37% were not initially recognized as malignant, this almost certainly contributing to the very poor survival figures in this series. Many lesions have a very variable appearance, with highly malignant-appearing and well-differentiated zones, the latter more often on the periphery. Adequate sampling is therefore essential. Poorly differentiated tumours may be difficult to distinguish from other sarcomas, spindle-cell carcinomas and melanoma. Immunohistological stains for endothelial markers may be very useful in these cases (see Chapter 3).

Haemangiopericytoma

Very few haemangiopericytomas have been reported in the breast, generally in adults but occasionally in children. Jiminez-Ayala et al. (1991) reported a case in a male. As in other sites most are benign, but a few are malignant. Although histological features do not always predict biological behaviour, malignant variants usually exhibit frequent mitoses, cellular pleomorphism, haemorrhage and necrosis. Arias-Stella and Rosen (1988) described five patients, all women aged between 47 and 57 years. Tumour size varied from 32 to 190 mm, with a mean of 90 mm. Three were treated by mastectomy and two by local excision, all remaining disease-free after 3–144 months of follow-up.

Eight previously reported cases were also reviewed. Patient age ranged from 33 to 67 years and tumour size from 10 to 290 mm. Three patients were treated by mastectomy and five by local excision. All remained disease-free after a follow-up period ranging from 16 to 276 months (mean 84 months). The authors concluded that haemangiopericytoma is a low-grade form of breast sarcoma regardless of size. They recommended that initial treatment should be complete local excision with breast conservation except in very large tumours, for which mastectomy is needed. Complete local excision is usually adequate.

As in other sites the crucial point of distinction from angiosarcoma is that the small, ovoid cells that comprise the tumour are situated around the vascular channels, which are lined by normal endothelial cells. The neoplastic cells show immunopositivity for actin and vimentin and negativity for factor VIII rag, desmin and myoglobin. On ultrastructural examination they exhibit elongated interdigitating cytoplasmic processes, pinocytotic vesicles, diffusely dispersed fine filaments and sparse intracellular organelles. The cells are surrounded by interrupted basal lamina. Features of smooth muscle differentiation are lacking (Mittal *et al.*, 1986).

Other sarcomas of the breast

Sarcomas other than angiosarcomas account for fewer than 1% of all primary malignant mammary tumours and usually occur in older women. Although some may develop from phyllodes tumours, most appear to arise *de novo*. Pain and skin retraction are not uncommon clinical features, in addition to the presence of a mass. Regional lymph node metastasis is uncommon, and spread is usually to the lungs and bones.

Macroscopically, they are not infrequently large, often showing areas of haemorrhage, necrosis and cyst formation

In a series of breast sarcomas reported by Norris and Taylor (1968) (which excluded angiosarcoma and malignant lymphoma), all 32 cases were essentially spindle-cell sarcomas of varying atypia but some showed metaplasia towards various specific mesenchymal elements. Thus 11 were partly myxoid, 5 contained osteoid and cartilage, 1 bone, 1 striated muscle, 1 smooth muscle and 3 liposarcomatous areas. One tumour was regarded as a dermatofibrosarcoma protuberans but arose deep within the breast rather than from the overlying skin. Although prognosis was difficult to predict, Norris and Taylor found that pushing margins and minimal atypia were associated with a low risk of recurrence or death. There was no strong association between prognosis and mitotic activity, but any tumour with more than five mitoses per 10 high-power fields appeared capable of metastasizing. Of the 32 tumours, 12 recurred, all within 14 months, and 8 patients died, all within 5 years.

Although the specific mesenchymal elements in Norris and Taylor's series seem to form minor components in otherwise undifferentiated spindle-cell tumours, there are other reported cases of pure sarcomas of specific histogenesis identical to those seen in other parts of the body. Most are composed of tissues normally present in the breast, but others such as *chondrosarcoma* (Beltaos and Banerjee, 1979), *osteogenic sarcoma* (Jernstrom *et al*, 1963) and *rhabdomyosarcoma* (Oberman, 1965), may be composed of heterologous elements. In the last of these it is important to ensure that the tumour has not arisen from the pectoral muscle. Oberman (1965) reported a case of *malignant mesenchymoma* composed of spindle cells, stellate cells and myxoid zones as well as foci of osteoid, bone, cartilage and neoplastic adipose tissue. Pollard *et al.* (1990) included single cases of *clear cell sarcoma*, *neurogenic sarcoma* and *alveolar soft part sarcoma* in their series of 25 cases.

Fibrosarcoma/malignant fibrous histiocytoma is the most common histological type, accounting for 15 of the 25 cases of breast sarcoma reported by Pollard *et al.* The subtypes were giant cell, fibrous, myxoid and inflammatory. The so-called stromal sarcomas described by Berg *et al.* (1962) are part of this group of tumours. Some have followed irradiation for breast carcinoma (Langham *et al.*, 1984; Lemson *et al.*, 1996). Jones *et al.* (1992) divided them into two grades. The high-grade tumours exhibited marked nuclear atypia and at least 5 mitotic figures per 10 high-power fields or moderate nuclear atypia and 6 or more mitoses per 10 high-power fields. All the low-grade lesions had 5 or fewer mitoses per 10 high-power fields, the average being 2. Thirty-one per cent of patients with a high-grade lesion died of tumour and 13% were alive with disease. Twenty-five per cent developed distant metastases. All patients with a low-grade lesion were free of tumour at last contact, despite recurrence in more than half. None of the tumours had metastasized.

Myofibrosarcoma (myofibroblastic sarcoma) is composed of cells showing myofibroblastic differentiation and is the malignant counterpart of the myofibroblastoma (*see* p. 292). The cells are spindle-shaped and usually arranged in fascicles surrounded by dense hyaline collagen. There is sometimes a storiform appearance, the cells occasionally being more pleomorphic. On immunostaining they exhibit positivity for vimentin, smooth muscle actin and fibronectin, and negativity for desmin, laminin and type IV collagen. Electron microscopy reveals abundant rough endoplasmic reticulum, myofilaments with focal densities and the fibronexus junctions and fibronectin fibrils that characterize myofibroblasts (Taccagni *et al.*, 1997). Some of the tumours labelled as stromal sarcomas, fibrosarcomas or simply undifferentiated spindle cell sarcomas before the extensive use of immunohistochemistry may have been myofibrosarcomas. They generally have a rather indolent course, but some exhibit very aggressive behaviour.

Liposarcoma, unlike lipoma, is a very rare breast tumour, although it appears to be the most common after malignant fibrous histiocytoma, accounting for 6 of the 25 cases reported by Pollard *et al.* (1990). Ii *et al.* (1980) gleaned 42 cases from the literature and added one of their own, including ultrastructural findings. They estimated that liposarcomas account for between 0.001 and 0.03% of all breast tumours and that only 0.8–1.9% of all liposarcomas arise in the breast. The age range of their patients was 18–76, with a mean of around 47. One of the tumours occurred in a male. The size was immensely variable, ranging from 10 to 230 mm, but on the whole they tended to be large, with a mean size of about 750 mm. Of the 32 cases in which histological type was known, 19 were myxoid, 6 pleomorphic, 4 well differentiated and 3 mixed. As in other sites care should be taken to distinguish the well-differentiated types from the much more common lipomas. About one quarter of the patients had pre-existing or co-existing fibroadenoma or phyllodes tumours, suggesting a possible histogenetic relationship. Eight of the 13 patients on whom follow-up information was available were tumour-free after 5 years. Local recurrence was seen in 15% of cases overall, but this figure rose to 60% in those treated by a local excision; 12.5% recurred after simple mastectomy and 7. 1 % after radical mastectomy.

The largest single series of breast liposarcomas to date is probably that of Austin and Dupree (1986) from the Armed Forces Institute of Pathology, comprising 20 cases: 13 pure and 7 arising in phyllodes tumours. The tumours in both groups exhibited similar age range and size to those included in the study of Ii *et al.* Five of the pure liposarcomas were well differentiated, 4 myxoid and 4 pleomorphic. Of the 7 arising in phyllodes tumours, 2 were well differentiated and 5 pleomorphic. Round cell liposarcoma was not encountered in either group. Four of the pure tumours recurred, of which three metastasized and two resulted in the death of the patient. One of the phyllodes-related tumours recurred and was lost to follow-up. Features associated with recurrence were the pleomorphic pattern and infiltrative margins. In contrast recurrence-free survival was associated with the well-differentiated pattern and circumscription. Complete excision with tumour-free margins is essential, but mastectomy is not necessary unless required to achieve complete removal. Axillary lymph node metastases were not encountered. Metastatic sites included the lungs, heart and bones. Two males were included in the study and remained tumour-free. The better prognosis in men may be explained by an earlier presentation.

Leiomyosarcoma of the breast is even less common than leiomyoma, and only a few cases have been reported. Only 1 of the 25 breast sarcomas reported by Pollard *et al.* was a leiomyosarcoma. The age range in the recorded cases is 49–77 years. Some have occurred in the nipple (Lonsdale and Widdison, 1992) and some in males. As in other parts of the body, it may be difficult to distinguish benign and malignant smooth muscle tumours. The number of mitoses has been considered by many authors to be the most important feature of malignancy, but the cut-off has varied greatly from one study to another. Barnes and Pietruszka (1977), Chen *et al.* (1981) and Nielsen (1984) considered 10, 3 and 2 mitoses per 10 high-power fields respectively to be indicative of unfavourable behaviour.

Boscaino *et al.* (1994) reported two smooth muscle tumours diagnosed as benign on initial histological examination that recurred as unequivocal leiomyosarcoma in one case and smooth muscle tumour of uncertain prognosis in the other. Both patients were alive and well 6 years and 3 years 4 months after their recurrence. The authors considered features indicative of malignancy to be necrosis, cellularity, cytological atypia and more than four mitoses per 10 high-power fields. Lesions lacking these features but exhibiting 1–3 mitoses per 10 high-power fields were regarded as intermediate, benign tumours being those without mitoses or any of the other adverse histological features. Given the present uncertainty this is probably a good rule of thumb. Leiomyosarcomas tend to be larger, but size is not a reliable criterion by itself. Like leiomyosarcomas, leiomyomas may also be cystic and poorly circumscribed (Chen *et al.*, 1981).

TUMOURS OF LYMPHOID AND HAEMOPOIETIC CELLS

Malignant lymphoma

Malignant lymphoma of the breast may be primary or, more usually, secondary. Primary cases should exhibit neither disease elsewhere at presentation nor evidence of origin from adjacent tissues such as intramammary lymph nodes or overlying skin. They are consequently rare, in two series accounting for only 0.12% and 0.3% of all breast malignancies (Mambo *et al.*, 1977; Bobrow *et al.*, 1993). Even among the extranodal lymphomas, the breast is an uncommon site, accounting for fewer than 2% of cases.

There appear to be two major groups of case. The first is bilateral at presentation, associated with pregnancy or recent childbirth and spreading widely to involve the central nervous system, ovaries, gastrointestinal tract or endocrine organs but not the lymph nodes. The second accounts for the majority (over 80%) of cases, affects older women, has a more variable clinical course (depending on the histological appearance and clinical stage) and presents like breast carcinoma as a unilateral mass of highly variable size (Hugh *et al.*, 1990). The former group has the histological appearance of Burkitt's lymphoma, although the lesions are rarely apparently of T-lymphoblastic type, as evidenced by the development of leukaemia or a mediastinal mass (Carbone *et al.*, 1982; Mambo *et al.*, 1977). The latter group exhibits greater histological variation, although nearly all cases are of B-cell phenotype and most are of diffuse large cell type (Fig. 14.8).

Cohen and Brooks (1991) reported 35 cases of breast lymphoma, including 16 considered to be primary. Ten cases were of diffuse large-cell type, 5 were composed of mixed small and large cells (2 follicular, and 3 diffuse), and 1 was a small lymphocytic lymphoma. All but one of the cases studied immunohistochemically were found to be of B-cell origin, the other being a T-cell lymphoma. The authors considered the tumours to be lymphomas of mucosa-associated lymphoid tissue in view of the frequent presence of lymphoepithelial lesions in the ducts and lobules.

Aozasa *et al.* (1992) reported 19 cases, of which one was bilateral. A wide range of histological types was encountered, diffuse large-cell type being the most common and accounting for 12 cases. Only one follicular lymphoma was encountered.

In their study of nine patients, Bobrow *et al.* (1993) found eight to be B-cell lymphomas using immunohistochemistry. Seven were of the high-grade centroblastic/polymorphic type using the modified Kiel classification (Lennert, 1981). One was a follicular centrocytic/centroblastic lymphoma and the other a true histiocytic lymphoma. None of the cases was CD30 positive and none exhibited a t[14;18] translocation using the polymerase chain reaction on formalin-fixed, paraffin-embedded sections, in keeping with the lack of follicular architecture in all but one case. Two of the four cases studied were oestrogen

14.8 Diffuse large B-cell lymphoma of the breast (REAL classification). (a) The lack of stroma, the circumscribed margin and the preservation of fat spaces at the periphery help to distinguish it from carcinoma (H&E, × 50). (b) Higher-power view showing that the cells are less cohesive than in breast carcinoma and have a higher nuclear-to-cytoplasmic ratio and more prominent nucleoli. There is also less stroma. Note the presence of tingible body macrophages, particularly in the upper part of the picture. The tumour stained positively for B-cell markers (H&E).

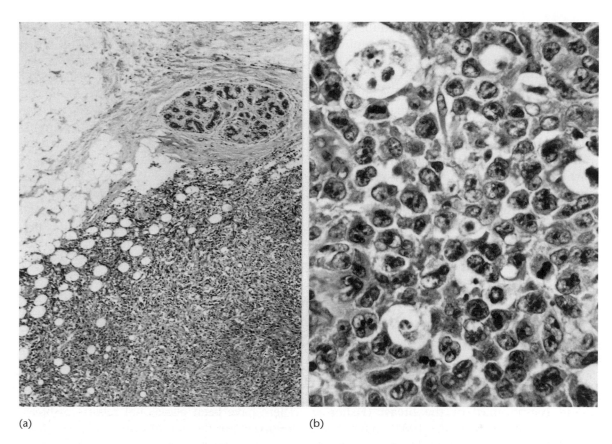

(a) (b)

receptor positive. One of these had previously been reported by Millis *et al.* (1988) as responding to tamoxifen. Oestrogen receptor positivity was also found in two of the cases reported by Hugh *et al.* (1990).

The 9 cases reported by Mattia *et al.* (1993) showed a different spectrum of histological type: 2 were small lymphocytic lymphomas with plasmacytoid differentiation, 6 were follicular and the ninth was a small non-cleaved cell (Burkitt-like) lymphoma, the only tumour regarded being as of high grade. All, however, were of B-cell type on immunohistochemical staining. These authors found double the number of secondary breast lymphomas in their files. These 18 cases were more commonly high grade but were also predominantly of B-cell type, follicular lymphomas comprising the majority.

Possible reasons for the differences are diagnostic inconsistency, the relatively small number of cases studied and that, in old archival cases, low-grade tumours may not have been recognized as neoplastic, particu-

larly if molecular investigations were unavailable.

An interesting aspect of Aozasa's study was that there was evidence of lymphocytic mastopathy (sclerosing lymphocytic lobulitis, *see* p. 278) in the neighbouring breast in eight (42%) of the cases, as evidenced by: (1) intralobular, perilobular and perivascular lymphocytic infiltrates associated with lobular atrophy and sclerosis; (2) the absence of histological findings compatible with fibrocystic disease or periductal mastitis/duct ectasia; (3) the predominance of B cells among the infiltrating lymphocytes, and (4) the expression of HLA-DR antigens by the involved epithelium. None of the patients, however, had clinical evidence of autoimmune disease.

It is clearly vital to distinguish malignant lymphoma of the breast from carcinoma in view of the fundamentally different management. Distinction may be especially difficult in intraoperative frozen sections, and it is best to defer the diagnosis if in doubt. Problems are most likely to arise in separating diffuse large cell lymphomas from medullary and atypical medullary carcinomas. Lymphomas usually exhibit less stroma and less of a tendency to grow in 'packets' than carcinomas. Tingible body macrophages are more common in breast lymphomas, and the presence of adjacent *in situ* carcinoma is, of course, strong evidence of epithelial origin. Immunohistological staining using the usual epithelial and lymphoid markers usually clinches the diagnosis.

The prognosis of primary lymphoma of the breast has varied in different studies, but actuarial survival appears to be about 50% over 5 years (DeCosse *et al.*, 1962; Mambo *et al.*, 1977). Tumour size and axillary node involvement do not appear to have the same prognostic significance as they do with carcinoma, but, as in non-mammary sites, prognosis is related to histological type and the stage of the disease.

'Pseudolymphoma'

'Pseudolymphomas' of the breast (Fisher *et al.*, 1979; Merino *et al.*, 1981) have been described as irregular, nodular, non-encapsulated masses that histologically exhibit an effacement of the normal architecture by a dense infiltrate of mature lymphoid cells, often forming reactive follicles and accompanied by histiocytes and plasma cells. The lymphocytes comprise a mixture of T and B cells, the latter staining for both κ and λ immunoglobulin light chains. A molecular genetic analysis of two cases undertaken by Knowles *et al.* (1989) showed two immunoglobulin gene rearrangements in each, suggesting that they were lymphoid hyperplasias containing immunophenotypically occult oligoclonal B-cell expansions. Rearrangements of the T-cell antigen receptor, *bcl-1*, *bcl-2* and *c-myc* genes were not detected, and no evidence of Epstein–Barr virus infection was found. Whether such cases carry a higher risk of developing malignant lymphoma has not been established; both patients had a benign clinical course over a limited follow-up period. The two patients reported by Fisher *et al.* (1979) and Merino *et al.* (1981) were receiving treatment

for hypertension. Strle *et al.* (1996) described 43 cases of lymphocytoma of the breast resulting from infection with *Borrelia burgdorferi*, the causative agent of Lyme disease.

The use of the term 'pseudolymphoma' is no longer advisable as it has been used to describe a variety of hyperplastic, inflammatory and immunological disorders and low-grade lymphomas. Three of the 35 cases of lymphoma reported by Cohen and Brooks (see above) were originally diagnosed as pseudolymphoma. As in other sites particular care should be taken to exclude the possibility of mantle zone lymphoma, in which the neoplastic cells often surround reactive germinal centres.

It should be noted that the nipple and areola are relatively common sites for the so-called cutaneous B-cell pseudolymphoma (lymphocytoma cutis or Spiegler–Fendt sarcoid) (McKee, 1996).

Granulocytic sarcoma

There have been occasional reports of breast involvement by granulocytic sarcoma. Both patients reported by Pascoe (1970) were known to be suffering from chronic granulocytic leukaemia, and in each case the breast lesion was followed by a blast crisis in the marrow. The patient of Kelch *et al.* (1990) experienced a relapse of acute myeloblastic leukaemia in the breast following allogeneic bone marrow transplantation. In the case reported by Sears and Reid (1976), however, the breast lesion was the first manifestation of acute myeloblastic leukaemia, detected in the marrow 4 months later.

Granulocytic sarcoma may strongly resemble malignant lymphoma in tissue sections and is frequently incorrectly diagnosed. There may also be a resemblance to carcinoma, particularly of the infiltrative lobular type. Enzyme histochemical staining for naphthol ASD-chloroacetate esterase can be performed on formalin-fixed, paraffin-embedded sections and is generally positive in granulocytic sarcoma, even if only in a few cells (Fig 14.9). Immunostaining for products of myeloid cells such as myeloperoxidase may also be very helpful.

14.9 Granulocytic sarcoma. (a) This low-power view shows an infiltration of the breast by monotonous cells, sparing the epithelial structures. (b) High-power view of the same lesion stained histochemically for naphthol ASD-chloroacetate esterase. Note the red reaction product in many of the tumour cells. This patient presented with a breast mass and developed marrow disease 2–3 months later.

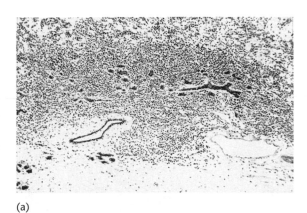
(a)

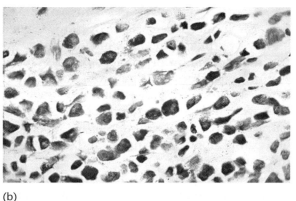
(b)

Follicular dendritic cell tumour

It is very rare for these tumours to occur in the breast (for a review, see Al-Nafussi, 1999). They are composed of spindle cells arranged in a fascicular or storiform growth pattern and intimately admixed with lymphocytes. Perivascular lymphocytes are also seen. There is usually little nuclear pleomorphism, but scattered multinucleated giant cells are frequent. Mitotic figures are highly variable. Immunostaining is positive for CD21, CD35 and vimentin. The tumour usually behaves as a low-grade sarcoma, recurring locally in about one third of cases. About one quarter of cases develop distant metastases.

Other malignant lymphohaemopoietic tumours

Breast involvement may occur in Hodgkin's disease, plasma cell myeloma and the various forms of histiocytosis but is rarely the presenting feature.

TUMOURS ARISING FROM THE BREAST SKIN

Tumours may arise from the skin of the breast, including that of the nipple; several cases of basal cell carcinoma of the nipple have been reported (e.g. Lupton and Goette, 1978). The diagnosis is usually obvious, but problems may sometimes arise, particularly with adnexal tumours, which may be mistaken for superficial breast carcinomas or nipple adenomas, particularly of the syringomatous variant (*see* p. 242). Poorly differentiated sweat gland carcinomas

are very rare but may bear a strong resemblance to breast carcinoma (Fig. 14.10).

The problem of distinguishing malignant melanoma from breast carcinoma exhibiting melanocyte colonization is discussed on p. 30.

METASTATIC TUMOURS IN THE BREAST

The breast is an uncommon site for metastases, accounting for 0.5–1.2% of all breast malignancies (Sandison, 1959; Hajdu and Urban, 1972). The correct identification of metastatic lesions is, however, very important in order to avoid unnecessary mutilating surgery.

Hajdu and Urban (1972) studied 51 malignant tumours metastatic to the breast, seven of which occurred in men. Of these, 18 were metastatic carcinomas, 14 malignant melanomas (Fig. 14.11), 16 malignant

14.10 Sweat gland carcinoma arising from the skin of the axillary tail of the breast. An *in situ* component is seen in the sweat gland coils at the bottom of the picture. Note the strong resemblance of the infiltrative component to breast carcinoma. Sweat gland tumours of this type are, fortunately, uncommon. A normal hair follicle is present at the top left of the picture (H&E).

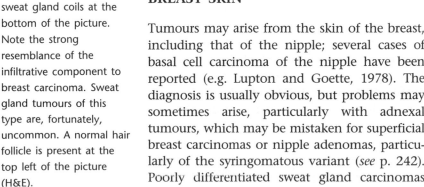

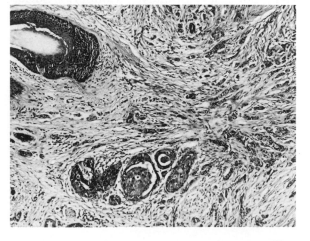

lymphomas (see above) and 3 myosarcomas. The carcinomas were derived from a wide variety of primary sites, of which the lung was the most common. The melanomas were all cutaneous and many arose from sites distant from the breast. In 16 cases the breast metastasis was the first presentation of the disease. Clinically, the tumours were often superficial and multinodular. Nipple retraction and discharge were rare.

Metastatic carcinomas may also occur in children, although they are excessively rare. Beattie *et al.* (1990) reported a case of metastatic alveolar rhabdomyosarcoma; on reviewing the literature, they noted that metastasizing medulloblastoma and glioblastoma had been previously reported.

An adequate history is essential as most patients will already be known to have tumours elsewhere; problems may arise, however, where there is a long time interval between the appearance of the primary tumour and the metastasis. Suspicion should be aroused with any breast tumour not conforming to any of the more common appearances described in Chapter 11. The presence of *in situ* carcinoma or atypical hyperplasia in the breast surrounding the tumour is highly suggestive of local origin, but it must be remembered that a metastatic carcinoma may on rare occasions invade and spread along the mammary ducts and lobules. Frozen section diagnosis should be deferred if there is any reasonable doubt about the origin of the tumour.

Conventional special stains may be of help. The presence of significant elastosis is indicative of a primary tumour. Alcian blue–periodic acid–Schiff stains may reveal the presence of intracytoplasmic target-like inclusions, which, although not pathognomonic of breast carcinoma, are more likely to occur in tumours of mammary origin. Masson-Fontana stains are of value in diagnosing metastatic melanomas.

Immunostaining for oestrogen and progesterone receptors may be useful in identifying primary breast tumours. It should be noted, however, that immunopositivity for oestrogen receptors is not entirely specific for carcinomas of the breast and female genital tract,

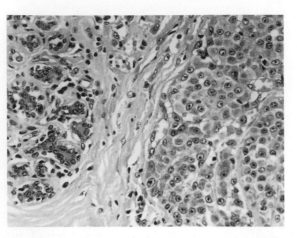

14.11 Metastatic amelanotic malignant melanoma. A residual breast lobule is seen on the left. Although it is not possible to diagnose melanoma confidently from this photograph, there should be strong suspicions about the non-mammary origin of the tumour as it does not resemble any of the more common types, as seen in Chapter 11. There is some cytological resemblance to medullary carcinoma, but the lymphoid infiltrate is lacking.

occasionally being found in tumours from a variety of other sites. The immunopositivity of some lymphomas is discussed above. In their large study using the anti-oestrogen receptor antibodies 1D5 and 6F11, however, Kaufmann *et al.* (1998) found no positivity of any of 22 pancreatic, 23 colonic or 27 renal carcinomas. Ten per cent of lung carcinomas were positive using the usual labelled streptavidin–biotin detection system, but this rose to 46% using 6F11 if the very sensitive tyramide signal amplification system was used. Between 3% and 9% of gastric carcinomas were positive depending on the detection system, and 67–71% of ovarian carcinomas were stained. Staining with antibodies hPRa3, 10A9 and a DAKO polyclonal antiserum was restricted to breast and ovarian tumours.

Kaufmann *et al.* (1996) found that combined immunostaining for oestrogen receptor and gross cystic disease fluid protein-15 (GCDFP-15) had a sensitivity and specificity for identifying breast carcinoma of 0.83 and 0.98 respectively. Wick *et al.*, (1998), however, found GCDFP-15 immunopositivity in a significant proportion of salivary and sweat gland carcinomas. Furthermore, 25% of salivary and 18% of sweat gland carcinomas were positive for progesterone receptors (antibody 1A6), and 32% of salivary carcinomas positive for oestrogen receptor (1D5). No sweat gland carcinomas were positive for oestrogen receptors.

Immunostaining for oestrogen receptors, progesterone receptors and GCDFP-15 may thus be of value in distinguishing breast from other carcinomas, but caution needs to be exercised and clinical features taken into account. Very sensitive detection systems are best avoided. In the author's experience breast carcinomas are almost always positive for epithelial membrane antigen, so a negative result should arouse suspicion. Immunostaining for prostatic acid phosphatase and prostate-specific antigen has been successfully used to distinguish between primary carcinoma of the male breast and metastasis from the prostate, a distinction that may otherwise prove difficult (Naritoku and Taylor, 1983).

REFERENCES

Al-Nafussi A. (1999) Spindle cell tumours of the breast. *Histopathology*, **35**, 1–13.

Aozasa K., Ohsawa M., Saeki K., Horiuchi K., Kawano K., Taguchi T. (1992) Malignant lymphoma of the breast. Immunologic type and association with lymphocytic mastopathy. *Am. J. Clin. Pathol.*, **97**, 699–704.

Arias-Stella J., Rosen P.P. (1988) Hemangiopericytoma of the breast. *Mod. Pathol.*, **1**, 98–103.

Austin R.M., Dupree W.B. (1986) Liposarcoma of the breast: a clinicopathologic study of 20 cases. *Hum Pathol.*, **17**, 906–13

Badwe R.A., Hanby A.M., Fentiman I.S., Chaudary M.A. (1991) Angiosarcoma of the skin overlying an irradiated breast. *Breast Cancer Res. Treat.*, **19**, 69–72.

Barnes L., Pietruszka M., (1977) Sarcomas of the breast: a clinicopathologic analysis of ten cases. *Cancer*, **40**, 1577–85.

Beattie M., Kingston J.E., Norton A.J., Malpas J.S. (1990) Nasopharyngeal rhabdomyosarcoma presenting as a breast mass. *Pediatr. Haematol. Oncol.*, **7**, 259–63.

Beltaos E., Banerjee T.K. (1979) Chondrosarcoma of the breast: report of two cases. *Am. J. Clin. Pathol.*, **71**, 345–9.

Berg J.W., DeCosse J.J., Fracchia A.A., Farrow J. (1962) Stromal sarcomas of the breast: a unified approach to connective tissue sarcomas other than cystosarcoma phyllodes. *Cancer*, **15**, 418–24.

Bobrow L.G., Richards M.A., Happerfield L.C. *et al.* (1993) Breast lymphomas: a clinicopathologic review. *Hum. Pathol.*, **24**, 3, 274–8.

Boscaino A., Gerrara G., Orabona P., Donofrio V., Staibano S., De Rosa G. (1994) Smooth muscle tumors of the breast: clinicopathologic features of two cases. *Tumori*, **80**, 241–5.

Carbone A., Volpe R., Tirelli U. *et al.* (1982) Primary lymphoblastic lymphoma of the breast. *Clin. Oncol.*, **8**, 367–73.

Chen K.T.K., Kirkegaard D.D., Bocian J.J. (1980) Angiosarcoma of the breast. *Cancer*, **46**, 368–71.

Chen K.T.K., Kuo T., Hoffmann K.D. (1981) Leiomyosarcoma of the breast: a case of long survival and late hepatic metastasis. *Cancer*, **47**, 1883–6.

Cohen P., Brooks J.J., (1991) Lymphomas of the breast. A clinipathological and immunohistochemical study of primary and secondary cases. *Cancer*, **67**, 1359–69.

Davies J.D., Riddell R.H. (1973) Muscular hamartomas of the breast. *J. Pathol.*, **111**, 209–11.

DeCosse J.J., Berg J.W., Fracchia A.A., Farrow J.H. (1962) Primary lymphosarcoma of the breast: a review of 14 cases. *Cancer*, **15**, 1264–8.

Donnell R.M., Rosen P.P., Lieberman P.H. *et al.* (1981) Angiosarcoma and other vascular tumors of the breast: pathologic analysis as a guide to prognosis. *Am. J. Surg. Pathol.*, **5**, 629–42.

Dworak O., Reck T., Greskotter K.R., Kockerling F. (1994) Hamartoma of an ectopic breast arising in the inguinal region. *Histopathology*, **24**, 169–71.

Fisher C.J., Hanby A.M., Robinson L., Millis R.R. (1992) Mammary hamartoma – a review of 35 cases. *Histopathology*, **20**, 99–106.

Fisher E.R., Palekar A.S., Paulson J.D. , Colinger R. (1979) Pseudolymphoma of breast. *Cancer*, **44**, 258–63.

Givens S.S., Ellerbroek N.A., Butler J.J., Libhitz H.I., Hortobagyi G.N., McNeese M.D. (1989) Angiosarcoma arising in an irradiated breast: a case report and review of the literature. *Cancer*, **11**, 2214–16

Haagensen C.D. (1971) *Diseases of the Breast*. London, W. B. Saunders.

Hajdu S.I., Urban J.A. (1972) Cancers metastatic to the breast. *Cancer*, **29**, 1691–6.

Hamels J., Blondiau P., Mirgaux M. (1981) Cutaneous angiosarcoma arising in a mastectomy scar after therapeutic irradiation. *Bull. Cancer (Paris)*, **68**, 353–6.

Hoda S.A., Cranor M.L., Rosen P.P. (1992) Hemangiomas of the breast with atypical histological features: further analysis of histological subtypes confirming their benign character. *Am. J. Surg. Pathol.*, **16 (6)**, 553–60.

Hugh J.C., Jackson F.I., Hanson J., Poppema S. (1990) Primary breast lymphoma. An immunohistologic study of 20 new cases. *Cancer*, **66**, 2602–11

Ii K., Hizawa K., Okazaki K., Morimoto T., Uyama Y. (1980) Liposarcoma of the breast – fine structural and histochemical study of a case and review of 42 cases in the literature. *Tokushima J. Exp. Med.*, **27**, 45–56.

Jernstrom P., Lindberg L., Meland O.N. (1963) Osteogenic sarcoma of the mammary gland. *Am. J. Clin. Pathol.*, **40**, 521–6.

Jiminez-Ayala M., Diez-Nau M.D., Larrad A. *et al.* (1991) Hemangiopericytoma in a male breast. Report of a case with cytologic, histologic and immunochemical studies. *Acta Cytol.*, **35**, 234–8.

Jones M.W., Norris H.J., Wargotz E.S., Weiss S.W. (1992) Fibrosarcoma – malignant fibrous histiocytoma of the breast: a clinicopathological study of 32 cases. *Am. J. Surg. Pathol.*, **16** (7), 667–74.

Kaufmann O., Deidesheimer T., Muehlenberg M., Deicke P., Dietel M. (1996) Immunohistochemical differentiation of metastatic breast carcinomas from metastatic adenocarcinomas of other common primary sites. *Histopathology*, **29**, 233–40.

Kaufmann O., Kother S., Dietel M. (1998) Use of antibodies against estrogen and progesterone receptors to identify metastatic breast and ovarian carcinomas by conventional immunohistochemical and tyramide signal amplification methods. *Mod. Pathol.*, **11**, 357–63.

Kelch B.P., Bulova S.I., Crilley P. *et al.* (1990) An unusual extramedullary relapse of acute nonlymphocytic leukaemia after allogeneic bone marrow transplantation. *Am. J. Clin. Oncol.*, **13** (3), 238–43.

Knowles D.M., Athan E., Ubriaco A. *et al.* (1989) Extranodal noncutaneous lymphoid hyperplasias represent a continous spectrum of B-cell neoplasia: demonstration by molecular genetic analysis. *Blood*, **73**, 1635–45.

Krishnan M.M.S., Krishnan R. (1982) An unusual breast lump: neurilemmoma. *Aust. N.Z. J. Surg.*, **52**, 612–13.

Langham M.R., Scott-Mills A., DeMay R.M., O'Dowd C.J., Grathwohl M.A., Shelton-Horsley J. (1984) Malignant fibrous histiocytoma of the breast. *Cancer*, **54**, 558–63.

Lemson M.S., Mud H.J., Wijnmaalen A.J., Giard R.W.M. (1996). Post-radiation fibrosarcoma of the breast. *Breast*, **5**, 368–71.

Lennert K., (1981) Classification of non-Hodgkin's lymphoma. In Lennert K. (ed.), *Histopathology of Non-Hodgkin's Lymphomas (on Kiel Classification)*. Berlin, Springer.

Linnell F., Ostberg G., Soderstrom J. (1979) Breast hamartomas: an important entity in mammary pathology. *Virchows Archiv A, Pathol. Anat. Histol.*, **383**, 253–64.

Lonsdale R.N., Widdison A. (1992) Leiomyosarcoma of the nipple. *Histopathology*, **20**, 537–9.

Lupton G.P., Goette D.K. (1978) Basal cell carcinoma of the nipple. *Arch. Dermatol.*, **114**, 1845.

Mambo N.C., Burke J.S., Butler J.J. (1977) Primary malignant lymphomas of the breast. *Cancer*, **39**, 2033–40.

Marsh W.L., Lucas J.G., Olsen J. (1989) Chondrolipoma of the breast. *Arch. Pathol. Lab. Med.*, **113**, 369–71.

Mattia A.R., Ferry J.A., Harris N.L. (1993) Breast lymphoma. A B-cell spectrum including the low grade B-cell lymphoma of mucosa associated lymphoid tissue. *Am. J. Surg. Pathol.*, **17**, 574–87.

McKee P.H. (1996) In *Pathology of the Skin*. 2nd edn. London, Mosby-Wolfe.

Merino M.J., Joyner R.E., Graham, A. (1981) Pseudolymphoma of the breast. *Diagn. Gynecol. Obstet.*, **3**, 315–18.

Millis R.R., Bobrow L.G., Rubens R.D. *et al.* (1988) Histocytic lymphoma of breast responds to tamoxifen. *Br. J. Cancer*, **58**, 808–9.

Mittal K.R., Gerald W., True L.D. (1986) Hemangiopericytoma of the breast: report of a case with ultrastructural and histochemical findings. *Hum. Pathol.*, **17**, 1181–3.

Mulcare R. (1968) Granular cell myoblastoma of the breast. *Ann. Surg.*, **168**, 262–8.

Naritoku W.Y., Taylor C.R. (1983) Immunohistologic diagnosis of 2 cases of metastatic prostate cancer to breast. *J. Urol.*, **130**, 365–7.

Nascimento A.G., Karas M., Rosen P.P., Caron A.G. (1979) Leiomyoma of the nipple. *Am. J. Surg. Pathol.*, **3**, 151–4.

Nielsen B.B., (1984) Leiomyosarcoma of the breast with late disemination. *Virchows Archiv, Pathol. Anat.*, **403**, 241–5.

Norris H.J., Taylor H.B. (1968) Sarcomas and related mesenchymal tumors of the breast. *Cancer*, **22**, 22–8.

Oberman H.A. (1965) Sarcomas of the breast. *Cancer*, **18**, 1233–43.

Oberman H.A. (1989) Hamartomas and hamartoma variants of the breast. *Semin. Diagn. Pathol.*, **6**, 135–45.

Pascoe H.R. (1970) Tumors composed of immature granulocytes occurring in the breast in chronic granulocytic leukemia. *Cancer*, **25**, 697–704.

Pollard S.G., Marks P.V., Temple L.N., Thompson H.H. (1990) Breast sarcoma: a clinicopathologic review of 25 cases. *Cancer*, **66**, 941–4.

Rosen P.P., Ridolfi R.L. (1977) The perilobular hemangioma: a benign microscopic vascular lesion of the breast. *Am. J. Clin. Pathol.*, **68**, 21–3.

Rosen PP, Kimmel M, Ernsbergern D. (1988) Mammary angiosarcoma: the prognostic significance of tumor differentiation. *Cancer*, **62**, 2145–51.

Sandison A.T. (1959) Metastatic tumours in the breast. *Br. J. Surg.*, **47**, 54–8.

Sears H.F., Reid J. (1976) Granulocytic sarcoma: local presentation of a systemic disease. *Cancer*, **37**, 1808–13.

Stout A.P. (1943) Hemangio-endothelioma: a tumor of blood vessels featuring vascular endothelial cells. *Ann. Surg.*, **118**, 445–64.

Strle F., Maraspin V., Pleterski-Rigler D. *et al.* (1996) Treatment of borrelial lymphocytoma. *Infection*, **24**, 82–6.

Taccagni G., Rovere E., Masullo M., Christensen L., Eyden B. (1997) Myofibrosarcoma of the breast: review of the literature on myofibroblastic tumours and criteria for defining myofibroblastic differentiation. *Am. J. Surg. Pathol.*, **21**, 489–96.

Umansky C., Bullock W.K. (1968) Granular cell myoblastoma of the breast. *Ann. Surg.*, **168**, 810–17.

Wick M.R., Ockner D.M., Mills S.E., Ritter J.H., Swanson P.E. (1998) Homologous carcinomas of the breasts, skin and salivary glands. A histologic and immuno-histochemical comparison of ductal mammary carcinoma, ductal sweat gland carcinoma, and salivary duct carcinoma. *Am. J. Clin. Pathol.*, **109**, 75–84.

15 Miscellaneous lesions

HYPERKERATOSIS OF NIPPLE AND AREOLA

Hyperkeratosis of the nipple and areola is a rare disorder, taking several forms. The naevoid form has been the subject of several reports (Garcia, 1973; Mehregan and Rahbari, 1977) and is characterized by bilateral, uniform, verrucose hyperpigmentation of both the nipples and areolae. It usually occurs in women in their second or third decade, sometimes beginning in mid-pregnancy. Coots (1996) has described a case in a male.

Macroscopically, there are numerous pigmented, friable papules, usually 1–3 mm in size. Histologically, the lesions are polypoid and exhibit hyperkeratosis, sometimes with plugging but little acanthosis. There is variable increase in pigmentation in the basal layer but without an increase in the number of junctional melanocytes. Melanophages may be present in the upper dermis, especially if epidermal pigmentation is marked. The papillary dermis may exhibit oedema and telangiectasia with focal perivascular lymphocytic infiltration.

The cause of the condition is not known. A possible hormonal aetiology is suggested by an onset in pregnancy in some female patients and by a case report of a 66-year-old man in whom the condition was associated with gynaecomastia following orchidectomy and diethylstiboestrol therapy for carcinoma of the prostate.

Hyperkeratosis of the nipple and areola may also be associated with either the sex-linked or the acquired form of ichthyosis. This may be bilateral and occurs in both sexes. Unilateral hyperkeratosis may also occur as a result of involvement of the nipple and areola by an epidermal naevus. Finally, bilateral involvement of the nipple by acanthosis nigricans has also been reported (Forman, 1943; Schwartz, 1978).

ECZEMA OF THE NIPPLE

Bilateral eczema of the nipple may be seen as part of an atopic eczema or contact dermatitis caused by clothing. Unilateral eczema of the nipple has also been described and may lead to an erroneous clinical diagnosis of Paget's disease. Histologically, there are the usual epidermal acanthosis and spongiosis but no evidence of malignant cells. Graham (1972) described two cases of unilateral eczema of the nipple in teenage girls, the cause of which was not elucidated.

FIBROMATOSIS OF THE BREAST

Fibromatosis rarely involves the breast but may cause considerable diagnostic difficulties. Most cases are solitary lesions, but the

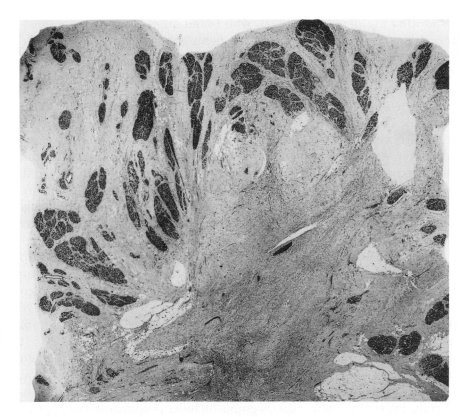

15.1 Fibromatosis of the breast. There is a stellate fibroblastic zone infiltrating and replacing the breast epithelium and stroma. Note the distortion of breast lobules at the periphery of the lesion (H&E).

breast may sometimes be involved in Gardner's syndrome (Haggitt and Booth, 1970; Rosen *et al.*, 1978; Gump *et al.*, 1981). Some cases have involved the pectoral muscles, suggesting the possibility of a musculoaponeurotic rather than a breast origin. A wide age range from 14 to 80 years has been reported (Gump *et al.*, 1981; Rosen and Ernsberger, 1989). Some cases are bilateral, either synchronous or metachronous (Rosen and Ernsberger, 1989).

Macroscopically, the lesion is firm and irregular, and may strongly resemble an infiltrating breast carcinoma. Clinically, the occasional presence of skin or nipple retraction may strengthen this resemblance, and the mammographic appearances may also be indistinguishable from those of carcinoma. Size is highly variable, ranging from 10 to 100 mm in Rosen and Ernsberger's (1989) series.

Histologically, fibromatosis of the breast has the same appearance as in other parts of the body. It is a progressive, non-encapsulated, infiltrative fibroblastic growth (Fig. 15.1) with a marked tendency to recur locally but with no capacity for distant metastasis. It is distinguished from spindle-cell sarcomas and carcinomas by the lack of cytological features of malignancy. The cells are thus less densely packed and exhibit little nuclear hyperchromatism or pleomorphism (Fig. 15.2). Mitotic figures are uncommon, and abnormal forms are not seen. Foci of mononuclear cell infiltration may be encountered (Fig. 15.2). Ossification was reported in one case reported by Mayers *et al.* (1994) but is extremely rare. Fibromatosis may grow around normal ducts and lobules, preserving them within the

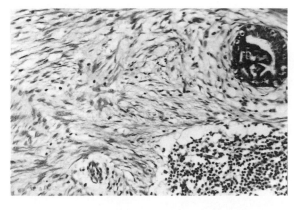

15.2 Fibromatosis of the breast. The lesion is less cellular than a fibrosarcoma and exhibits neither cytological atypia nor significant mitotic activity. There is sparing of a duct at the top right of the picture. Note the focus of mononuclear cells at the bottom right (H&E).

proliferating mass. This is another useful point of distinction from fibrosarcoma, in which normal structures are more likely to be replaced. The retention of normal epithelial structures within the spindle-cell proliferation may produce an appearance reminiscent of phyllodes tumour, although the characteristic growth pattern of the latter is not seen.

The distinction of fibromatosis from reactive fibrosis is equally important in view of the tendency of fibromatosis to replace tissues and recur. Scars from various causes are less cellular and tend to be associated with the presence of lipid-laden macrophages, chronic inflammatory cell infiltration and haemosiderin deposition. It should be noted that keloid-type collagen fibres are occasionally seen in fibromatosis. Other conditions entering into the differential diagnosis are fibrous histiocytoma and nodular fasciitis. The former is distinguished by its greater polymorphism, particularly the presence of giant cells, and the latter by the characteristic plump, mitotically active spindle cells, myxoid stroma and rapid growth rate.

Intraoperative frozen section diagnosis may be very difficult. In the nine cases of Gump *et al.* (1981) on which frozen sections were performed, only three were reported as fibroproliferative lesions. One was thought to be a phyllodes tumour and one a scirrhous carcinoma, the diagnosis being deferred in the remaining four.

As complete excision appears to be the key to successful treatment, the pathologist should assess the excision margins with some care. Wargotz *et al.* (1987) reported 20 cases of fibromatosis treated by local excision, of which five recurred. The excision margins were involved in all recurrent cases. Specific histological features such as size, cellularity, atypia and mitotic figures were not helpful in predicting recurrence. Recurrent cases may require radical surgery. Very occasional examples of spontaneous regression have been reported.

NODULAR FASCIITIS

The breast is a very uncommon site for nodular fasciitis: one case was reported by Mokbel *et al.*

(1994), who found another nine in the literature. The patients have ranged in age from 36 to 59 years and the length of history from 2 days to 6 months, although the majority of lesions appear to have been present for less than 3 months. Like fibromatosis, nodular fasciitis may closely resemble carcinoma both clinically and radiologically, forming a hard, infiltrative mass that is often spiculated on mammography. Furthermore, growth is rapid, and cytological examination may reveal sufficient cellular pleomorphism to suspect malignancy. In other cases the clinical features may be more like those of a fibroadenoma.

The lesions are histologically identical to those arising in the soft tissues, being composed of plump but cytologically benign spindle cells separated by myxoid connective tissue and usually arranged in a storiform growth pattern. Mitoses may be frequent, but abnormal forms are not seen. There is often zoning with a fibrous centre and vascular, cellular periphery. Histologically, the differential diagnosis includes fibromatosis (see above), fibrous histiocytoma, myofibroblastoma and the cellular phase of scarring following surgery. The condition is almost invariably cured by local excision, and recurrence should prompt a reconsideration of the diagnosis.

MULTINUCLEATED MAMMARY STROMAL GIANT CELLS

This phenomenon, described by Rosen (1979), consists of localized groups of hyperchromatic multinucleated cells (somewhat resembling those of a fibrous histiocytoma) within the mammary stroma (Fig. 15.3). The abnormality

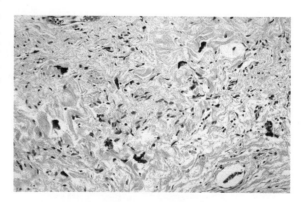

Fig.15.3 Mammary stromal giant cells. The characteristic pleomorphic multinucleate cells form a small focus that extends throughout most of the stroma in this field (H&E).

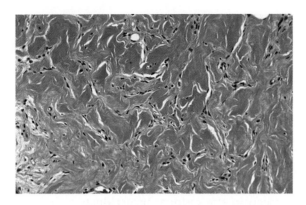

Fig.15.4
Pseudoangiomatous hyperplasia. There is a zone of dense collagenous fibrosis containing irregularly distributed spindle cells, many of which lie on either side of elongated spaces (H&E).

is visible at low magnification and usually limited to a low-power field, but multiple separate foci may occur. The cells are usually found in the collagenous portions of the interlobular stroma, the adipose tissue being rarely involved. There is no accompanying inflammation or foreign material. The cells are sometimes distorted by the surrounding collagen and resemble invasive carcinoma. Mucin stains are negative. Immunohistochemical staining confirms that the cells are stromal and that they exhibit no evidence of epithelial differentiation.

In Rosen's series the lesion was found in 4.5% of 200 consecutive mastectomy specimens removed for carcinoma, as well as in breast tissue from patients with no evidence of malignancy. The multinucleated cells were usually not adjacent to the malignant neoplasm. There was a striking clustering of cases within the 40–50-year age group, suggesting some relationship to an impending menopause. There was no relationship to parity, hormone usage or family history of breast carcinoma.

PSEUDOANGIOMATOUS STROMAL HYPERPLASIA

Pseudoangiomatous stromal hyperplasia (PASH) may present as a well-circumscribed mass in the breast or as an irregular zone of thickening, usually clinically palpable but occasionally impalpable and detectable by mammography (Vuitch et al., 1986; Powell et al., 1995). It is bilateral in only a small proportion of cases. In the study of Powell et al., the

size ranged from 12 to 120 mm and patient age from 14 to 67, with a mean of 37. PASH may also occur focally or extensively in a variety of breast lesions in which stromal proliferation is a feature, for example fibroadenomas and phyllodes tumours. In particular, it was reported in over two thirds of hamartomas by Fisher et al. (1992), raising the possibility that some cases, particularly the well-circumscribed examples, may be regarded as PASH by some workers and as hamartomas exhibiting PASH by others.

Histologically, the process strongly resembles a vascular proliferation, consisting of complex anastomosing channels lined by slender spindle cells and separated by coarse bundles of collagen that often appear hyalinized (Fig 15.4). Some lesions exhibit a greater degree of proliferation in which the spindle cells form fascicles obliterating the pseudoangiomatous lumina. The change often expands the intralobular stroma and diffusely involves the interlobular stroma. The epithelium of the ducts and lobules is variably hyperplastic, and myoepithelial cells may be prominent. Some cases have been misdiagnosed as angiosarcoma, although the spindle cells do not show atypia or mitotic activity, even in the more cellular examples. Furthermore, they exhibit no evidence of endothelial differentiation on ultrastructural or immunohistological examination (see below). There is no evidence of recent or old haemorrhage, and the spaces do not contain erythrocytes. They are discernible in frozen sections, indicating that they are not an artefact of formalin fixation or paraffin embedding.

Thirty-eight of 40 patients reported by Powell et al. were treated by excisional biopsy; incisional biopsy alone was undertaken in one prepubertal girl, and one patient underwent bilateral mastectomy. Follow-up was for 0.6–11 years (mean 4.5 years), during which six patients experienced a recurrent lesion. Five had ipsilateral recurrences, one in association with contralateral disease. The other developed contralateral change without ipsilateral recurrence.

Detailed immunostaining was undertaken by Powell et al. (1995), who found positivity for vimentin, smooth muscle actin and CD34 and negativity for factor VIII rag, Ulex, cyto-keratins and S100. The positivity for CD34 was found in nearly all cases and should not be misinterpreted as evidence of vascular differentiation as these antibodies are not endothelium specific. Powell *et al.* concluded that the spindle cells lining the spaces are probably myofibroblasts. Intriguingly, immunopositivity of the spindle cells for oestrogen or progesterone receptors or both was observed in a significant proportion of cases.

Badve and Sloane (1995) observed the phenomenon in the male breast in cases of gynaecomastia, particularly those of interme-diate cellularity. They concluded that the change might represent a phase in the maturation of breast stroma that has under-gone recent proliferation.

SPONTANEOUS NECROSIS OF THE BREAST IN PREGNANCY AND LACTATION

This is a well-recognized uncommon condition that may occur in a fibroadenoma or in breast tissue showing no evidence of a pre-existing lesion. Lucey (1975) described five cases and reviewed the findings from previous studies.

The condition presents as a circumscribed breast lump that may be tender. Although there is a wide variation in size, most lesions are between 10 and 20 mm. They are usually solitary, although two or three masses may occasionally be found; bilateral lesions are rare. There appears to be a disproportionately high incidence in Negroes.

Histologically, there is a central zone of coagulative necrosis surrounded by lympho-cytes, plasma cells, haemosiderin-laden macrophages and fibrosis, the proportion depending on the age of the lesion. Lucey found intimal fibrous thickening or organizing thrombi in arteries and veins in 3 of 5 cases and suggested that the lesions have a vascular cause. Other authors have failed to find any vascular abnormality and have suggested a relative vascular insufficiency resulting from the increased metabolic demands of

pregnancy. Reticulin stains may show the well-preserved outlines of lactating breast lobules in the necrotic zone. This appearance and the well-circumscribed nature of the lesions have led to the conclusion that they are infarcted adenomas. Most lumps are, however, not removed until the postpartum period, when the surrounding breast has involuted and would contrast markedly with the non-involuted architecture in the necrotic zone. Foci of squamous metaplasia may occasionally be seen in the residual breast ducts.

NECROSIS OF THE BREAST ASSOCIATED WITH ANTICOAGULANTS

Necrosis of the subcutaneous and soft tissues is a rare complication of treatment with coumarin derivatives or sodium warfarin but not, apparently, heparin. The disorder occurs most commonly in middle-aged or elderly obese women, particularly in sites rich in subcutaneous fat, such as the buttocks, thighs and breasts (Verhagen, 1954). The onset is rapid, occurring about 3–10 days after begin-ning treatment at the usual dosage. The disor-der progresses inexorably even if the drug is discontinued. The first manifestations are pain and bruising, which become extensive and lead to the formation of bullae filled with serosanguinous fluid. Gangrene, sloughing and scarring eventually supervene. Mastectomy is often necessary.

Histologically, there is extensive necrosis, and some authors have found acute necrotiz-ing vasculitis of the small and medium-sized arteries, as well as venous thromboses (Davis *et al.*, 1972).

The pathogenesis is not clearly understood. One explanation is that the lesions result from simple haemorrhage due to the intended pharmacological effect of the drug. Another is that the necrosis may be yet another manifestation of the original coagu-lation disorder for which the anticoagulants were given. The third possibility is a hyper-sensitivity reaction. The distribution of lesions and the lack of an association with heparin would seem to militate against the first two possibilities.

VASCULAR DISEASE IN THE BREAST

The breast may be involved in generalized vascular disorders or may, very rarely, be the sole or predominant site of the lesions. Waugh (1950) reported a patient with bilateral breast lumps caused by giant cell arteritis. Histologically, the involved vessels showed fragmentation and necrosis of the media associated with a granulomatous inflammation consisting of lymphocytes, plasma cells, histiocytes, multinucleate giant cells and a few eosinophils. No extramammary lesions became apparent during a 16-month follow-up period.

McCarty *et al.* (1968) described a patient who developed multiple bilateral tender breast lumps. Histologically, the lesions resembled polyarteritis nodosa; there was fibrinoid necrosis of vessel walls associated with neutrophil, eosinophil and monocyte infiltration. Systemic features were absent, but the condition responded to prednisolone.

Pambakian and Tighe (1971) described two patients with Wegener's granulomatosis in whom the predominant lesions lay in the breast. All three cases reported by Jordan *et al.* (1987) presented with a breast mass thought clinically to be a carcinoma. The breast lesion and other manifestations of Wegener's developed concomitantly in one patient, but in the other two the breast involvement preceded an unequivocal diagnosis at other sites.

Mondor's disease (Mondor, 1939; Haagensen, 1971) is a superficial thrombophlebitis of the chest wall that usually occurs in middle-aged women but may also be seen in men. The aetiology is unknown, but some cases have followed vigorous exertion. Clinically, the lesion presents as a tender subcutaneous cord, often in the lateral aspect of the breast. The condition usually resolves without treatment in 4–8 weeks. Histological examination shows bland venous thrombosis, the degree of organization depending on the age of the lesion.

Infarction of the breast may also be seen in diabetes, with carbon monoxide poisoning and after trauma.

A focal medial calcification of arteries in the breast is not uncommon and is of uncertain significance. It is frequently observed in screening mammograms.

CHANGES DUE TO RADIOTHERAPY AND CHEMOTHERAPY

The main abnormalities in the non-neoplastic epithelium of the breast after radiotherapy are atrophy and cytological atypia (Fig. 15.5). The lobules show a reduction in both the size and the number of acini and an increase in the amount fibrous stroma. Interlobular ducts may also show a reduction in size and number. In many cases the epithelium appears to be affected more than the myoepithelium, so that the latter may appear more prominent or even abut the lumen (Fig. 15.5). The lobular changes may be similar to those seen in the normal process of involution. The epithelial atypia may be pronounced (Fig. 15.5) but can generally be distinguished from *in situ* carcinoma by its focal nature, the atypical cells being interspersed with non-atypical cells or gaps resulting from cell loss. The associated atrophy and lack of multilayering are other useful points of distinction. An increased expression of p53 and Ki67 may be seen for up to 5 years after irradiation (Poeze *et al.*, 1998).

Changes are also seen in the stroma. The fibroblasts may show pleomorphism, the nuclei being of variable size and either hyper- or hypochromatic. In the latter case they may have a indistinct outline, giving a 'smudged' appearance (Girling *et al.*, 1990). Multinucleate forms are sometimes seen. The

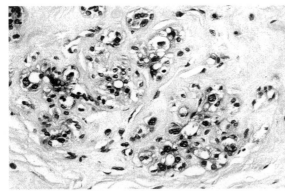

Fig.15.5 Normal lobule following radiotherapy. Note the pronounced atypia and extensive loss of epithelial cells. In some places myoepithelial cells abut the lumen. In contrast to *in situ* carcinoma, the atypical cells are sparsely distributed and interspersed with non-atypical cells. There is also intralobular fibrosis (H&E).

275

ground substance exhibits fibrosis with or without elastosis. Fat necrosis may be encountered. Girling *et al.* (1990) described a distinctive type of fat necrosis around iridium wire implants. This comprised an irregular rim of relatively acellular fibrous tissue lined by fibrin and surrounded by a zone of fat necrosis, giving the overall appearance of a cyst.

Blood vessels may show a variety of changes, involving both arteries and veins. In small to medium-sized vessels the most prominent change is usually subintimal fibrous thickening, sometimes with severe occlusion of the lumen. In arteries the elastic lamina may be fragmented. There may be nuclear pleomorphism and hyperchromatism of the endothelial cells, particularly in the capillaries.

Changes somewhat similar to those induced by irradiation have been noted following combination chemotherapy, but these appear to be less severe and consistent. Kennedy *et al.* (1990) noted cytological atypia and cellular loss in ducts and lobules after treatment with cyclophosphamide, doxorubicin, methotrexate and 5-fluorouracil. In another study undertaken by the author, no change was seen in the non-neoplastic breast after chemotherapy with mitozantrone, methotrexate and mitomycin C, despite striking histological effects on the tumours (unpublished data). It thus appears that the effects of chemotherapy on the normal breast are dependent on the choice and dosage of the drugs used.

CHANGES DUE TO TAMOXIFEN

There are very few publications on the effects of tamoxifen on the non-neoplastic breast. Hurst *et al.* (1998) reported the regression of cysts in association with tamoxifen treatment. Uehara *et al.* (1998) studied 24 premenopausal women undergoing biopsy for fibroadenoma. Twelve received 20 mg per day for 10 consecutive days beginning on the thirteenth day of the menstrual cycle, the other 12 receiving no treatment. The fibroadenomas were removed between days 23 and 26 of the cycle, along with a small amount of surrounding tissue. The nuclear volume and mitotic activity of the non-lesional epithelial cells were significantly reduced in the treated group. In another study from the same group, tamoxifen was found to reduce the number of lysosomes in the breast epithelial cells (Facina *et al.*, 1997). In experimental rats and mice tamoxifen has been shown to induce atrophy and block developmental growth of the breast (Sourla *et al.*, 1997; Kafkasli *et al.*, 1998).

CHANGES DUE TO SILICONE IMPLANTS

Most implants currently used for breast augmentation comprise a silicone elastomer bag or shell containing silicone gel or saline, free silicone liquid no longer being used. Following implantation, they become surrounded by a fibrous capsule that varies from a thin flexible membrane to a thick zone of dense collagen. If sufficiently extensive, the capsule may give rise to contracture of the prosthesis and clinical deformity. The capsule typically has three zones (Fig. 15.6) (Kasper, 1998). The inner layer consists of epithelioid cells, often arranged in a palisade, in direct contact with the implant and surrounded by basement membrane. These cells have round-to-ovoid nuclei with inconspicuous nucleoli and abundant eosinophilic cytoplasm. Their precise nature is not certain, but they appear to be of macrophage origin. On electron microscopic examination, there are two main cell types: phagocytic cells with prominent mitochondria, phagocytic vacuoles, intermediate filaments and filopodia, and secretory-like cells, having prominent endoplasmic reticulum, occasional vesicles and Golgi

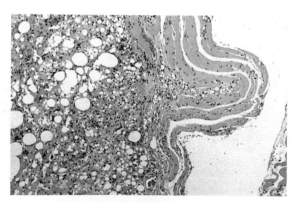

Fig 15.6 Breast tissue surrounding a silicone prosthesis. On the right is a zone of dense collagen, which was in contact with the implant. No synovial-type lining is seen in this field. The outer zone on the left consists of adipose tissue containing globules of silicone, a few chronic inflammatory cells and many vacuolated histiocytes (H&E).

complexes and fewer vacuoles (van Diest *et al.*, 1998). These changes are often called synovial metaplasia, although there are no true synovial cells.

The middle layer comprises dense collagen that often contains globules of silicone. The outer zone consists of well-vascularized adipose tissue containing chronic inflammatory cells, including histiocytes with foamy cytoplasm. Fat necrosis and giant cell reactions to foreign material, such as silicone granulomas, may also be seen. Calcification may be present, particularly around implants that have been present for many years. The synovial-like membrane at the interface with the prosthesis may be flat or villous (Hameed *et al.*, 1995). In the latter case the appearance may resemble detritic synovitis, a reactive process seen around failed orthopaedic devices. Histiocytes, lymphocytes and multinucleate giant cells may infiltrate the villous processes.

The silicone in the breast usually results from gel bleed rather than capsular rupture. Gel bleed is almost invariable and results from a leakage of silicone into the tissues through microscopic pores in the elastomer envelope. Rupture is characterized by nodular tumour-like aggregates of siliconomas, often surrounding large lake-like accumulations of free silicone. The ensuing fibrosis may produce hard lumps and cause considerable distortion of the breast. A large number of lymphocytes and plasma cells may be present around ruptured implants but should not be interpreted as evidence of an immune response. Silicone granulomas may be seen some distance from the implant as a result of the ability of silicone to migrate within the breast. Regional lymph nodes sometimes contain globules of silicone, usually within the cytoplasm of macrophages. Clinical lymphadenopathy may occur if the deposits are extensive enough. The migration of silicone to more distant sites in the body may rarely occur.

Some of the pathological features vary according to the type of implant. Capsules surrounding smooth-surfaced implants have a smooth contour, whereas those around the currently favoured rough-surfaced implants tend to exhibit knob-like projections. Most foreign material is non-polarizing silicone in either liquid or solid form. The former appears as vacuoles, whereas the latter has a curvilinear appearance and is derived from the elastomer bag. Only the latter is demonstrable around saline-filled implants. Polyurethane was previously a constituent of the bags of some prostheses and may be demonstrated in and around the capsules as triangular refractile crystals in histological sections. Dacron or talc may be seen around older implants.

There have been suggestions that breast silicone implants may be associated with generalized illnesses often resembling collagen vascular disorders, but rigorous investigations have concluded that there is an absence of evidence that they cause systemic disease (Rosenbaum, 1998; Sturrock *et al.*, 1998). Similarly, there is no evidence that silicone implants are associated with an increased incidence of breast cancer.

CHANGES DUE TO NEEDLING PROCEDURES

Lee *et al.* (1994) performed a retrospective study of 184 consecutive breast excision specimens from patients with a history of fine needle aspiration. Effects definitely attributable to fine needle aspiration were identified in 17 and included haemorrhage with or without organization in 6, haemosiderin deposition in 7, near destruction of the lesion in 3 and implantation of benign epithelium in 1. Those showing haemorrhage were taken 2–32 days after needling and those exhibiting haemosiderin deposition between 14 and 101 days. The cases in which there was near destruction of the lesion were associated with coagulative necrosis or haematoma and presented significant diagnostic problems. One was thought to be a fibroadenoma, one a papilloma and the third a ductal carcinoma *in situ*. Immunostaining of the devitalized areas for myoepithelial cells was useful in excluding malignancy. The case with displaced benign epithelium was an intraductal papilloma in which scattered epithelial cells exhibiting mild atypia and occasional mitoses formed nests and tubules without lobular grouping in a crescent-shaped zone around the main lesion. Immunostaining was useful in demonstrating a layer of myoepithelial cells around the infiltrative-looking cells. Accurate diagnosis was thus jeopardized by fine needle aspiration in 4 of the 184 cases.

Other authors have reported a displacement of tissue after biopsy and localization procedures. Youngson *et al.* (1994) described 29 surgical breast specimens in which histological examination revealed fragments of benign or malignant epithelium displaced in stroma or in lymphatic or blood vascular lumina following fine needle aspiration, needle core biopsy, needle localization biopsy, suture placement or infiltration with local anaesthetic. A microscopically identifiable needle track was often, but not always, present. The phenomenon presented little diagnostic problem in benign lesions or invasive tumours but caused significant difficulties in cases of *in situ* carcinoma. In view of the rarity of the problem, Youngson *et al.* continued to regard intravascular tumour as evidence of invasion in cases which otherwise appeared to be pure ductal carcinoma *in situ*. Eliciting a history of a needling procedure is clearly important in arriving at the correct interpretation when direct evidence cannot be seen in the histological sections.

The biological and prognostic implications of traumatic malignant epithelial displacement are uncertain. Berg and Robbins (1962) found no difference in 15-year survival between mastectomy patients diagnosed by aspiration biopsy and those diagnosed by open biopsy. Kopans *et al.* (1988) found no evidence of local recurrence that could be attributed to needle localization in 74 patients. The problem with this type of study is that it is probable that any residual carcinoma in the needle track would subsequently have been excised. Nevertheless, it seems unlikely that, by displacing malignant epithelium, needling gives rise to clinically significant metastases that would not otherwise have developed. Eriksson *et al.* (1984) aspirated tumours in mice and found that seeding occurred only under extreme test conditions and that needling was in any case not associated with an increase in death rate from tumour dissemination.

SCLEROSING LYMPHOCYTIC LOBULITIS

Patients with this condition generally present with breast lumps and sometimes pain. Macroscopically, the appearances are variable; there may be an ill-defined zone of fibrosis or a fairly well defined fibrotic nodule. In some cases there may be no discernible gross abnormality.

The lesion is thought to have an autoimmune basis and is characterized by dense, poorly defined zones of collagenous sclerosis and foci of chronic inflammatory cell infiltration around vessels and within lobules, where they are associated with glandular atrophy and intralobular sclerosis (Fig. 15.7). The vessels may show endothelial swelling, but there is no evidence of vasculitis. The changes have been likened to those seen in Sjögren's

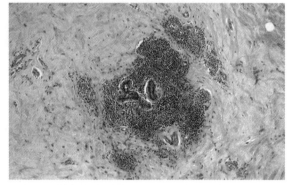

(a)

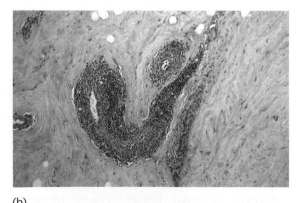

(b)

Fig.15.7 Sclerosing lymphocytic lobulitis. (a) There is dense lymphocytic infiltrate within and around an atrophic lobule. (b) A different field from the same section, showing a similar infiltrate around a collection of small blood vessels. Note the dense stromal sclerosis in each picture (H&E).

syndrome, Hashimoto's thyroiditis and pancreatic 'insulinitis'. Recurrences occasionally occur in the same or contralateral breast and tend to show increasing epithelial atrophy and resolving inflammation.

Immunophenotyping has shown that most of the infiltrating leucocytes are B lymphocytes, with a smaller number of T cells, plasma cells and histiocytes. Although occasional multinucleate cells may be seen, granulomata are not encountered. The breast epithelial cells in the vicinity of the infiltrates express a detectable amount of HLA-DR antigens, a feature that is seen in the normal breast only in pregnancy and lactation. Of those patients whose HLA status has been determined, a disproportionate number have been HLA-DR3, 4 or 5.

A significant number of patients suffer from, or have a family history of, type 1 diabetes mellitus (Soler and Khardori, 1984). The condition thus appears to be identical to that which has been termed diabetic mastopathy (Tomaszewski et al., 1992). In diabetic patients the condition is more common in those with long-standing disease with complications such as nephropathy, retinopathy and neuropathy. Less commonly, the condition is associated with Hashimoto's thyroiditis. Circulating autoantibodies have been detected in about half the cases, usually of the smooth muscle, parietal cell or thyroid microsomal types (Lammie et al., 1991).

ROSAI–DORFMAN DISEASE

Also known as sinus histiocytosis with massive lymphadenopathy, this condition was first described in young patients with greatly enlarged lymph nodes but has since been reported in various extranodal sites, including a few cases in the breast. Hammond et al. (1996) reported the case of 67-year-old woman with a painless, 50 mm, ill-defined mass in the breast suggestive of malignancy on mammography. Histologically, the lesion comprised neutrophil polymorphs, plasma cells, lymphocytes and histiocytes with large vesicular and sometimes multiple nuclei and often prominent nucleoli. These cells had copious foamy, finely granular or densely eosinophilic cytoplasm, often exhibited phagocytosis of lymphocytes and/or plasma cells and were S100 positive on immunostaining.

AMYLOIDOSIS OF THE BREAST

Amyloid deposition in the breast has been infrequently described. It may occur as a solitary mass or as multiple bilateral deposits associated with the amyloidosis of other organs. The latter type may be associated with a plasma cell dyscrasia (Hardy et al., 1979) or systemic disease such as rheumatoid arthritis (Sadeghee and Moore, 1974).

Fernandez and Hernandez (1973) and Walker et al. (1982) have described cases of mammary amyloidosis presenting as a solitary, firm, tender mass. In each study there was no evidence of amyloid deposition elsewhere or of any systemic disease. The amyloid was located around ducts and blood vessels as well as free within the stroma. The material showed green dichroism on Congo red staining and exhibited metachromasia with crystal violet. Ultrastructural studies have shown the characteristic appearance of amyloid. Giant cells, lymphocytes, plasma cells and lymphoplasmacytoid cells often surround the deposits. The ultrastructural demonstration of amyloid within plasma cells suggests a possible derivation from immunoglobulin.

NON-INFECTIOUS GRANULOMAS IN THE BREAST

Fat necrosis

Fat necrosis usually follows trauma, including surgery and needling procedures. It has also been described after radiation therapy (Girling et al., 1990; Coyne et al., 1996). A history of trauma cannot always be obtained in non-iatrogenic cases, which occur more frequently in obese subjects. Focal ischaemia has been suggested as a cause.

Histologically, the necrosis leads to the breaking up of adipocytes, from which fat is liberated and taken up by macrophages that acquire copious vacuolated cytoplasm.

Crystals of lipid may also be seen. The necrotic tissue and lipid material may become surrounded by a giant cell granulomatous reaction that later becomes fibrotic (Fig. 15.8). Deposits of haemosiderin are usually demonstrable, and this, together with the large number of lipophages, serves to distinguish the condition from infective granulomas. Special stains for organisms are negative. In the later sclerotic phases of the process, the lesion feels hard and irregular and may resemble a carcinoma on both clinical palpation and macroscopic pathological examination.

Membranous fat necrosis is a term used to describe a type of fat necrosis characterized by the formation of cysts lined by a membrane with the histochemical features of ceroid (Poppiti *et al.*, 1986). Two forms were noted by Coyne *et al.* (1996): cystic and non-cystic. The former comprised what appeared to be the ghost outlines of adipocytes surrounded by a thick membrane, which was eosinophilic on H&E staining but better demonstrated by oil red O. The latter was more characteristic, consisting of fibrous-walled cysts ranging from 2 to 15 mm in diameter also lined by oil red O-positive membranes. The membranes in both types were frequently undulating. The two types of membranous fat necrosis may co-exist with each other and with usual-type fat necrosis. In Coyne's series membranous fat necrosis was seen after surgery, needling procedures and irradiation.

Foreign body granulomas

Most foreign body granulomas in the breasts are caused by the introduction of prosthetic materials for cosmetic purposes. Symmers (1968) collected a series of cases of foreign body mastitis resulting from a wide range of compounds, including paraffin wax, beeswax, silicone (see above), shellac, silk, putty, spun glass and epoxy resin. Granulomatous reactions have also been seen with polyethylene and polyurethane (Cocke *et al.*, 1975). Oily compounds may produce the typical appearance of an oleogranuloma, rounded empty spaces being surrounded by histiocytes with vacuolated cytoplasm and multinucleate giant cells.

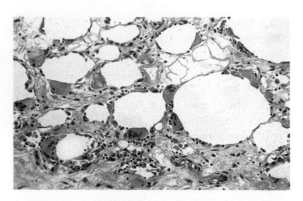

Fig.15.8 Fat necrosis. Fat globules are surrounded by foreign body-type giant cells, lymphocytes and fibrous tissue (H&E).

Trichogranulomatous mastopathy

Goepel (1980) described a case of bleeding from the nipple due to fragments of hair within the breast ducts. There was focal ulceration of the ductal epithelium and bleeding into the lumen. A foreign body giant cell reaction was seen in the periductal tissue where the hair fragments had penetrated the duct wall.

Sarcoidosis

The breast is very rarely involved in sarcoidosis, usually only when other organs are involved (Ross and Merino, 1985). The histological appearances are similar to those seen elsewhere.

Granulomas associated with vascular disease

These are described on p. 275.

Granulomatous mastitis

This is an uncommon and curious condition of unknown aetiology. It occurs in young parous women and presents as a firm tender lump that may be mistaken for carcinoma. All the cases described by Kessler and Wolloch (1972) and Fletcher *et al.* (1982) occurred within 6 years of pregnancy. Histologically, there are discrete, non-caseating granulomata composed of epithelioid histiocytes, giant cells, eosinophils and neutrophils confined to the breast lobules (Fig. 15.9). Damage to the ductular epithelium may also be seen, and there may be neutrophils within the lumina.

The condition may respond to steroids and be associated with a high incidence of postoperative wound infection. It appears to be a

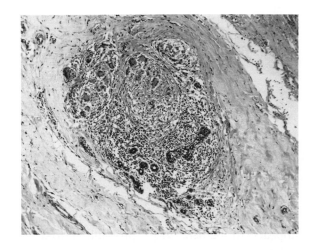

15.9 Granulomatous mastitis. Several non-caseating giant cell granulomata are seen within a breast lobule (H&E).

distinct disease entity as neither organisms nor foreign body material have been identified and patients give no history of trauma or sarcoidosis. Fletcher *et al.* (1982) suggested that the finding of polymorphs in some of the ductular lumina might indicate a primary damage, by some unknown agent, to the epithelium, resulting in a leakage of contents and a subsequent granulomatous response in the surrounding stroma.

MAMMARY DUCT FISTULA (RECURRING SUBAREOLAR ABSCESS)

This condition presents as an eccentric subareolar lump that tends to rupture spontaneously onto the surface of the areola (Patey and Thackray, 1958). Periods of discharge from a small orifice on the areola tend to alternate with periods of quiescence. The lesion does not heal spontaneously, surgical excision being necessary.

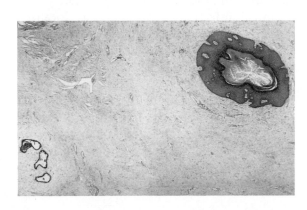

15.10 Mammary duct fistula. On the right is a main subareolar duct exhibiting squamous metaplasia and luminal occlusion by debris and cornified epithelial cells. On the left are normal subareolar ducts (or one duct cut in several places) lined by normal two-layered epithelium (H&E).

Histologically, there is a fistulous track lined by granulation tissue extending from the surface of the areola to a main subareolar mammary duct that exhibits extensive squamous metaplasia (Fig. 15.10). The lumen of the duct is often occluded by debris and cornified epithelial cells. It is not certain whether ductal changes are secondary to the inflammation or the cause of it. Patey and Thackray (1958) favoured the latter explanation, suggesting that the duct may be congenitally abnormal and that the resulting blockage gives rise to a susceptibility to chronic infection.

BACTERIAL INFECTION

Acute pyogenic infection

Most cases of acute pyogenic mastitis occur as a complication of lactation. *Staphylococcus aureus* is the most common pathogen and often produces a breast abscess if antibiotics are not given promptly. The infection may be confined to one segment of the breast. Cases of acute lactational mastitis caused by *Streptococcus pyogenes* have also been reported and tend to exhibit less well localized inflammation. The organisms usually appear to enter the breast from the infant's nasopharynx by a crack in the nipple.

Breast abscesses resulting from *Bacteroides* spp. and *Salmonella typhi* have also been reported in nulliparous women (Barrett and MacDermot, 1972; Hale *et al.*, 1976).

Tuberculosis

Tuberculosis rarely involves the breast, and its incidence has declined considerably in recent years. Ikard and Perkins (1977) found tuberculosis in 0.025% of cases of surgically treated breast disease in Nashville, Tennessee, in the 20-year period up to 1977. A higher incidence, however, could be expected in the economically less well developed parts of the world. The disease usually occurs in women of childbearing age and appears to be more common in parous women. Occasional cases have been reported in males. Tuberculosis may occur in association with AIDS.

Mammary tuberculosis may be primary or secondary; the infection may reach the breast by the haematogenous or lymphatic routes, or sometimes by direct extension from a lesion in the pleura or rib cage.

There are two main pathological forms of the disease: the more usual nodular form and the less common sclerosing type (McKeown and Wilkinson, 1952; Ikard and Perkins, 1977). In the former there are one or multiple discrete nodules composed of giant cell granulomata that eventually undergo caseation to form fluctuant abscesses that may lead to sinus formation. The sclerosing type occurs more commonly in older women and is characterized by a marked fibrous reaction around the granulomata, some of which may become completely hyalinized. Initially there are multiple hard nodules in the breast, but there may later be extensive fibrous replacement of the gland, which may become contracted and distorted. The additional presence of *peau d'orange* and nipple retraction may strengthen the clinical resemblance of this form of tuberculosis to breast carcinoma. Tuberculosis may spread within the breast along the ductal system, and the ducts involved may exhibit epithelial proliferation, necrosis and periductal fibrosis.

As in any other site it is important for the pathologist to identify acid-fast bacilli before making a confident diagnosis as there are many other forms of granulomatous breast disease (see below). Some of the decreased incidence of mammary tuberculosis has been because of the adoption of stricter diagnostic criteria.

There have been several reports of coincident mammary tuberculosis and breast carcinoma, but there is no evidence of a causal relationship.

Leprosy

Although extremely rare, leprosy has been described in the breast and may even present as a mass clinically resembling a carcinoma (Furniss, 1952).

Syphilis

Syphilis may involve the breast in the form of gummatous mastitis that tends to ulcerate. A primary chancre may occasionally develop because of infection acquired by kissing or nursing a child with congenital syphilis (Symmers, 1978).

FUNGAL INFECTION

Actinomycosis

Actinomycosis of the breast is a rarity but appears to be the most common fungal infection of the breast in Great Britain. It may occur as a primary lesion or secondary to disease in the lung by extension through the thoracic cage. In the primary cases the nipple appears to be the most probable portal of entry.

The clinical presentation is usually as a hard lump in the breast, often close to the nipple. Retraction of the nipple may be present and the regional lymph nodes enlarged. The lesion may be painful, but there is usually neither pyrexia nor any elevation of local skin temperature. The clinical picture may thus be strongly suggestive of carcinoma, and, indeed, mastectomy is occasionally performed in error (Gogas *et al.*, 1972). Histologically, there are intercommunicating zones of necrosis and abscess formation containing the characteristic colonies of the fungus. The regional lymph nodes may exhibit intense reactive hyperplasia.

Other fungal infections

Other fungi that have been reported to infect the breast include *Histoplasma capsulatum*, *Blastomyces dermatitidis*, *Cryptococcus neoformans*, *Rhizopus* sp. and *Paracoccidioides brasiliensis* (Symmers, 1968; Salfelder and Schwarz, 1975). Most of these cases have been described in North or South America.

Fungal infections may occur as localized masses within the breast or as part of a disseminated infection, usually in immunosuppressed patients. *Candida* sp. are occasionally encountered in the latter situation. The inflammatory response is usually poor or absent in such subjects. Sometimes, however, fungi may be associated with a marked granulomatous response, which may result in masses or 'pseudotumours' that may be clinically misinterpreted as true neoplasms.

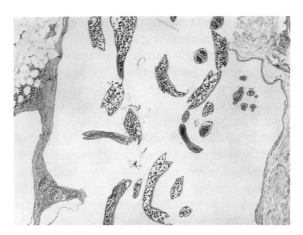

15.11 Filarial worms in dilated deep dermal lymphatics of the breast (H&E).

PARASITIC DISEASE

There have been occasional reports, particularly from the Indian subcontinent, of breast lumps caused by filariasis (Chandrasoma *et al*, 1977; Mukherjee *et al.*, 1977) (Fig. 15.11). Histologically, the worms are usually surrounded by an inflammatory infiltrate of eosinophils, lymphocytes and plasma cells. Foreign body giant cell granulomata may also be seen, and old lesions may exhibit considerable fibrosis. An involvement of the regional lymph nodes, rather than the breast itself, may give rise to breast enlargement and *peau d'orange*.

Rare examples of hydatid disease and cysticercosis (Symmers, 1978) have been reported.

VIRUS INFECTION

There are very few reports of virus infection of the breast. Quinn and Lofberg (1978) reported a case of herpes simplex infection of both nipples in a mother after her 8-day-old breast-fed baby had died of disseminated herpes simplex infection.

MUCOVISCIDOSIS

The breast in mucoviscidosis may show very poor lobular development with some small acinar structures surrounded by markedly thickened and hyalinized basement membrane (Ward, 1972). The interlobular ducts and interlobular stroma appear normal.

OCHRONOSIS

Ochronosis is part of a clinical syndrome characterized by the presence of homogentisic acid in the urine and the deposition of pigment within the soft tissues. It is caused by the presence of an autosomal recessive allele resulting in homogentisic acid oxidase deficiency. The ochronotic pigment may be deposited in the breast as well as in many other sites. There may be concomitant fibrosis and epithelial atrophy, resulting in firm breast masses. The pigment is yellow-brown in H&E-stained sections and may have a diffuse or finely particulate appearance. It is found in smooth muscle and endothelial cells, as well as free within the stroma. The pigment gives staining reactions similar to melanin, being positive with Masson-Fontana and negative with Perls', periodic acid–Schiff and oil red O stains (Lefer and Rosier, 1979).

CHANGES IN REGIONAL LYMPH NODES

The significance of metastatic breast carcinoma in regional nodes is discussed in Chapter 12.

Reactive changes in lymph nodes draining carcinomas

The regional lymph nodes in patients with breast carcinoma may show reactive changes, particularly in the form of sinus histiocytosis and follicular hyperplasia. These changes are usually more pronounced in the nodes of the axilla than in other groups draining the breast. The once generally held belief that tumours excite an immune response that is beneficial to the host stimulated many studies investigating the relationship between changes in the nodes draining breast carcinomas and the course of the disease. The results (like those obtained in studies of lymphoid infiltration in the primary tumour) have been conflicting.

The most widely studied change is sinus histiocytosis. Some workers have found a direct relationship between sinus histiocytosis and survival independent of nodal metastases and the appearance of the primary tumour

(Black *et al.*, 1955), but others have failed to confirm the relationship (Berg, 1956). It has also been claimed that sinus histiocytosis may be related to prognosis only in patients whose tumours exhibit an irregular border or poor differentiation or if there are axillary metastases (DiRe and Lane, 1963; Silverberg *et al.*, 1970). In the most comprehensive study, Fisher *et al.* (1983) examined the lymph nodes from 472 patients undergoing radical mastectomy. They found that survival was not related to the absence or presence of any type of sinus reaction.

There are several possible explanations for these divergent findings. The definition of sinus histiocytosis has varied in terms of the number and type of cells that the sinuses contain (Black and Kwon, 1978; Hartveit, 1982). Mixed patterns may be seen in the same patient or even in the same node. Reactive changes are not evenly distributed throughout the nodes in the same group, finding them being heavily dependent on the number examined. Fisher *et al.* (1983) found that sinus histiocytosis was related to the duration of symptoms and Friedell *et al.* (1983) that it was more common in Japanese than British women, suggesting that racial and/or geographical factors may be important. Finally, it is often forgotten that the axillary nodes drain other sites, particularly the upper limb, and that reactive changes do not necessarily reflect events taking place in the breast.

Follicular hyperplasia with germinal centre formation is a less common change and has attracted less attention. The findings are as inconclusive as those in sinus histiocytosis, for similar reasons.

The lymph nodes draining mammary carcinoma may contain an increased number of mast cells. Thoresen *et al.* (1982) found that the increase occurred largely in node-positive patients in both the tumour and non-tumour-bearing nodes, but this has not been substantiated. Granulomata may rarely be encountered in nodes draining carcinomas of the breast as well as of other organs (Syrjanen, 1981). Their significance is not understood, but they appear to represent a reaction to some aspect of the tumour. It is important to exclude other causes; the granulomata are usually non-necrotizing and thus resemble those of sarcoidosis rather than tuberculosis.

In conclusion a variety of reactive changes may occur in lymph nodes draining mammary carcinomas, but it is very doubtful that they provide the pathologist with any reliable indication of prognosis. Although breast carcinoma is often associated with lymphoreticular responses in both the primary tumour and the regional nodes, the precise nature of the interaction between the tumour and the cells of the lymphoid system is still very poorly understood.

Similarity of sinus histiocytosis and metastatic carcinoma

Metastases from breast carcinoma may remain confined to the sinusoids rather than invading the lymph node substance. This phenomenon may be mistaken for sinus histiocytosis. It appears to occur more frequently with infiltrating lobular carcinomas, in which the relatively bland cytological appearance of the tumour cells may strengthen the resemblance (Fig. 15.12). Attention to cytological detail usually resolves the problem, but immunostaining with histiocytic and epithelial markers may be needed in difficult cases.

The occurrence of sinus histiocytes with signet-ring morphology was first documented by Gould *et al.* (1989) in axillary lymph nodes from a patient with insulin-dependent diabetes mellitus and breast cancer. These signet-ring histiocytes may easily be mistaken for metastatic carcinoma, but they lack cytological atypia and exhibit positivity for histiocytic markers and negativity for cytokeratins (Fig. 15.13).

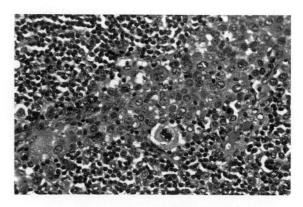

15.12 Metastatic lobular carcinoma confined within a sinusoid of an axillary lymph node, producing a resemblance to sinus histiocytosis. The tumour cells are more pleomorphic than those in the breast. Note the atypical mitosis in the lower centre of the field (H&E).

15.13 Signet-ring sinus histiocytosis. (a) Note the presence of numerous signet-ring cells filling the sinus on the right of the picture. (b) Immunostain for CD68 revealing that the cells are histiocytes. Immunostains for epithelial markers were negative. (Case kindly supplied by Dr Nikiforos Apostolikas.)

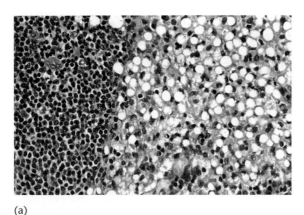

(a)

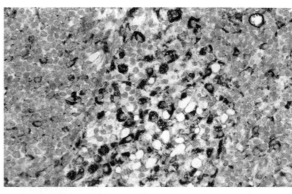

(b)

Guerrero-Medrano *et al.* (1997) found such cells in lymph nodes from 1% of axillary dissection specimens. They were generally negative for mucin and fat, but the vacuoles sometimes contained granular material on electron microscopy.

Ectopic naevus cells

Benign naevus cells may be seen in lymph nodes. They are, however, extremely rare: Ridolfi *et al.* (1977) found them in 0.33% of mastectomy specimens, and Fisher *et al.*(1994) found none in 518 lymph nodes from 41 consecutive axillary clearances using immunostaining for S100. They are usually arranged in small clusters and are cytologically indistinguishable from the cells of ordinary dermal naevi (Fig. 15.14). Their small, uniform, normochromic nuclei distinguish them from metastatic carcinoma, although problems may be encountered with invasive lobular carcinomas (Fisher *et al.*,

15.14 Ectopic naevus cells in an axillary lymph node. The cells are similar to those seen in ordinary cutaneous naevi, and Fontana stains were focally positive. Note that the cells lie in the capsule outside the peripheral sinus (H&E).

1994). About half the cases contain melanin, immunostaining revealing positivity for S100 and negativity for cytokeratins. Another point of distinction is their location in the lymph node capsule rather than in the peripheral sinus, although collections of cells may rarely be seen in the substance of the node.

The origin of these cells is obscure. Aberrant migration from the neural crest in embryological development and 'benign metastasis' after the completion of development have been suggested (Johnson and Helwig, 1969). The absence of cells from the peripheral sinus would seem to argue against the latter mechanism.

Very rare cases have been reported of blue naevi arising in lymph node capsules (Lamovec, 1984).

Breast tissue inclusions

Ectopic breast tissue inclusions in the axillary nodes are even rarer than naevus cells. They may be misinterpreted as metastases, particularly from tumours exhibiting significant tubular differentiation. The inclusions usually take the form of tubules composed of a double layer of cytologically normal cells. Myoepithelial cells can be demonstrated by immunostaining for smooth muscle actin (Fisher *et al.*, 1994). The normal architecture of lobules and interlobular ducts is rarely, if ever, perfectly reproduced (Figs 15.15 and 15.16). The epithelium may reflect changes occurring in the breast. Turner and Millis (1980) described a patient in whom the lymph node inclusions showed epithelial hyperplasia

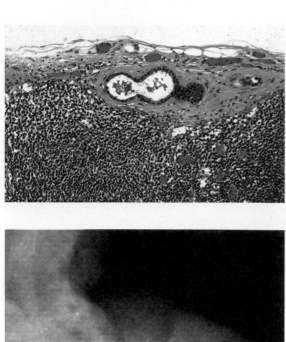

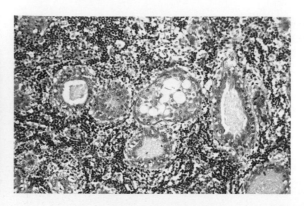

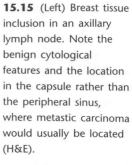

15.15 (Left) Breast tissue inclusion in an axillary lymph node. Note the benign cytological features and the location in the capsule rather than the peripheral sinus, where metastic carcinoma would usually be located (H&E).

15.16 (Right) Another node in which the inclusions exhibit some intraluminal proliferation (H&E).

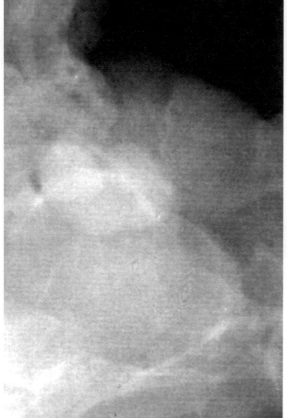

(a)

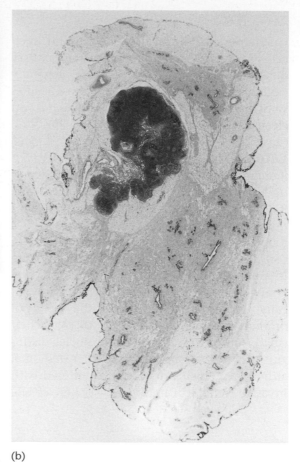

(b)

15.17 Intramammary lymph node detected by mammography. (a) The clinical radiograph shows a well-circumscribed mass resembling a fibro-adenoma. (b) Low-power view of the histological section showing a normal lymph node (H&E).

similar to that seen in the breast. Edlow and Carter (1973) found inclusions showing apocrine and squamous-lined cysts as well as structures resembling normal lobules. Walker and Fechner (1982) described a case of papillary carcinoma that appeared to have arisen in ectopic breast tissue within an axillary lymph node.

Intramammary lymph nodes

It is usual to find a small number of lymph nodes in the axillary tail of the breast; they may also be encountered elsewhere in the gland. Although usually solitary, they are occasionally multiple, as many as nine having been reported involving all four quadrants of the same breast (Egan and McSweeney, 1984). Jadusingh (1992) found 7 intramammary nodes in 5 of 533 routinely examined benign and malignant surgical breast specimens. Four appeared normal, 2 exhibited slight sinus histiocytosis and 1 contained metastatic carcinoma and benign glandular inclusions.

Intramammary lymph nodes may be palpable (Dawson et al., 1987) but are usually detected incidentally in pathological specimens or by mammography, where they appear as well-circumscribed nodules resembling small fibroadenomas (Fig. 15.17). The size has been reported to vary from 3 to 30 mm, but they do not generally exceed 10 mm in size.

Reactive or neoplastic conditions primarily involving the lymph nodes may thus present as a breast mass. Local invasion of the intramammary nodes by a laterally situated carcinoma of the breast should be distinguished from true nodal metastasis.

REFERENCES

Badve S., Sloane J.P. (1995) Pseudoangiomatous hyperplasia of the male breast. *Histopathology*, **26**, 463–6.

Barrett G.S., MacDermot J. (1972) Breast abscess: a rare presentation of typhoid. *Br. Med. J.*, **2**, 628–9.

Berg J.W. (1956) Sinus histiocytosis: a fallacious measure of host resistance to cancer. *Cancer*, **9**, 935–9.

Berg J.W., Robbins G.F. (1962) A late look at the safety of aspiration biopsy. *Cancer*, **15**, 826–7.

Black M.M., Kwon C.S. (1978) Prognostic factors. In Gallagher H.S., Leis H.P., Snyderman R.K. *et al.* (eds) *The Breast*. St Louis, C.V. Mosby.

Black M.M., Opler S.R., Speer F.D. (1955) Survival in breast cancer cases in relation to the structure of the primary tumor and regional lymph nodes. *Surg. Gynecol. Obstet.*, **100**, 543–51.

Chandrasoma P.T., Mendis K.N., Kumararatne D.S. (1977) Microfilarial granuloma of the breast in a patient with tropical pulmonary eosinophilia. *Am. J. Trop. Med. Hyg.*, **26**, 570–1.

Cocke W.M., Leathers H.K., Lynch J.B. (1975) Foreign body reactions to polyurethane covers of some breast prostheses. *Plastic Reconstr. Surg.*, **56**, 527–30.

Coots N.V. (1996) A man with nevoid hyperkeratosis of the areola. *Cutis*, **57**, 354–6.

Coyne J.D., Parkinson D., Baildam A.D. (1996) Membranous fat necrosis of the breast. *Histopathology*, **28**, 61–4.

Davis C.E., Wiley W.B., Faulconer R.J. (1972) Necrosis of the female breast complicating oral anticoagulant treatment. *Ann. Surg.*, **175**, 647–56.

Dawson P.M., Shousha S., Burn J.I. (1987). Lymph nodes presenting as breast lumps. *Br. J. Surg.* **74**, 1167–8.

DiRe J.J., Lane N. (1963) The relation of sinus histiocytosis in axillary lymph nodes to surgical curability of carcinoma of the breast. *Am. J. Clin. Pathol.*, **40**, 508–15.

Edlow D.W., Carter D. (1973) Heterotopic epithelium in axillary lymph nodes: report of a case and review of the literature. *Am. J. Clin. Pathol.*, **59**, 666–73.

Eriksson O., Hagmar B., Ryd W. (1984) Effects of fine-needle aspiration and other biopsy procedures on tumour dissemination in mice. *Cancer*, **54**, 73–8.

Facina G., de Lima G.R., Simoes M.J., Novo N.F., Gebrim L.H. (1997) Estrogenic activity of tamoxifen on normal mammary parenchyma in the luteal phase of the menstrual cycle. *Int. J. Gynaecol. Obstet.*, **56**, 19–24.

Fernandez B.B., Hernandez F.J. (1973) Amyloid tumor of the breast. *Arch. Pathol.*, **95**, 102–5.

Fisher C.J., Hanby A.M., Robinson L., Millis R.R. (1992). Mammary hamartoma – a review of 35 cases. *Histopathology*, **20**, 99–106.

Fisher C.J., Hill S., Millis R.R. (1994) Benign lymph node inclusions mimicking metastatic carcinoma. *J. Clin. Pathol.*, **47**, 245–7.

Fisher E.R., Kotwal N., Hermann C., Fisher B. (1983) Types of tumor lymphoid response and sinus histiocytosis: relationship to five-year, disease-free survival in patients with breast cancer. *Arch. Pathol. Lab. Med.*, **107**, 222–7.

Fletcher A., Magrath I.M., Riddell R.H., Talbot I.C. (1982) Granulomatous mastitis: a report of seven cases. *J. Clin. Pathol.*, **35**, 941–5.

Forman L. (1943) Acanthosis nigricans with discrete warts and marked mucous membrane changes in a patient with vitiligo. *Proc. Roy. Soc. Med.*, **36**, 611.

Friedell G.H., Soto E.A., Kumaoka S., Hirota T., Hayward J.L., Bulbrook R.D. (1983) Pathology of primary tumors and axillary lymph nodes in British and Japanese women with breast cancer. *Breast Cancer Res. Treat.*, **3**, 165–9.

Furniss A.L. (1952) Leproma in female breast presenting as carcinoma. *Ind. Med. Gaz.*, **87**, 304.

Garcia R.L. (1973) Verrucose areolar hyperpigmentation of pregnancy. *Arch. Dermatol.*, **107**, 774.

Girling A.C., Hanby A., Millis R.R. (1990) Radiation and other changes in breast tissue after conservation treatment for carcinoma. *J. Clin. Pathol.* **43**, 152–6.

Goepel J.R. (1980) Trichogranulomatous mastopathy: an unusual cause of bleeding from the nipple. *Postgrad. Med. J.*, **56**, 850–1.

Gogas J., Sechas M., Diamantis S., Sbokos C. (1972) Actinomycosis of the breast. *Int. Surg.*, **57**, 664–5.

Gould E., Perez J., Albores-Saavedra J., Legaspi A. (1989) Signet ring cell sinus histiocytosis: a previously unrecognised condition mimicking metastatic adenocarcinoma in lymph nodes. *Am. J. Clin. Pathol.*, **92**, 509.

Graham D.F. (1972) Eczema of the nipple. *Trans. St John's Hosp. Derm. Soc.*, **58**, 98–9.

Guerrero-Medrano J., Delgado R., Albores-Saavedra J. (1997) Signet-ring sinus histiocytosis. A reactive disorder that mimics metastatic adenocarcinoma. *Cancer*, **80**, 277–85.

Gump F.E., Sternschein M.J., Wolff M. (1981) Fibromatosis of the breast. *Surg. Gynecol. Obstet.*, **153**, 57–60.

Haagensen C.D. (1971) *Diseases of the Breast*, 2nd edn. London, W.B. Saunders.

Haggitt R.C., Booth J.L. (1970) Bilateral fibromatosis of the breast in Gardner's syndrome. *Cancer*, **25**, 161–6.

Hale J.E., Perinpanayagam R.M., Smith G. (1976) Bacteroides: an unusual cause of breast abscess. *Lancet*, **ii**, 70–1.

Hameed M.R., Erlandson R., Rosen P.P. (1995) Capsular synovial-like hyperplasia around mammary implants similar to detritic synovitis. *Am. J. Surg. Pathol.*, **19**, 433–8.

Hammond L.A., Keh C., Rowlands D.C. (1996) Rosai–Dorfman disease of the breast. *Histopathology*, **29**, 582–4.

Hardy T.J., Myerowitz R.L., Bender B.L. (1979) Diffuse parenchymal amyloidosis of lungs and breast. *Arch. Pathol. Lab. Med.*, **103**, 583–5.

Hartveit F. (1982) The sinus reaction in the axillary nodes in breast cancer related to tumour size and nodal state. *Histopathology*, **6**, 753–64.

Hurst J.L., Mega J.F., Hogg J.P. (1998) Tamoxifen-induced regression of breast cysts. *Clin. Imaging*, **22**, 95–8.

Ikard R.W., Perkins D. (1977) Mammary tuberculosis: a rare modern disease. *Southern Med. J.*, **70**, 208–12.

Jadusingh I.H. (1992) Intramammary lymph nodes. *J. Clin. Pathol.*, **45**, 1023–206.

Johnson W.T., Helwig E.B. (1969) Benign nevus cells in the capsule of lymph nodes. *Cancer*, **23**, 747–53.

Jordan J.M., Rowe W.T., Allen N.B. (1987) Wegener's granulomatosis involving the breast. Report of three cases and review of the literature. *Am. J. Med.*, **83**, 159–64.

Kafkasli A., Erdem F., Muezzinoglu B., *et al.* (1998) Side effects of tamoxifen in oophorectomized rats. *Gynecol. Obstet. Invest.*, **45**, 93–8.

Kasper C.S. (1998) Pathology of breast implant capsules. *Semin. Breast Dis.*, **1**, 168–75.

Kennedy S., Merino M.J., Swain S.M., Lippman M.E. (1990) The effects of hormonal and chemotherapy on tumoral and nonneoplastic breast tissue. *Hum. Pathol.*, **21**, 631–7.

Kessler E., Wolloch Y. (1972) Granulomatous mastitis: a lesion clinically simulating carcinoma. *Am. J. Clin. Pathol.*, **58**, 642–6.

Kopans D.B., Gallagher W.J., Swann C.A. *et al.* (1988) Does preoperative needle localization lead to an increase in local breast cancer recurrence? *Radiology*, **167**, 667–8.

Lammie G.A., Bobrow L.G., Staunton M..D.M., Levison D.A., Page G., Millis R.R. (1991) Sclerosing lymphocytic lobulitis of the breast -evidence for an autoimmune pathogenesis. *Histopathology*, **19**, 13–20.

Lamovec J. (1984) Blue nevus of the lymph node capsule. *Am. J. Clin. Pathol.*, **81**, 367–72.

Lee KC., Chan J.K.C., Ho L.C. (1994) Histologic changes in the breast after fine-needle aspiration. *Am. J. Surg. Pathol.*, **18**, 1039–47.

Lefer L.G., Rosier R.P. (1979) Ochronosis in the breast. *Am. J. Clin. Pathol.*, **71**, 349–52.

Lucey J.J. (1975) Spontaneous infarction of the breast. *J. Clin. Pathol.*, **28**, 937–43.

Mayers M.M., Evans P., MacVicar D. (1994) Ossifying fibromatosis of the breast. *Clin. Radiol.*, **49**, 211–2.

McCarty D.J., Imbrigia J., Hung J.K. (1968) Vasculitis of the breasts. *Arthritis Rheum.*, **11**, 796–803.

McKeown K.C., Wilkinson K.W. (1952) Tuberculous disease of the breast. *Br. J. Surg.*, **39**, 420–9.

Mehregan H., Rahbari H. (1977) Hyperkeratosis of nipple and areola. *Arch. Dermatol.*, **113**, 1691–2.

Mokbel K.M., Benson J.R., Fisher C., Baum M. (1994) Nodular fasciitis. II. A rare cause of a lump in the breast in a 44-year-old woman. *Breast*, **3**, 50–1.

Mondor H. (1939) Tronculite sous-cutanée subaigue de la paroi thoracique antero-laterale. *Mem. Acad. Chir.*, **65**, 1271–8.

Mukherjee D.R., Gupta A., Sengupta P. (1977) Solitary filarial breast lump. *J. Ind. Med. Assoc.*, **69**, 36–8.

Pambakian H., Tighe J.R. (1971) Breast involvement in Wegener's granulomatosis. *J. Clin. Pathol.*, **24**, 343–7.

Patey D.H., Thackray A.C. (1958) Pathology and treatment of mammary duct fistula. *Lancet*, **ii**, 871–3.

Poeze M., von Meyenfeldt M.F., Peterse J.L. *et al.* (1998) Increased proliferative activity and p53 expression in normal glandular breast tissue after radiation therapy. *J. Pathol.*, **185**, 32–7.

Poppiti R.J., Margulies M., Cabello B., Rywlin A.M. (1986) Membranous fat necrosis. *Am. J. Surg. Pathol.*, **10**, 62–9.

Powell C.M., Cranor M.L., Rosen P.P. (1995) Pseudoangiomatous stromal hyperplasia (PASH): a mammary stromal tumour with myofibroblastic differentiation. *Am. J. Surg. Pathol.*, **19**, 270–7.

Quinn P.T., Lofberg J.V. (1978) Maternal herpetic breast infection: another hazard of neonatal herpes simplex. *Med. J. Aust.*, **3**, 411–12.

Ridolfi RL, Rosen PP, Thaler H. (1977) Nevus cell aggregates associated with lymph nodes: estimated frequency and clinical significance. *Cancer*, **39**, 164–71.

Rosen P.P. (1979) Multinucleated mammary stromal giant cells: a benign lesion that simulates invasive carcinoma. *Cancer*, **44**, 1305–8.

Rosen P.P., Ernsberger D. (1989) Mammary fibromatosis – a benign spindle-cell tumor with significant risk for local recurrence. *Cancer*, **63**, 1363–9.

Rosen Y., Papasozomenos S.C., Gardner B. (1978) Fibromatosis of the breast. *Cancer*, **41**, 1409–13.

Rosenbaum J.T. (1998) Silicone-associated disease: a SAD chapter in American medicine. *Semin. Breast Dis.*, **1**, 205–4.

Ross M.J., Merino M.J. (1985) Sarcoidosis of the breast. *Hum. Pathol.*, **16**, 185–7.

Sadeghee S.A., Moore S.W. (1974) Rheumatoid arthritis, bilateral amyloid tumors of the breast, and multiple cutaneous amyloid nodules. *Am. J. Clin. Pathol.*, **62**, 472–6.

Salfelder K., Schwarz J. (1975) Mycotic 'pseudotumors' of the breast: report of four cases. *Arch. Surg.*, **110**, 751–4.

Schwartz R.A. (1978) Hyperkeratosis of nipple and areola. *Arch. Dermatol.*, **114**, 1844–5.

Silverberg S.G., Chitale A.R., Hind A.D., Frazier A.B., Levitt S.H. (1970) Sinus histiocytosis and mammary carcinoma: study of 366 radical mastectomies and an historical review. *Cancer*, **26**, 1177–85.

Soler N.G., Khardori R. (1984) Fibrous disease of the breast, thyroiditis, and cheiroarthropathy in type I diabetes mellitus. *Lancet* 1, 193–5.

Sourla A., Luo S., Labrie C., Belanger A., Labrie F., (1997) Morphological changes induced by 6-month treatment of intact and ovariectomized mice with tamoxifen and the pure antiestrogen EM-800. *Endocrinology*, **138**, 5605–17.

Sturrock R.D., Batchelor J.R., Harpwood V. *et al.* (1998) *Silicone Gel Implants: The Report of the Independent Review Group*. London, .

Symmers W. StC. (1968) Silicone mastitis in 'topless' waitresses and some other varieties of foreign-body mastitis. *Br. Med. J.*, **3**, 19–22.

Symmers W. StC. (1978) Rarer infections of the breasts. In *Systemic Pathology*, 2nd edn. London, Churchill Livingstone.

Syrjanen K.J. (1981) Epithelioid cell granulomas in the lymph nodes draining human cancer: ultrastructural findings of a breast cancer case. *Diagn. Histopathol.*, **4**, 291–4.

Thoresen S., Tangen M., Hartveit F. (1982) Mast cells in the axillary nodes of breast cancer patients. *Diagn. Histopathol.*, **5**, 65–7.

Tomaskewski J.E., Brooks J.S.J., Hicks D., Livolsi V.A. (1992). Diabetic mastopathy: a distinctive clinicopathologic entity. *Hum. Pathol.*, **23**, 780–6.

Turner D.R., Millis R.R. (1980) Breast tissue inclusions in axillary lymph nodes. *Histopathology*, **4**, 631–6.

Uehara J., Nazario A.C., Rodrigues de Lima G., Simoes M.J., Juliano Y., Gebrim L.H. (1998) Effects of tamoxifen on the breast in the luteal phase of the menstrual cycle. *Int. J. Gynaecol. Obstet.*, **62**, 77–82.

Van Diest P.J., Beekman W.H., Hage J.J. (1998). Pathology of silicone leakage from breast implants. *J. Clin. Pathol.*, **51**, 493–7.

Verhagen H. (1954) Local haemorrhage and necrosis of the skin and underlying tissues, during anticoagulant therapy with dicumarol or dicumacyl. *Acta Med. Scand.*, **148**, 453–67.

Vuitch M.F., Rosen P.P., Erlandson R.A. (1986) Pseudoangiomatous hyperplasia of mammary stroma. *Hum. Pathol.*, **17** (2), 185–91.

Walker A.N., Fechner R.E. (1982) Papillary carcinoma arising from ectopic breast tissue in an axillary lymph node. *Diagn. Gynecol. Obstet.*, **4**, 141–5.

Walker A.N., Fechner R.E., Callicott J.H. (1982) Amyloid tumor of the breast. *Diagn. Gynecol. Obstet.*, **4**, 339–41.

Ward A.M. (1972) The structure of the breast in mucoviscidosis. *J. Clin. Pathol.*, **25**, 119–22.

Wargotz E.S., Norris H.J., Austin R.M., Enzinger F.M. (1987) Fibromatosis of the breast: a clinical and pathological study of 28 cases. *Am. J. Surg. Pathol.*, **11** (1), 38–45.

Waugh T.R. (1950) Bilateral mammary arteritis: report of a case. *Am. J. Pathol.*, **26**, 85–61.

Youngson B.J., Cranor M., Rosen P.P. (1994) Epithelial displacement in surgical breast specimens following needling procedures. *Am. J. Surg. Pathol.*, **18** (9), 896–903.

16 The male breast

INTRODUCTION

The male breast resembles that of the prepubertal female, consisting of ducts of interlobular size lined by epithelial and myoepithelial cells embedded in a fibroadipose stroma. Lactiferous sinuses are absent, and there is no formation of terminal duct–lobular units (Fig. 16.1). Lobular lesions such as cysts, sclerosing adenosis and atypical lobular hyperplasia are thus virtually unknown in the male. Apocrine metaplasia has, however, occasionally been found in otherwise normal male breasts (Andersen and Gram, 1982a). The author is

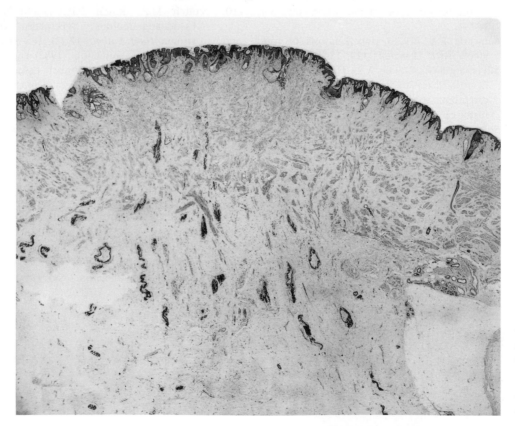

16.1 Normal male breast. The epithelium consists entirely of widely spaced, two-layered ducts without lobule formation. Note the large number of smooth muscle bundles superficially (H&E).

unaware of any convincing examples of fibroadenoma in the male breast, although these and other lobular lesions could conceivably occur in breasts exhibiting gynaecomastia with lobule formation (see below). Reingold and Ascher (1970) and Pantoja *et al.* (1976) reported cases of phyllodes tumour in males, both with gynaecomastia.

Ductal lesions such as duct ectasia (Tedeschi and McCarthy, 1974) and intraduct papilloma (Simpson and Barson, 1969; Giltman, 1981) are occasionally reported, and hyperplasia of usual type frequently forms part of the spectrum of changes in gynaecomastia (see below).

Tumours and other lesions not specific for the breast may occur in males and females, and are discussed individually in Chapters 14

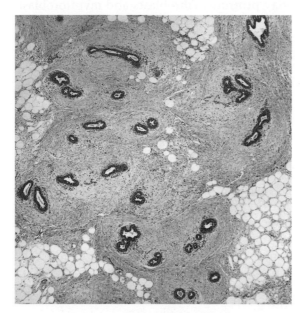

16.2 Active phase of gynaecomastia. The stroma shows increased cellularity, particularly around the ducts, which exhibit dilatation and hyperplasia of usual type (H&E).

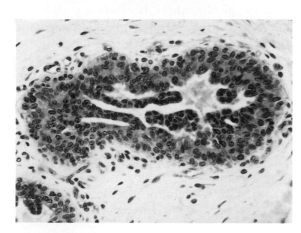

16.3 Detail of Fig. 16.2 showing hyperplasia of usual type (H&E).

and 15. Sarcomas occurring in males may have a better prognosis in view of their earlier presentation.

The two most common lesions in the male breast are gynaecomastia and carcinoma; these are discussed in more detail below.

GYNAECOMASTIA

The term gynaecomastia is used to describe the benign, non-neoplastic enlargement of male breast tissue. The clinical and histological appearances are somewhat variable, and some of the features of gynaecomastia may also be found in normal breasts at autopsy (Andersen and Gram, 1982a). Problems may thus arise in defining the condition precisely at the histological level, a situation similar to that seen with benign epithelial alterations in the female breast (see Chapter 6).

Clinically, the breast may be well formed, resembling that of a young adolescent female in appearance and consistency. Alternatively, there may be a firm, mobile, discoid subareolar plaque (Hamer, 1975). The age incidence is bimodal, peaks occurring in adolescence and middle age. About 75% of cases are unilateral, and about 25% regress spontaneously.

Gynaecomastia may be associated with other endocrine disorders, such as hyperthyroidism, pituitary disorders and tumours of the adrenal, testis and prostate. The association with prostate carcinoma is especially likely to occur with endocrine therapy. Other disorders that have been associated with gynaecomastia include Klinefelter's syndrome, malnutrition, diabetes and many chronic debilitating, cardiac, pulmonary, renal and hepatic disorders. A number of drugs, including chlorpromazine, spironolactone, amphetamines and digitalis, have also been linked with gynaecomastia (Hamer, 1975).

The histological changes in gynaecomastia have been divided into the active, inactive and intermediate phases (Bannayan and Hajdu, 1972; Andersen and Gram, 1982b). In the active type (Figs 16.2 and 16.3), the ducts are increased in number and usually exhibit some degree of dilatation. Intraductal epithelial proliferation is seen and is essentially similar in appearance to hyperplasia of usual type in the female. The stroma is cellular, vascular and often myxoid, particularly around the ducts. There may be an increase in the number of lymphocytes and plasma cells.

In the inactive form there is neither a perceptible increase in the number of ducts nor evidence of significant epithelial hyperplasia. The stroma is hyalinized and usually extensively replaces the mammary adipose tissue. There are no special features in the periductal stroma. About one third of cases show an appearance intermediate between these of the active and inactive forms.

Multinucleated stromal giant cells, similar to those seen in the female breast, may occasionally be encountered in gynaecomastia (Campbell, 1992). Pseudoangiomatous hyperplasia may also be observed. As this change is usually seen in the intermediate phase, it has been suggested that it may represent a stage in the maturation of newly formed breast stroma (Badve and Sloane, 1995).

These different histological forms of gynaecomastia appear to be related to the duration of symptoms rather than aetiology. Andersen and Gram (1982b) found no examples of the active form in patients who had had symptoms for more than 12 months.

True lobules, indistinguishable from those seen in the normal female breast, have occasionally been reported in gynaecomastia, and some have exhibited secretory changes not unlike those seen in pregnancy. Most cases with lobular development have occurred in patients with prostate carcinoma on long-term stilboestrol therapy (Schwartz and Wilens, 1963).

Foci of atypical hyperplasia verging on cribriform intraduct carcinoma were seen in 7% of the cases reported by Andersen and Gram (1982b). This change appears to be incidental as the same authors found a similar incidence in an unselected autopsy series (1982a). Clinically undisclosed atypical hyperplasia and ductal carcinoma *in situ* thus occur in a small proportion of otherwise normal males as well as females. There is no convincing evidence that gynaecomastia is precancerous (see below).

Ultrastructural studies (Hassan and Olaizola, 1979) of gynaecomastia have shown that the intraductal proliferation consists of epithelial and myoepithelial cells. The former exhibit surface microvilli and contain few mitochondria, inconspicuous Golgi apparatus and a number of short profiles of rough endoplasmic reticulum. Intracytoplasmic lumina have been observed in some cells, and occasional cells containing tonofilaments and keratohyaline-like granules have been observed. (Squamous metaplasia at the histological level has also been seen in otherwise normal breasts at autopsy; see Andersen and Gram, 1982b.) The basement membrane around the ducts may show splitting and exhibit occasional small gaps through which epithelial cells may protrude. Fibroblasts and myofibroblasts may be seen in the stroma.

MYOFIBROBLASTOMA

Most examples of this tumour have been described in men, a few of whom have had concomitant gynaecomastia (Wargotz *et al.*, 1987). An increasing number are, however, being described in women (Hamele-Bena *et al.*, 1996). The age at presentation ranges from about 40 to 85 years, with an average in the early 60s. Clinically, the tumour appears as a solitary, nodular, mobile, painless, well-demarcated mass. The size is usually less than 30 mm, but Ali *et al.* (1994) have reported a case of giant myofibroblastoma that measured 100 mm and weighed 169 g.

Histologically, there is often a pseudocapsule. The cells are slender, spindle-shaped and arranged haphazardly or in swirling fascicles among broad bands of hyalinized collagen (Fig. 16.4). They generally have ovoid vesicular nuclei with one or two discernible nuclei. Mitoses are rare (up to two per 10 high-power fields). Necrosis and calcification are not seen. Stromal mast cells are generally conspicuous. Very occasional tumours contain mature cartilage or adipocytes, the case described by Magro *et al.* containing pleomorphic lipoma-like areas. A haemangiopericytoma-like

16.4 (a) Myofibroblastoma showing groups of benign spindle cells separated by bundles of coarse collagen fibres (H&E). (b) The same tumour immunostained for androgen receptors, showing extensive nuclear positivity. This tumour was also positive for oestrogen and progesterone receptors.

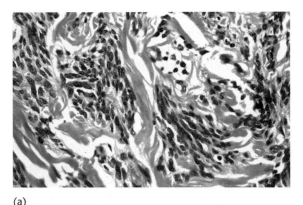

(a)

(b)

pattern similar to that seen in solitary fibrous tumours has also been described in some cases (Magro *et al.*, 1999) and it has indeed been argued that myofibroblastomas of the breast should be regarded as solitary fibrous tumours (Damiani *et al* 1994). Typical smooth muscle cells are not usually present although leiomyoma-like areas were described in the case reported by Thomas *et al.* (1997). The myofibroblastic nature of the neoplastic cells is revealed by electron microscopy, on which myofilaments arranged in dense bodies or plaques are usually seen.

Immunostaining usually shows positivity for vimentin and smooth muscle actin, and about one third of cases are positive for desmin; S100 and cytokeratin staining is negative. Interestingly, the tumours are usually positive for androgen receptors (Fig. 16.4) (Morgan and Pitha, 1998), a situation analogous to the oestrogen and progesterone receptor positivity of pseudoangiomatous hyperplasia of the female breast. More recently, it has been recognized that myofibroblastomas may also express oestrogen and progesterone receptors.

A number of benign tumours enter into the differential diagnosis. Fasciitis is excluded by its non-encapsulated, stellate outline, plumper cells and generally mucoid stroma. Fibromatosis is also poorly circumscribed, and the cells are not clustered. Nerve sheath tumours usually exhibit more slender cytoplasmic processes and irregular nuclei and, in the case of neurilemmoma, Antoni A and B areas. They are also generally S100 positive. Leiomyomas are classically composed of cells

with blunt-ended nuclei and more copious amounts of deeply eosinophilic cytoplasm; furthermore, they show stronger and more diffuse desmin positivity. Malignant mesenchymal breast tumours (spindle cell sarcomas and carcinomas, malignant fibrous histiocytomas, etc.) exhibit greater cellularity, mitotic activity and pleomorphism as well as poorer circumscription and, frequently, necrosis. It should be noted that some sarcomas exhibit myofibroblastic differentiation.

Immunostaining for steroid receptors may be useful in resolving the differential diagnosis. Morgan and Pitha (1998) found smooth muscle tumours, fibromatosis, dermatofibrosarcoma protuberans and monophasic synovial sarcomas to be negative.

Inflammatory myofibroblastic tumour (inflammatory pseudotumour) rarely occurs in the breast (Pettinato *et al.*, 1988; Al-Nafussi, 1999). The myofibroblasts are admixed with inflammatory cells including plasma cells and eosinophils. The lesion is circumscribed, varies in greatly in size and is often associated with constitutional symptoms. It is considered to be a neoplasm as cases have been found to be clonal.

Three histological patterns have been described. The first consists of loosely arranged plump myofibroblasts in a vascular myxoid matrix with chronic inflammatory cells and eosinophils. The second is composed of more compact spindle cells and a variable number of inflammatory cells. The third has a scar-like appearance, being poorly cellular and exhibiting dense collagen and occasionally calcification and osseous metaplasia.

Inflammatory cells are sparse in this variant. Recurrence may occur after inadequate surgical excision.

ADENOMYOEPITHELIOMA

A case of adenomyoepithelioma presenting as a well-circumscribed 10 mm mass arising under the nipple in a 47-year-old man was described by Tamura *et al.* (1993). Histologically, there was a proliferation of spindle cells exhibiting fasciculated or storiform growth patterns around the mammary ducts. A few mitoses were seen. The spindle cells were positive for S100, cytokeratin and actin.

MALE BREAST CARCINOMA

About 1% of breast carcinomas occur in males, accounting for about 0.7% of all cancers in men (Holleb *et al.*, 1968). The incidence, unlike that of female breast cancer, does not appear to have increased over the past 40 years (see Crichlow and Galt, 1990). The disease is rare in young men, only 6% of sufferers being under the age of 40. The peak age incidence is about 5–10 years older than in females. Bilaterality is less common. A number of studies have found that the prognosis is worse for male than female breast cancer in terms of both overall and disease-free survival, even when corrected for stage at presentation (Ciatto *et al.*, 1990).

The aetiology, as in female breast carcinoma, is obscure, although there is an increased incidence in males who inherit mutations of the *BRCA-2* gene (Thorlacius *et al.*, 1995), and there appears to be a significantly increased risk in patients with Klinefelter's syndrome (Jackson *et al.*, 1965; Scheike *et al.*, 1973). Although breast carcinoma has been reported in males treated by irradiation for gynaecomastia (Crichlow, 1972), it is now generally accepted that gynaecomastia *per se* is not associated with an increased risk of malignancy.

The presenting symptom is usually of a lump in the breast, but there is occasionally nipple discharge or retraction. Skin infiltration and Paget's disease are more common in men, presumably because of the smaller size of the male breast. Melanin pigmentation has been reported in Paget's disease in the male, as it has in a small minority of cases in the female. These cases may mimic malignant melanoma both clinically and histopathologically (Stretch *et al.*, 1991).

All varieties of *in situ* and infiltrating female breast carcinoma (see Chapters 8 and 11) may also occur in the male and generally with a similar relative frequency (Treves and Holleb, 1955; Norris and Taylor, 1969; Simpson and Barson, 1969; Crichlow, 1974). Even secretory carcinomas have been described (Roth *et al.*,1988). Costa and Silverberg (1989) reported a case of oncocytic carcinoma. Two exceptions are lobular carcinoma *in situ*, which is very rare or non-existent, and carcinomas exhibiting neuroendocrine differentiation, which appear to be more common (Scopsi *et al.*, 1991; Alm *et al.*, 1992).

Scopsi *et al.* (1991) studied 134 consecutive male patients with breast cancer and found that 28 (20.8%) contained argyrophil cells, as detected by Grimelius staining. On immunostaining 17 of the 28 contained chromogranin B-positive cells, 4 of which also exhibited chromogranin A positivity. An ultrastructural examination of three cases revealed the presence of classic dense-core granules. Histologically, most tumours were expansile and highly cellular, with scanty fibrillary stroma. They were composed of uniform cells arranged in an organoid fashion with peripheral palisading as well as glandular and pseudofollicular structures. In half the cases alcianophilic material could be demonstrated within the cytoplasm of a minority of cells. Disease-free survival was comparable to that of patients with ordinary invasive ductal (nst, that is, no special type) carcinomas. In a later study Alm *et al.* (1992) found evidence of neuroendocrine differentiation in 45% of male breast carcinomas, as judged by immunopositivity for chromogranin. A proportion of cases were examined ultrastructurally, and dense-core granules were found.

At the time of writing there appear to be no convincing reports of lobular carcinoma *in situ* in males, although occasional examples of infiltrating lobular carcinoma have been reported. These tumours are cytologically indistinguishable from those seen in females and exhibit the same types of growth pattern, with single files and targetoid arrangements around ducts. In one case reported by Giffler and Kay (1976), there was also gynaecomastia with an incomplete formation of lobules, which contained cells similar to those of the infiltrating tumour. The appearances fell short of lobular carcinoma *in situ*, however. In Giffler and Kay's other case, there was no evidence of gynaecomastia.

The difference between lobular and ductal carcinoma is discussed in Chapters 8, 9 and 11, being based essentially on differences in cytology and growth pattern rather than on the precise point of origin from the glandular tree. Many ductal carcinomas in the female appear to arise from the terminal duct–lobular units, and, similarly, some lobular carcinomas may arise from small ducts proximal to the lobule. The occurrence of infiltrating lobular carcinoma in males, in whom lobular carcinoma *in situ* does not appear to occur, is further evidence that this tumour cannot be defined simply in terms of site of origin.

The prognosis of male carcinoma is related to the same histological factors as is that in females, particularly axillary lymph node involvement and tumour size and grade (Norris and Taylor, 1969).

Although the histological features of breast carcinoma in the male are similar to those in the female, some of the molecular characteristics appear to be different. Oestrogen receptor positivity is more frequent in carcinomas in the male, occurring in over 80% of tumours. This probably reflects the higher percentage of oestrogen receptor-positive cells in the male (Shoker *et al.*, 1999). As in the female there is a strong association between oestrogen receptor positivity and response to endocrine therapy (Friedman *et al.*, 1981). A similar proportion of tumours is positive for progesterone and androgen receptors (Rayson *et al.*, 1998). The reciprocal relationship between the oestrogen receptor and the epidermal growth factor receptor (EGFR) that characterizes female breast carcinoma does not appear to occur in the male as EGFR expression is also encountered in about three quarters of cases (Fox *et al.*, 1992). Rayson *et al.* (1998) found immunopositivity for c-erbB-2 in 29% of male breast carcinomas, for p53 in 21%, for cyclin D1 in 58% and for bcl-2 in 94%.

Loss of heterozygosity (allelic imbalance) is common in male breast cancer. Chuaqui *et al.* (1995) found a high incidence of loss of heterozygosity at two discrete loci on chromosome 8p.

REFERENCES

Ali S., Teichberg S., DeRisi D.C., Urmacher C. (1994) Giant myofibroblastoma of the breast. *Am. J. Surg. Pathol.*, **18**, 1170–76.

Alm P., Alumets J., Bak-Jensen E., Olsson H. (1992) Neuroendocrine differentiation in male breast carcinomas. *APMIS*, **100**, 720–6.

Al-Nafussi A. (1999) Spindle cell tumours of the breast. *Histopathology*, **35**, 1–13.

Andersen J.A., Gram J.B. (1982a) Gynecomasty: histological aspects in a surgical material. *Acta Pathol. Microbiol. Immunol. Scand.*, **90**, 185–90.

Andersen J.A., Gram J.B. (1982b) Male breast at autopsy. *Acta Pathol. Microbiol. Immunol. Scand.*, **90**, 191–7.

Badve S., Sloane J.P. (1995) Pseudoangiomatous hyperplasia of the male breast. *Histopathology*, **26**, 463–6.

Bannayan G.A., Hajdu S.I. (1972) Gynecomastia: clinicopathologic study of 351 cases. *Am. J. Clin. Pathol.*, **57**, 431–7.

Campbell A.P. (1992) Multinucleated stromal giant cells in adolescent gynaecomastia. *J. Clin. Pathol.*, **45**, 443–4.

Chuaqui R.F., Sanz-Ortega J., Vocke C. *et al.* (1995) Loss of heterozygosity on the short arm of chromosome 8 in male breast carcinomas. *Cancer Res.*, **55**, 4995–8.

Ciatto S., Iossa A., Pacini P. (1990) Male breast carcinoma: review of a multicenter series of 150 cases. *Tumori*, **76**, 555–8.

Costa M.J., Silverberg S.G. (1989) Oncocytic carcinoma of the male breast. *Arch. Pathol.*, **113**, 1396–9.

Crichlow R.W. (1972) Carcinoma of the male breast. *Surg. Gynecol. Obstet.*, **134**, 1011–19.

Crichlow R.W. (1974) Breast cancer in men. *Semin. Oncol.*, **1**, 145–52.

Crichlow R.W., Galt S.W. (1990) Male breast cancer. *Surg. Clin. North Am.*, **70**, 1165–77.

Damiani S., Miettinen M., Peterse J.L., Eusebi V. (1994) Solitary fibrous tumour (myofibroblastoma) of the breast. *Virchows Archiv*, **425**, 89–92.

Fox S.B., Day C.A., Rogers S. (1991) Lack of c-erbB-2 oncoprotein expression in male breast carcinoma. *J. Clin. Pathol.*, **44**, 960–1.

Fox S.B., Rogers S., Day C.A., Underwood J.C.E.(1992) Oestrogen receptor and epidermal growth factor receptor expression in male breast carcinoma. *J. Pathol.*, **166**, 13–18.

Friedman M.A., Hoffman P.G., Dandolos E.M., Lagios M.D., Johnston W.H., Siiteri, P.K. (1981) Estrogen receptors in male breast cancer: clinical and pathologic correlations. *Cancer*, **47**, 134–7.

Gatalica Z. (1997) Immunohistochemical analysis of apocrine breast lesions. Consistent over-expression of androgen receptor accompanied by the loss of estrogen and progesterone receptors in apocrine metaplasia and apocrine carcinoma *in situ*. *Pathol. Res. Pract.*, **193**, 753–8

Giffler R.F., Kay S. (1976) Small-cell carcinoma of the male mammary gland: a tumor resembling infiltrating lobular carcinoma. *Am. J. Clin. Pathol.*, **66**, 715–22.

Giltman L. (1981) Solitary intraductal papilloma of the male breast. *Southern Med. J.*, **74**, 774.

Hamele-Bena D., Cranor M.L., Sciotto C., Erlandson R., Rosen P.P. Uncommon presentation of mammary myofibroblastoma. *Mod. Pathol.*, **9**, 786–90.

Hamer D.B. (1975) Gynaecomastia. *Br. J. Surg.*, **62**, 326–9.

Hassan M.O., Olaizola M.Y. (1979) Ultrastructural observations on gynecomastia. *Arch. Pathol. Lab. Med.*, **103**, 624–30.

Holleb A.I., Freeman H.P., Farrow J.H. (1968) Cancer of male breast. I. *N.Y. State J. Med.*, **68**, 544–53.

Jackson A.W., Muldal S., Ockey C.H., O'Connor P.J. (1965) Carcinoma of male breast in association with the Kleinefelter syndrome. *Br. Med. J.*, **1**, 223–5.

Magro G., Fraggetta F., Torrisi A., Emmanuele C., Lanzafame S. (1999) Myofibroblastoma of the breast with hemangiopericytoma-like pattern and pleomorphic lipoma-like areas. Report of a case with diagnostic and histogenetic considerations. *Pathol. Res. Pract.*, **195**, 257–62.

Morgan M.B., Pitha J.V. (1998) Myofibroblastoma of the breast revisited: an etiologic association with androgens? *Hum. Pathol.*, **29**, 347–51.

Norris H.F., Taylor H.B. (1969) Carcinoma of the male breast. *Cancer*, **23**, 1428–35.

Pantoja E., Llobet R.E., Lopez E. (1976) Gigantic cystosarcoma phyllodes in a man with gynecomastia. *Arch. Surg.*, **111**, 611.

Pettinato G., Manivel J.C., Insabato A., De Chiara A., Petrella G. (1988) Plasma cell granuloma (inflammatory pseudotumor) of the breast. *Am. J. Clin. Pathol.*, **90**, 627–32.

Rayson D., Erlichman C., Suman V.J. *et al.* (1998) Molecular markers in male breast carcinoma. *Cancer*, **83**, 1947–55.

Reingold I.M., Ascher G.S. (1970) Cystosarcoma phyllodes in a man with gynecomastia. *Am. J. Clin. Pathol.*, **53**, 852–6.

Roth J.A., Discafani C., O'Malley M. (1988) Secretory breast carcinoma in a man. *Am. J. Surg. Pathol.*, **12**, 150–4.

Scheike O., Visfeldt J., Petersen B. (1973) Male breast cancer: breast carcinoma in association with the Klinefelter's syndrome. *Acta Pathol. Microbiol. Scand.*, **81**, 352–8.

Schwartz I.S., Wilens S.L. (1963) The formation of acinar tissue in gynecomastia. *Am. J. Pathol.*, **43**, 797–807.

Scopsi L., Andreola S., Saccozzi R. *et al.* (1991) Argyrophilic carcinoma of the male breast. *Am. J. Surg. Pathol.*, **15 (11)**, 1063–71.

Shoker B.S., Jarvis C., Sibson R., Walker C., Sloane J.P. (1999) Oestrogen receptor expression in the normal and pre-cancerous breast. *J. Pathol.*, **188**, 237–44.

Simpson J.S., Barson A.J. (1969) Breast tumours in infants and children: a 40-year review of cases at a children's hospital. *Can. Med. Assoc. J.*, **101**, 100–2.

Stretch J.R., Denton K.J., Millard P.R., Horak E. (1991) Paget's disease in the male breast clinically and histopathologically mimicking melanoma. *Histopathology*, **19**, 470–2.

Tamura G., Monma N., Suzuki Y., Satodate R., Abe H. (1993) Adenomyoepithelioma of the breast in a male. *Hum. Pathol.*, **24**, 678–81.

Tedeschi L.G., McCarthy P.E. (1974) Involutional mammary duct ectasia and periductal ectasia in a male. *Hum. Pathol.*, **5**, 232–6.

Thomas T.M., Myint A., Mak C.K., Chan J.K. (1997) Mammary myofibroblastoma with leiomyomatous differentiation. *Am. J. Clin. Pathol.*, **107**, 52–5.

Thorlacius S., Tryggvadottir L., Olafsdottir G.H. *et al.* (1995) Linkage to BRCA2 region in hereditary male breast cancer. *Lancet*, **346**, 544–5.

Treves N., Holleb A.I. (1955) Cancer of the male breast: a report of 146 cases. *Cancer*, **8**, 1239–50.

Wargotz E.S., Weiss S.W., Norris H.J. (1987) Myofibroblastoma of the breast. *Am. J. Surg. Pathol.*, **11**, 493–502.

Index

Note: page numbers in **bold** denote tables